MOVEMENT IS MEDICINE

The Potential for Self-Renewal is in Your Bones

By Suresha Hill, EdS, HSE, DOMTP

Somatic Intelligence - Volume 8

Movement is Medicine

The Potential for Self-Renewal is in Your Bones

By Suresha Hill, EdS, HSE, DOMTP

Cover image courtesy of Ahmad Odeh and Unsplash

ONE SKY
PRODUCTIONS

Movement is Medicine

The potential for self-renewal is in your bones

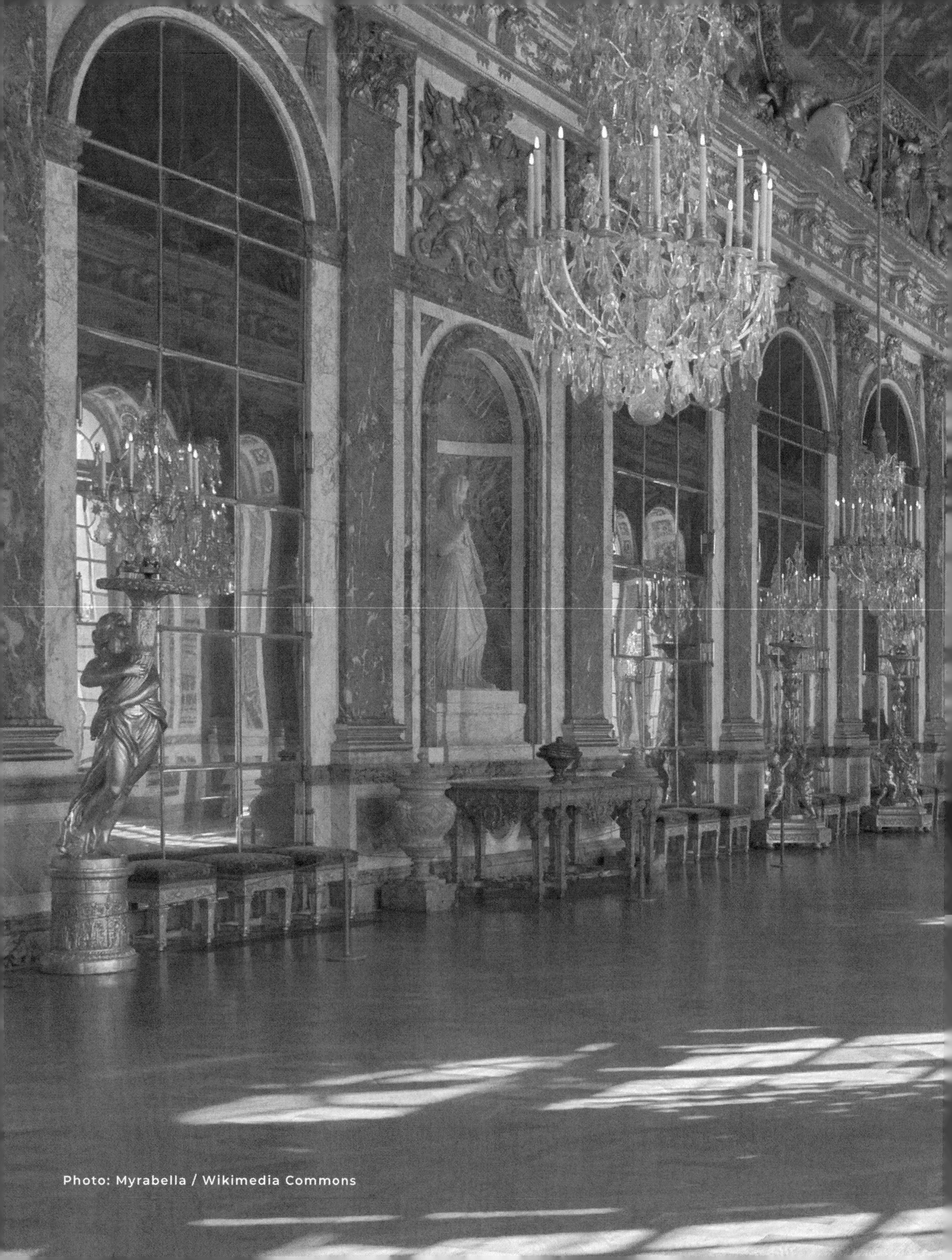

Photo: Myrabella / Wikimedia Commons

Acknowledgments

Many thanks to the inspirational teachers I've had throughout the years that have spawned a ceaseless process of inquiry and discovery. I offer much gratitude for the contributions of Dr. Tom Hanna has led to an endless exploration into the healing power of movement. The work of Dr. Paul Chauffeur, in particular, was most inspiring to deepen the journey of understanding more about the structure, function, significance, and capabilities of bone. I also want to express gratitude for the entities providing the variety of images as well as the photographers or science professionals who uploaded them to the sites that make them available to the public. This service has made a world of difference. Thanks again to Pexels and Pixabay and a very special thanks to Wikimedia Commons/Creative Commons.

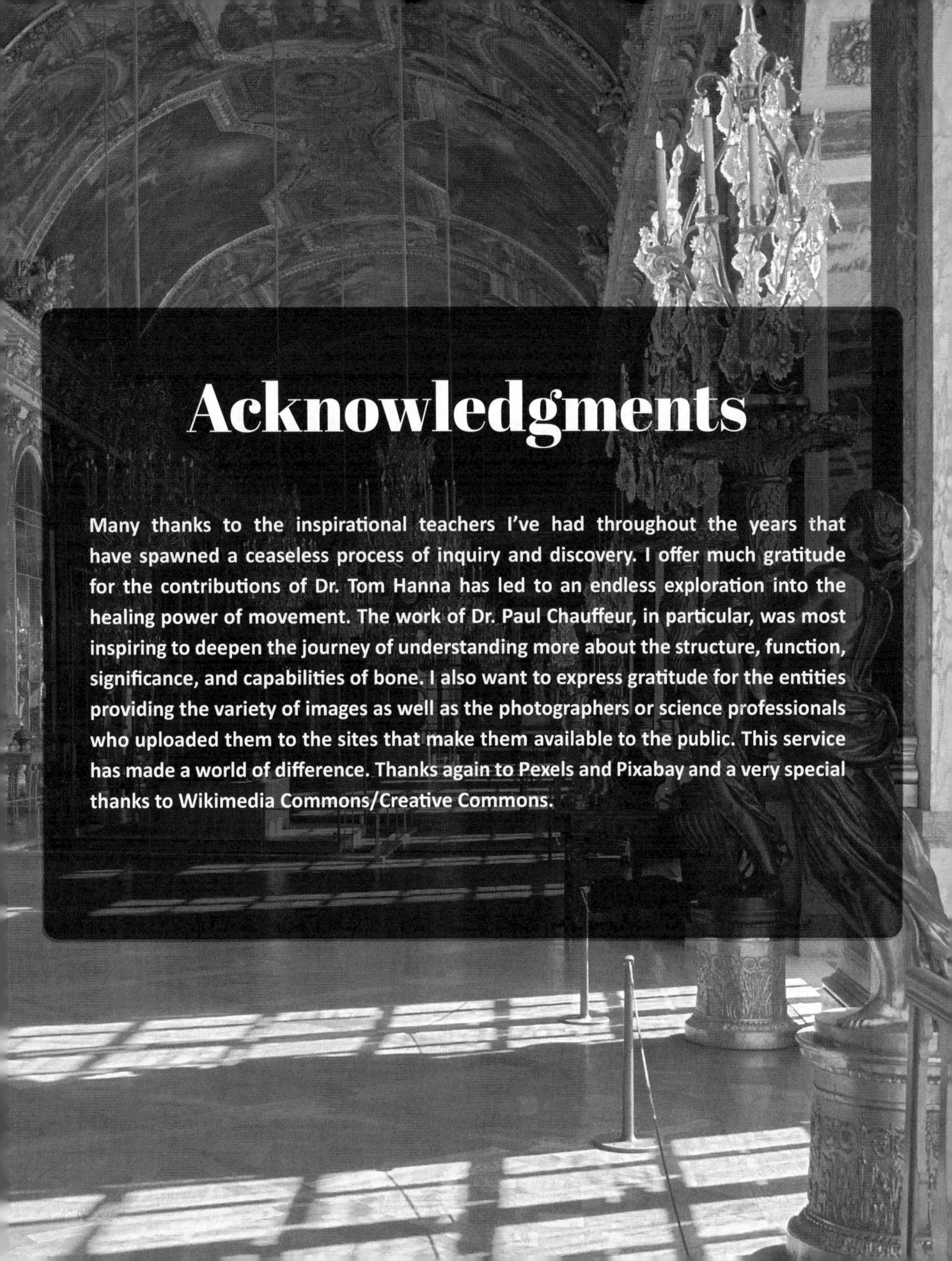

Preface

During the years spent working in a physical therapy clinic, I'd often questioned the phenomenon of chronic injuries - how did they come about? Why didn't they heal completely? Then I had an epiphany. I thought to myself, "This isn't happening in a vacuum! The body is telling itself to do that. If it can tell itself to do that, it can tell itself to do something else!" This began a 30-year journey to discover what language the body speaks. I needed to know how to intercept some of that communication and understand how to guide it in a more healthy direction.

Having started the quest for optimum healing 20 years prior to that, I'd already explored numerous methods to do that same thing for the mind and emotions. Initially, the course of study was in school psychology with a specialty in Systems Intervention and Prevention. The principles and concepts that we were applying to help children learn by avoiding conditions known to be unaligned with their well-being could also apply to adults and their bodies, I presumed. Children's ability to focus and learn depended upon the health of their mental, emotional, physical, and social/familial milieu. The optimal expression of their intelligence depended upon those key factors.

It's not so different for adults. The ability of our bodies to express optimum health depends upon the same key features. The ability of our bodies to learn needs a certain milieu for it to be able to communicate with itself and with the outside world. I began studying how the body learns and what language it uses to do so. My interest was peaked. Dr. Tom Hanna's training in Hanna Somatic Education (neuromuscular reeducation) in the 1990s got me started on the path to demystify chronic injuries and chronic pain in general.

Many in the training were there because they'd had incredible reversals of conditions they'd suffered from for years by working personally with Tom. That fact made me even more determined to understand the science behind the change. Tom's theory that, "The muscles don't do anything that the brain doesn't tell them to do" answered many of my questions but not all of them.

I was intuitively drawn to a distributed hierarchy. It seemed that the brain was just as much a receiver as a transmitter, and that the quality and accuracy of the input was critical to the accuracy of the output, which is dependent upon the milieu of the information processors everywhere in the body. Twenty-five years later and studies with several osteopaths along the way have led me to the views presented in this book, which I trust you'll find as fascinating as I have.

Foreword

Suresha Hill has a curious mind and I love it. In this, her eighth volume of the somatic intelligence series, Suresha explores the concept of movement as medicine and our bodies potential for self-renewal. She has done an exemplary job of bringing together the writings and teachings of many forward-thinking health practitioners from multiple fields, interweaving their messages in a very coherent fashion to present her own insights about how we influence our health.

As an osteopathic family physician and neuromusculoskeletal specialist, my job is to make complicated medicine simple so my patients can be well and their "to do list" is understandable and actionable. To this end, I strive to understand the complicated, and I found this book added a new layer to my experience. As you read this very thoughtful and insightful book you will explore the author's own journey to understand the concept of movement and its effect on health and well-being.

Because the foundational principle of osteopathy is based upon "our body's ability to heal itself," I know when I work to support my patient's, or my own optimal health, I must support this intrinsic healing mechanism. To do this I explain to patients that, as a team, we need to remove impediments to healing, provide the building blocks for healing, and get out of our own way to let healing occur. A key component of this process is movement and our system's response to it. Suresha ties together science and common sense to provide background to what we intrinsically know, "movement is life" and when we add intention to our daily activities, we can positively affect our well-being.

As you read this book, you will not only come across new concepts but also familiar concepts which may be presented in a different manner. Just like me, I hope you will feel both challenged and supported by the detailed evidence presented as you explore a deeper understanding of the body's intrinsic ability to heal.

This book is excellent, and anyone who reads it will have used their time wisely. I wish you all good health and if reading this book gives you even one new thought about how to influence your own health, then the journey will be worth it.

Dr Sean Moloney D.O.

San Anselmo CA

TABLE OF CONTENTS

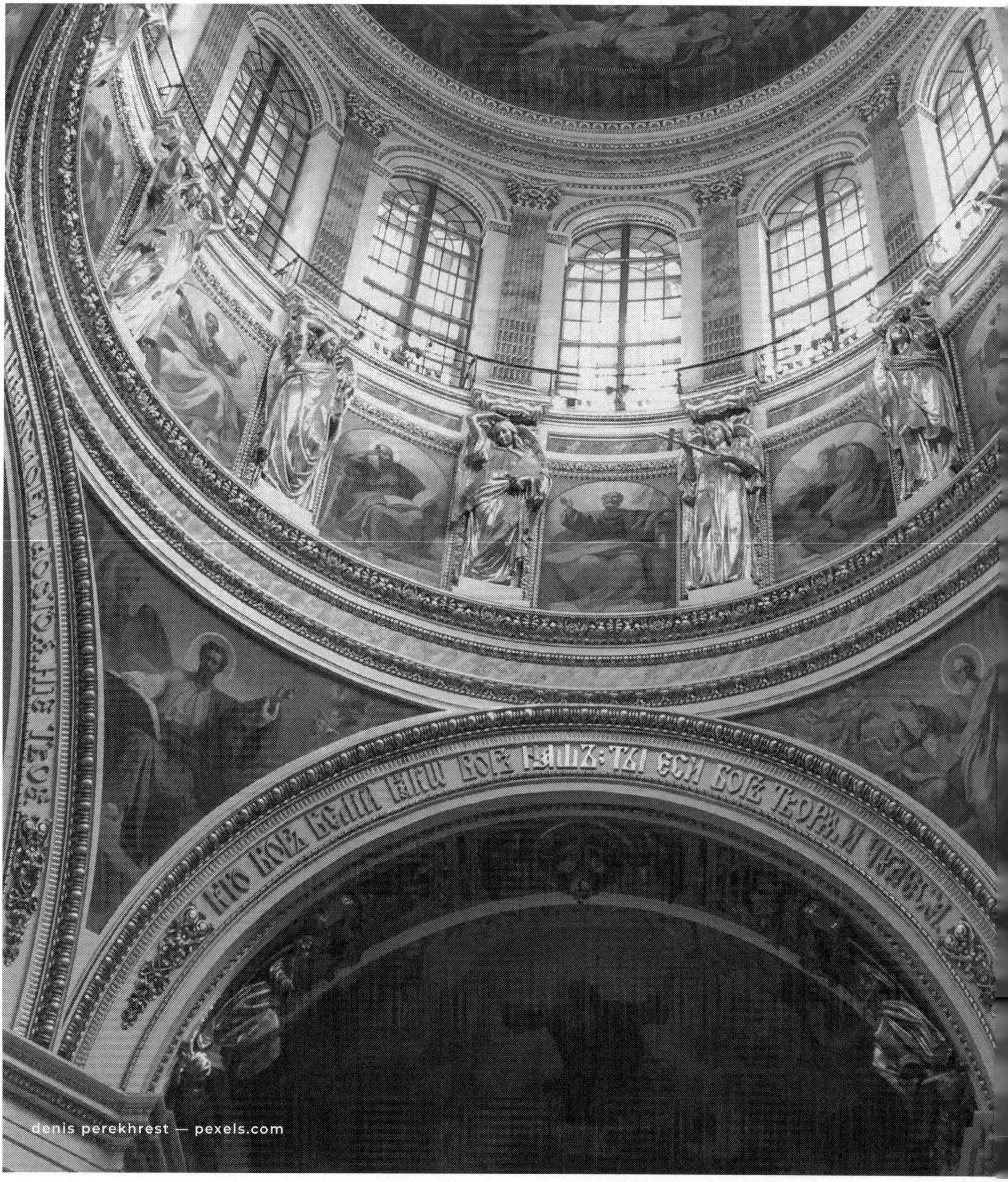

denis perekhrest — pexels.com

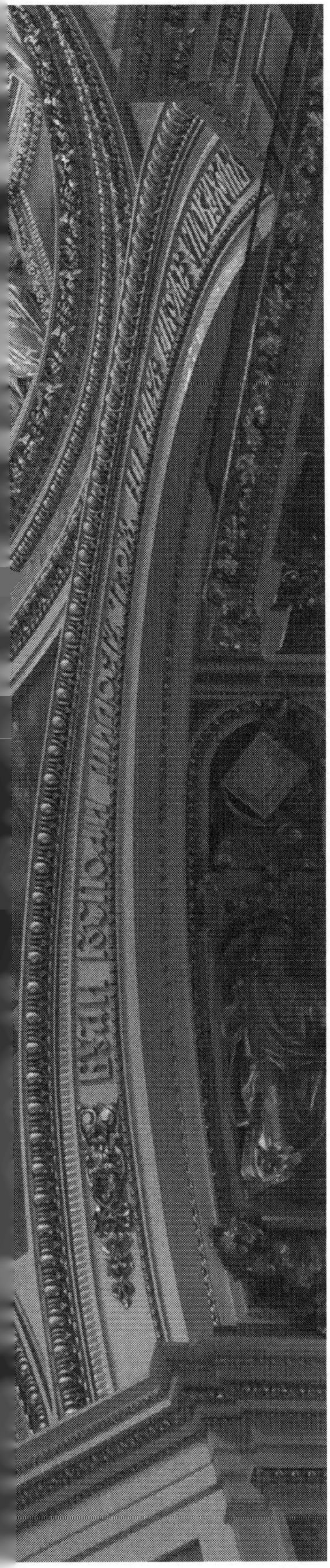

Introduction

The exquisite architecture of the body's design is unparalleled in its ability to be both supple and able to absorb and transmit tons of force using very small structures. It is an absolute marvel in so many ways! In every one of the prior Somatic Intelligence books I've written, I have emphasized the importance of communication as the way that change happens in the system. I also encouraged everyone to become a part of that conversation wherever you can; in whatever system you feel drawn to listen to.

Similar to significant features in a building, you may want to make sure your plumbing - fluid systems - are in optimum condition, or your wiring and insulation (nervous system). You'd want to make sure the framework, foundation, and support beams are plumb and sturdy, watching out for dry rot.

There are so many different types and levels of interaction happening inside of us, it's always fascinating and rewarding to tune into a different system. That way we can see what that form of communication will offer towards increased balance and integration. A few years ago I became interested in bones, and was impressed by their ability to create releases in soft tissue.

I assumed there was some degree of cross-talk that enabled these changes to happen, and there was, but there is so much more! Bones are talking to almost every system in the body, and are a significant contributor to our well-being. One somatic relationship that stands out as particularly useful and barely understood is the efficacy of bones and bone morphogenetic proteins. From what I've discovered about bones in recent years, I would honor them with the status of a brain. They bear the complex communication characteristics of a brain, and employ several neurotransmitters to help coordinate osteogenesis along with other functions. They not only communicate with numerous organs and glands, but also help to regulate their function; particularly the pancreas.

Bones have a nervous system, a vascular system, an endocrine system, an immune system, a detox function, along with storage and cognitive functions. The cognitive function is gaining more traction in recent years as Baby Boomers approach senior citizen status in great numbers. A 12-year Taiwan study in 2014 of over 66,000 patients with fractures and over 100,000 without, adjusting for age, sex, pre-existing dementia, urbanization, and co-morbidities as risk factors, those with fractures were found to have a 41% increased incidence of dementia compared to those without. [1] (Chun-Hao Tsa, et al, 2014)

Another study in 2014 found a parallel increase in osteoporosis and in disorders such as MS, ALS, Alzheimer's, and Parkinson's disease. At that time, it was estimated that there were at least 200 million people with osteoporosis worldwide, with nearly 25% of that number being in the United States. In general, the percentage of those affected is higher for women than for men in the populations being tested. All are over 50 years old in this study. [2](Per M Roos, 2014) It doesn't seem like this information has reached the public at large yet.

Gerosa and Lombardi assert that,

> *"Bone is highly innervated and hosts all nervous system branches; bone cells are sensitive to most neurotransmitters, neuropeptides and neurohormones that directly affect their metabolic activity. Besides the classical ones that support protection, hematopoiesis, storage for calcium and phosphate, multiple roles have emerged for bone tissue, definitely making it an organ." [3](Laura Gerosa and Giovanni Lombardi, 2021)*

Along with the structural support, detox, and bone remodeling functions we've come to appreciate bones for, they also participate in the alkaline/acid balance and blood sugar regulation for our bodies in ways that can significantly influence quality of life. They have also played a role in ancient times in a variety of ways that improve health. Iron Shirt Chi Kung, for example, recognizes that focusing on bone provides the fundamental strength that the frame needs for years to come.

Slow, deliberate movements, along with bone tapping, and other principles of this art activate the piezo-electric current that flows through bones. This current stimulates the osteoblast/bone-building aspect of bone remodeling. There have been anecdotal reports of osteoporosis being reversed using these methods. Harvard Medical School reports that the ancient practice of t'ai chi can improve sensory awareness, balance, focus, and limit damage from inflammation and bone loss. (Women's Health, 2021)

There may be many ways that we can benefit from a better understanding of the relationship that bones have with other structures and their functions. For example, one biochemical relationship shows that serotonin plays a role in the communication from the spine to the brain, which can influence idiopathic scoliosis during adolescence. There may be a way to intervene in biochemical or biomechanical messaging processes that can help thousands of teens avoid uncomfortable braces or surgery. There may be interruptions in accurate signaling from the spine or connective tissue based upon faulty alignment that can also be avoided.

As of 2000, 85% of people living in the U.S. had experienced back pain, costing billions annually for medical care and even more in work productivity. Psycho-emotional stressors on the skeleton and connective tissue can have widespread impacts. By some statistics, over 30% have experienced back and neck pain in the last 3 months. The majority of these are female, and about the same percentage have had this issue chronically for over five years. Most people believe it comes from stress or a bad mattress, a good portion from physical labor, and just as many from a sedentary job. The health field is ripe with a need for change in our approach to attaining well-being.

The potential of improving these statistics based upon formative embryological relationships is very exciting from my point of view! It is generally understood that everything is literally connected, and that a change anywhere in the system can potentially influence many other systems. The fact that certain tissue fields were formed at the same time in utero is particularly significant for movement practices as well as for manual therapy.

Change in the system is based upon complex signaling. From this perspective, utilizing the embryological signaling relationships can be very helpful in returning the system to balance quickly. Applying techniques that use the awareness of molecular cross-talk between systems are also helpful during an acute phase of any condition. Research and my own clinical experience will bear this out. Working therapeutically with bones can also provide a source of settling and calm, if not well-being for the entire system.

There are many theories concerning emotions or traumas being stored in the bones and joints. Bones are known by some to be a source of deep energy flows. Dr. Fritz Smith is one of the few practitioners offering a manual therapy approach that works directly with the energy he feels is present in bones as a source of potential balance for the entire system. A couple of his books, "Life in the Bones," and "Zero Balancing: Touching the Energy of Bones," describe the possible ways that accessing sensation and energy in bones can be of benefit for the entire system. It is surprisingly one of the quickest ways to a deep feeling of rest after one of these sessions.

Osteopathy embraces a holistic approach, as stated in part by Dr. Willis Haycock in Vol.2 of Osteopathy Principles & Practices, *"Early osteopathic writings in the first decades of the 1900s by Burns, Haycock, and Speransky, attribute most every dysfunction to a specific imbalance in a spinal segment which in turn irritates the nervous system, thereby carrying the disruption into the vascular and organ systems or into a neurodegenerative process."* {4}(Haycock, 2000)

The skin also deserves more attention as a significant player in the overall health and well-being of the system. It maintains countless interactions with other systems as well, and is often a reflection of the status of other organs. Embryologically, the ectoderm is responsible for the proliferation of cells that differentiate into the spinal cord, brain, heart, internal organs, soft tissue, and skeleton. There is no separation between the fields of function for any of these structures. Biomechanically, there are many proprioceptors in the skin that transmit tactile and kinesthetic information to the brain and adjacent cells, which makes it is an ideal organ to employ consciously in movement sequences as well as for manual therapies.

Andrew Taylor Still, Ida Rolf, Tom Myers, and John Barnes are credited with manual approaches related to fascia, our fine, interconnected web of inner skin. Marion Rosen, influenced by Elsa Gindler, was a physical therapist and movement educator who noticed emotional releases were availed using her approach to the skin. It makes sense that the skin being our first layer of defense could also apply in socio-emotional contexts, and the phrase about having a 'thick skin' could suggest that subconsciously we already know that this is happening.

Marion conceived of her method of movement as a 'work in' rather than a workout. She intended it to lubricate joints, expand the chest and ribs, release the diaphragm, lengthen the muscles, and support ongoing healthy aging along with injury recovery. Many of the early Somatic Pioneers in Europe discovered that a variety of health conditions were improved using the type of systemic communication that happens using mindful movement and conscious awareness. Massage, of course, has a variety of proven health benefits that happen through therapeutic contact with the skin.

Massage is not new. India is perhaps the first culture to use oils in Ayurvedic massage techniques going back 5000 years. "The Yellow Emperor's Classic Book of Internal Medicine" includes massage practices as early as 2700 B.C., and images in tombs of Egyptians giving each other massage date back as far as 2500 B.C. Egyptians are also credited with the beginnings of reflexology. The oldest known book written about massage is from China, called the "Cong-Fu of the Toa Tse," which was translated into French in the 1700's. {5} (Julie Onofrio, 2021)

In 1895, John Harvey Kellogg wrote in his book, "The Art of Massage," that:

> *"The physiologic research which has been applied to the methods of massage within recent years has clearly demonstrated the effectiveness of external manipulations as a means of influencing metabolic and other processes in the deeper parts of the organism. At present time, it may be said to be clearly established that every organ and every function of the body may be influenced by the producers of massage. Both the volume of the blood and the movement of blood in every internal viscus may be decidedly influenced in either direction by external manipulations."*

This text will elucidate the benefits of using skin as a source of communication for the rest of the system from an embryological and epigenetic perspective. The ectoderm was the initial signaling domain for migration and differentiation of the cells that form all other tissues and the regulation of their functions. So there could be ways that this inherent relationship can be utilized to create meaningful and lasting balance for the body. I maintain that this is so, and that how you approach this potential powerhouse can increase or decrease the therapeutic value. The more conscious intent there is in the approach to skin and bones in movement or manual therapy, the greater the possibilities for excellent outcomes.

The preventative potential has always been a main focus in presenting somatic intelligence principles and practices, as well as why they work. In this case, bringing awareness to the multiple functions of skin and its cross-talk with bone broadens the benefits even more.

There is science backing up every claim. Opening the discussion at the embryological/molecular level of influence can lead to improved health outcomes for all ages, and particularly for aging populations. Perhaps neuroplasticity can be extended to the brain in our bones, revealing more of a regenerative process than we thought possible. Ideally, the concepts of separation fade more and more into the web of inextricable, intelligent, somatic functionality that is always listening and responding.

This book will focus on the fact that cellular communication, particularly between skin and bone with other systems, is extremely useful therapeutically. Their shared transcription factors and pathways can facilitate deeper, epigenetic changes for greater well-being and healthier longevity. This means that averting the major diseases plaguing most people in our society is not only possible, but it's very likely to happen when you incorporate this information into your life.

Bear in mind, that any one aspect of a particular stage of development - a transcription pathway, an epigenetic consideration for dietary choices, a part of our anatomy, or its function, could entertain decades of study (and many have) and still not be completely understood. In fact, every research article I quoted stated that the mechanisms of action for that particular aspect of inquiry are yet to be fully understood. Articles written in 2009 may be outdated by 2015, so the field is changing quickly. I made efforts to search out the most recent thought in any area being covered. Nonetheless, what is currently 'known' is still exciting and very promising for future health outcomes even though it's still evolving. Scientifically and experientially verified, communicating with our bodies from a conscious tactile or kinesthetic level may be the most effective tool in any medicine chest.

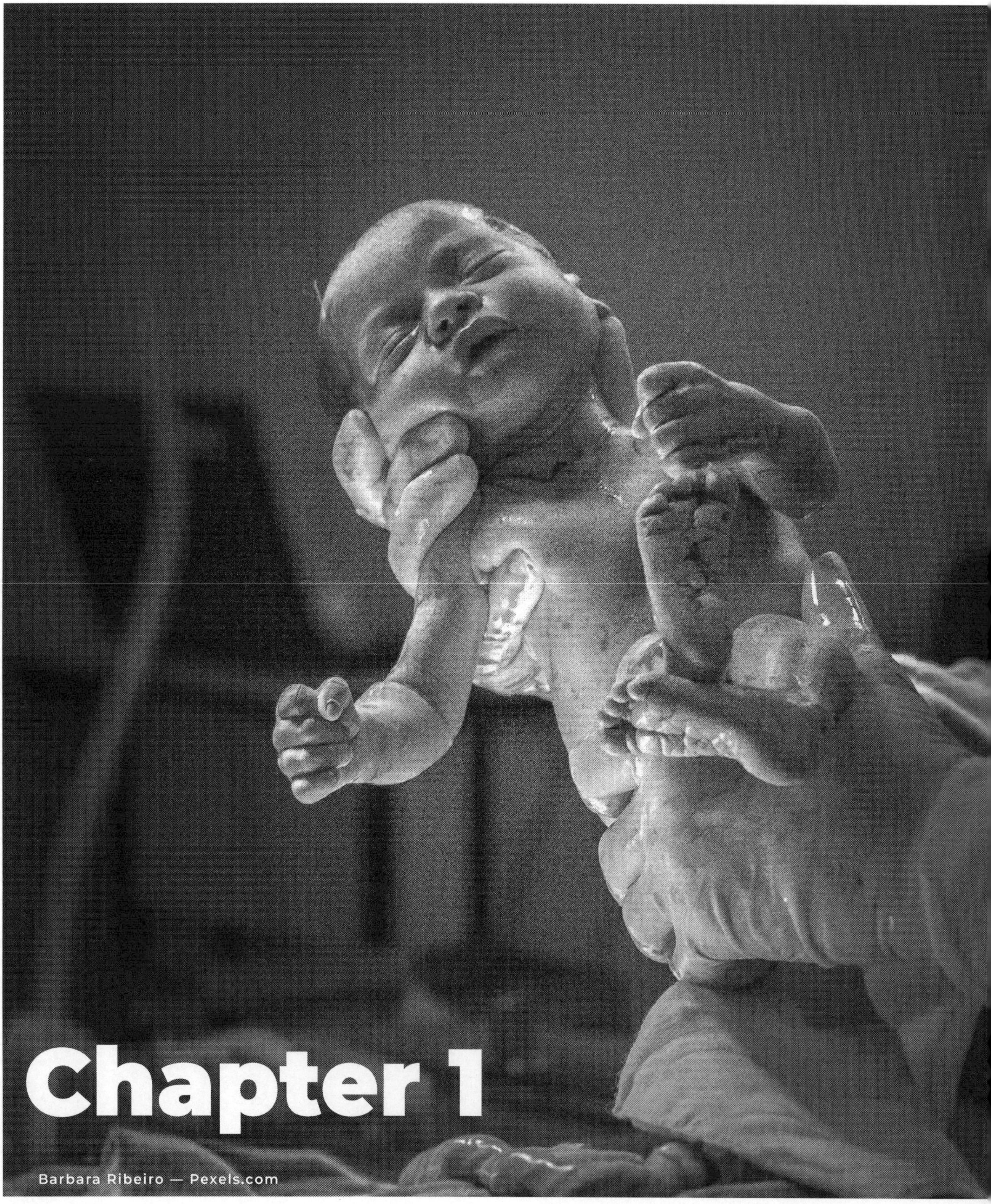

Chapter 1

Barbara Ribeiro — Pexels.com

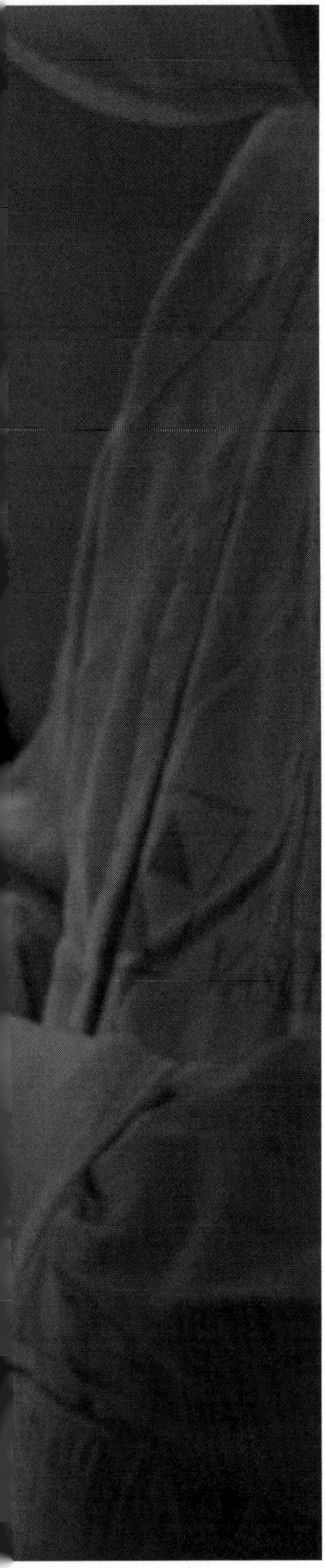

Primal Beginnings

It's good to begin with humbled awe and a Namaste to the miracle that instills a life-building capacity into a sperm and an egg. We can also appreciate that these tiny cells hold the coding that gives rise to a dynamic human being. Although we will focus on the structures that express their initial blueprint into very detailed specifications, that focus doesn't make the 'elephant in the room' any smaller: which is the fact that the structures themselves are expressing an exquisite, functional, adaptive, genius design that is imbued with responsive intelligence.

Mothers and scientists alike must spend their lifetimes mulling over the amazement of how it unfolds. That responsive intelligence is listening to many types and sources of input from inside and outside of the body. Some sources are biomechanical, but most are biochemical. The initial processes which determine that a particular organization will become human happen very quickly. This is all going on inside a woman's womb before she realizes that she's pregnant. After fertilization, the simplest of cellular structures rapidly divide from a single cell into a morula, (Fig. 1.0) which then compresses those 32 cells into a space the same size as the original single cell.

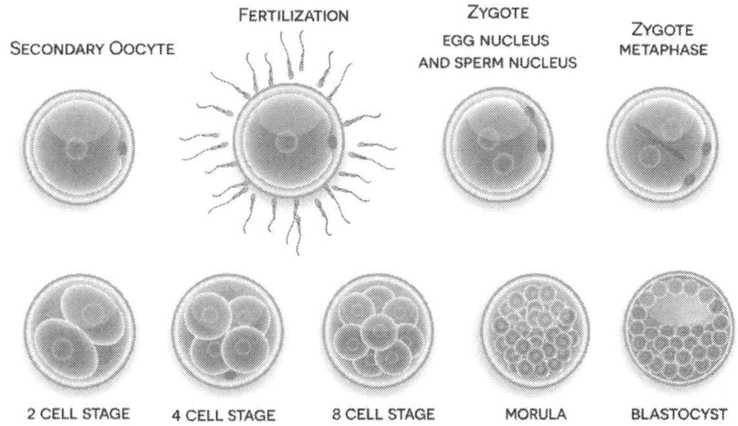

Fig. 1.0 – Initial stages of cell division after fertilization

BLASTULATION

A space called the amnion or amniotic cavity will eventually house the fetus. It's about 2 – 5mm in diameter. The head of a pin is about 2 mm. The space below it, called the coelom or yolk sac, later attaches to the outside of the fetus. (Fig.1.1) During this blastulation phase, the zona pellucida disintegrates and the inner cell mass begins to differentiate and migrate. This mass initially forms two new cell layers below the amnion. The upper layer, called the epiblast, is made of slightly elongated cells, and the hypoblast is just beneath it. These two layers form what is called a bilaminar disc, the most primitive layers of the ectoderm and endoderm. Following stem cell signaling at the caudal (tail) end of the blastula, some epiblast cells migrate into what is called the 'primitive streak'. This streak runs about 40% of the way through the middle of the blastula before it terminates into the primitive node at the other end of the streak.

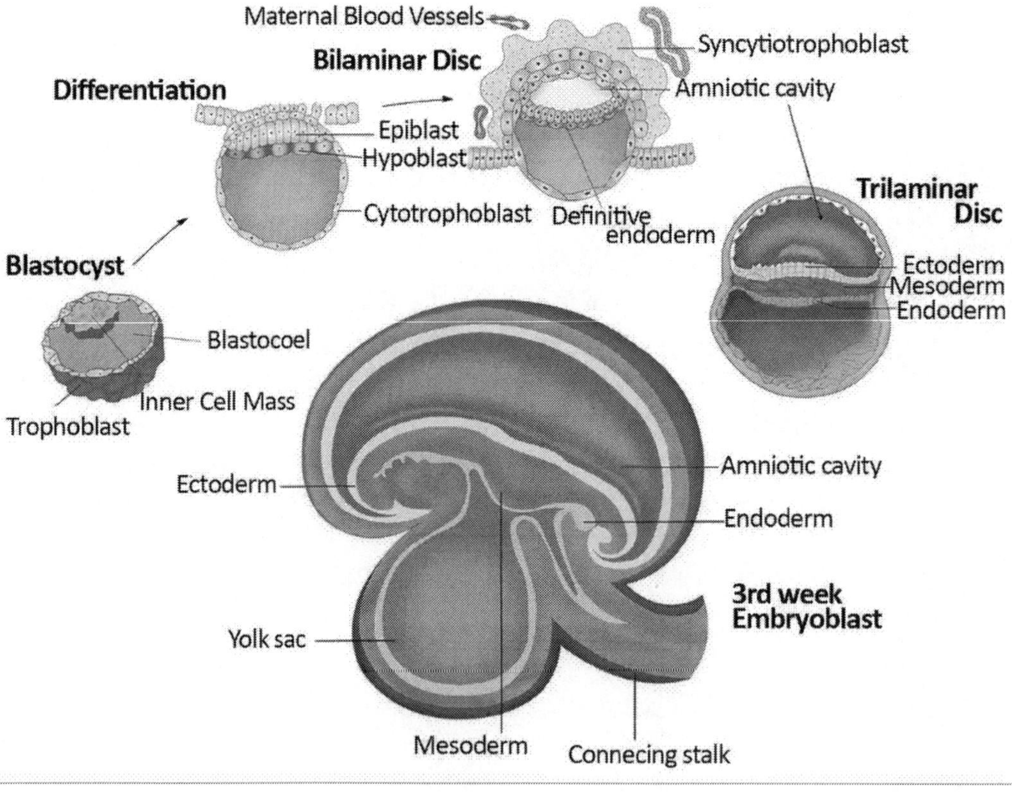

Fig. 1.1 Blastulation phase as the bilaminar becomes the trilaminar disc

A basic differentiation begins to occur whereby a zona pellucida forms as an outermost protective later on top of a ring of cells just inside of the zona pellucida called a trophoblast. The trophoblast separates from the inner cell mass that remains compressed, but moves to make room for a fluid that will serve as a form of nutrition for the growing mass. As the mass collects in one section, it is called a blastocyst or blastula. That mass will become the fetus.

The formation of the streak initiates the spatial organization of the body. The zones of caudal and cranial, right and left, and soon after, ventral and dorsal develop. This streak continues to thicken along a vertical line. Then, about a third of the way across the surface of the disc, the primitive node sinks within itself to form a primitive pit. (Fig. 1.2) Complex signaling from the pit directs the migrating cells as they drop in and curve around to form the **notochord**. The notochord then drives itself cranially towards a small circle The question remains in my mind as to which form of intelligence establishes the what, where, and how of all this signaling. A Higher Power?

GASTRULATION

Professor Jack Murphy, from the Philadelphia College of Osteopathic Medicine, finds that FGF-8 (fibroblast growth factor) participates in the increasingly complex signaling that directs the epiblast cells (ectoderm). Yes, but what created this FGF-8 and its ability to function? Okay, this is the last time I'll confront the gorilla in the womb. These cells invaginate the current layers of the blastocyst and form the endoderm beneath it. Spatial organizing messengers arise from the Nieuwkoop center of the disc. That causes genetic information from the nucleus to induce both neurulation and the dorsal placement of the mesoderm. (Gary C. Schoenwolf, PhD, 2021)

The conversion of the bilaminar disc into the trilaminar disc that represents the three germ layers is called gastrulation. (Fig. 1.2) As the upper (ectoderm) layer folds up and around into the anterior body wall, the lower (endoderm) layer folds down and forms the gut tube from the mouth to the anus. The membrane that develops toward the cranial end of the disc at the *prochordal plate* produces the buccopharyngeal membrane that forms at the back of the throat. At the caudal end of the disc, the **cloacal plate** forms a membrane that becomes the anus.

Several significant functions happen simultaneously during the third week. Around day 15, the notochord begins as a hollow tube. The tube secretes a protein called Shh (secretory or sonic hedgehog) that stimulates the organization and definitive commitment of other cells and their function. {6}(Ashwell, 2009) Shh is significant later in life. As the mesoderm cells continue to migrate, they further differentiate into paraxial, intermediate, and lateral plate mesoderm functions. (Fig. 1.2) Dr. Judith Ann Silverman, who is in the Department of Anatomy & Cell Biology at Columbia University, stated that these mesoderm divisions are placed adjacent to the neural tube. The neural tube has also been forming out of the ectoderm.

Additional differentiation happens in the mesoderm layer of cells around day 17. The lateral plate mesoderm subdivides into the splanchnic, somitic, and extra-embryonic cells. The mesenchymal cells of the splanchnic division form the lining around the chest, viscera, and abdominal cavities, as well as the smooth muscle cells of the heart, and endothelial cells of blood vessels. {7}(Yiangou, et al., 2019). Consider that tension or restrictions in one of these areas could potentially create tension or restrictions in any of the others. The intermediate mesoderm gives rise to the urogenital system, including the kidneys, gonads, reproductive duct systems, and accessory glands. Maintaining awareness of these initial groupings can inform where we look to explain or possibly resolve a restriction in any one of these related areas. For example, relieving restrictions in the parietal peritoneum could theoretically also improve conditions in the lining of blood vessels or heart.

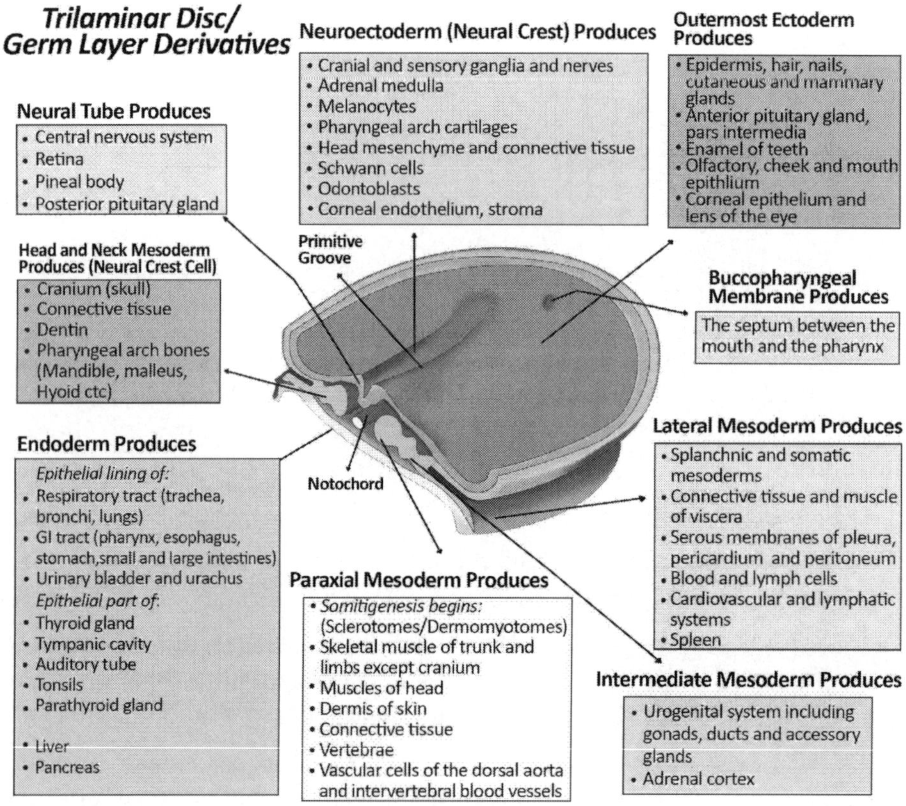

Fig. 1.2 There is no consensus among researchers as to exactly which structures arise according to a specific fate map, but this chart does represent the cumulative findings of several studies, such as Luis Williams, et al., 2012, Gilbert, 2000, Larsen, 2008, Ansari and Pillarisetty, 2021, Elshazzly, 2021, Garland and Pomerantz, 2012

All of the structures in the paraxial mesoderm, which are continually used in daily activities, exercises, and therapeutic modalities are derived from the same cells. Both manual and movement medicine make use of these shared signaling pathways and inherent interconnectedness to facilitate positive outcomes. The muscles of the limbs, skeleton, dermis, connective tissue, and significant blood vessels interact in such a way that the intentional, conscious motion — passive or active — of any of these systems will automatically signal the other structures and potentially improve their function.

Bordoni and Simonelli state,

"The fascia is any tissue that contains features capable of responding to mechanical stimuli. The fascial continuum is the result of the evolution of the perfect synergy among different tissues capable of supporting, dividing, penetrating, and connecting all the districts of the body, from the epidermis to the bone, involving all of the functions and organic structures.

The continuum constantly transmits and receives mechano-metabolic information that can influence the shape and function of the entire body.

Fascial cells derive from tissues developed from the mesoderm and partly from the neural crests of the ectoderm. A seamless web of connective tissues that covers, supports, and penetrates the viscera is part of the fascial system. Although the difference between the cells in different tissues is evident, their behavior in case of mechanical stress is very similar." {8}(Bordoni and Simonelli, 2018).

Including the epidermis (skin) in a conscious, intentional way during movement sequences or manual therapy approaches will automatically connect to the fascial system. It will further optimize messaging throughout the body, and therefore catalyze its balancing, integrative, resetting potentials. All of these points will be gone into in great detail in later chapters. Making a mental note now, while ingesting how these systems were brought into existence together, can set the stage for more fully digesting how they continue their regulatory role all throughout life.

The skin is directly related to the central nervous system where a great deal of feedback from peripheral stimuli is processed. Combining the epidermis with mesoderm components like muscle or connective tissue has already proven to be a very powerful therapeutic intervention. It can be particularly useful when there is an acute flare up or a new injury where many areas are sensitive to touch or to move. These structures are all capable of responding to slight changes, so gentle touch and micro movements could be more readily accepted by the body. In some cases it may be even more beneficial than strong stretching, large movements, or deep pressure.

There has been a great deal of study of these connections recently in hopes that more understanding will help develop and refine therapeutic interventions. Everything presented here will be a drop in the molecular bucket compared to the complexity of how even one system functions, but it's good to present a general idea so you can further explore and develop the relationships in your own body and practice.

NEURULATION

The ectoderm thickens to form the neural plate, the center of which both folds down into what becomes a neural groove. It then lifts itself as it wraps around to form the neural tube just above the notochord. (Fig. 1.3) Dr. Taube P. Rothman, from the Department of Clinical Pathology and Cell Biology at Columbia University, reports that the anterior part of the neural tube will evolve into the brain, while the caudal section develops into the spinal cord. The process by which the neural plate forms a neural tube is called neurulation.

The plate comes together and seals itself across the top, while a new layer is forming there that is called the neural crest. The neural crest gives rise to, among other structures, the central and peripheral nervous systems, the adrenal medulla, glial and Schwann cells, and dentine of the teeth. From this viewpoint, it's easy to see how stress could possibly cause weakness and grinding of the teeth, and even cavities.

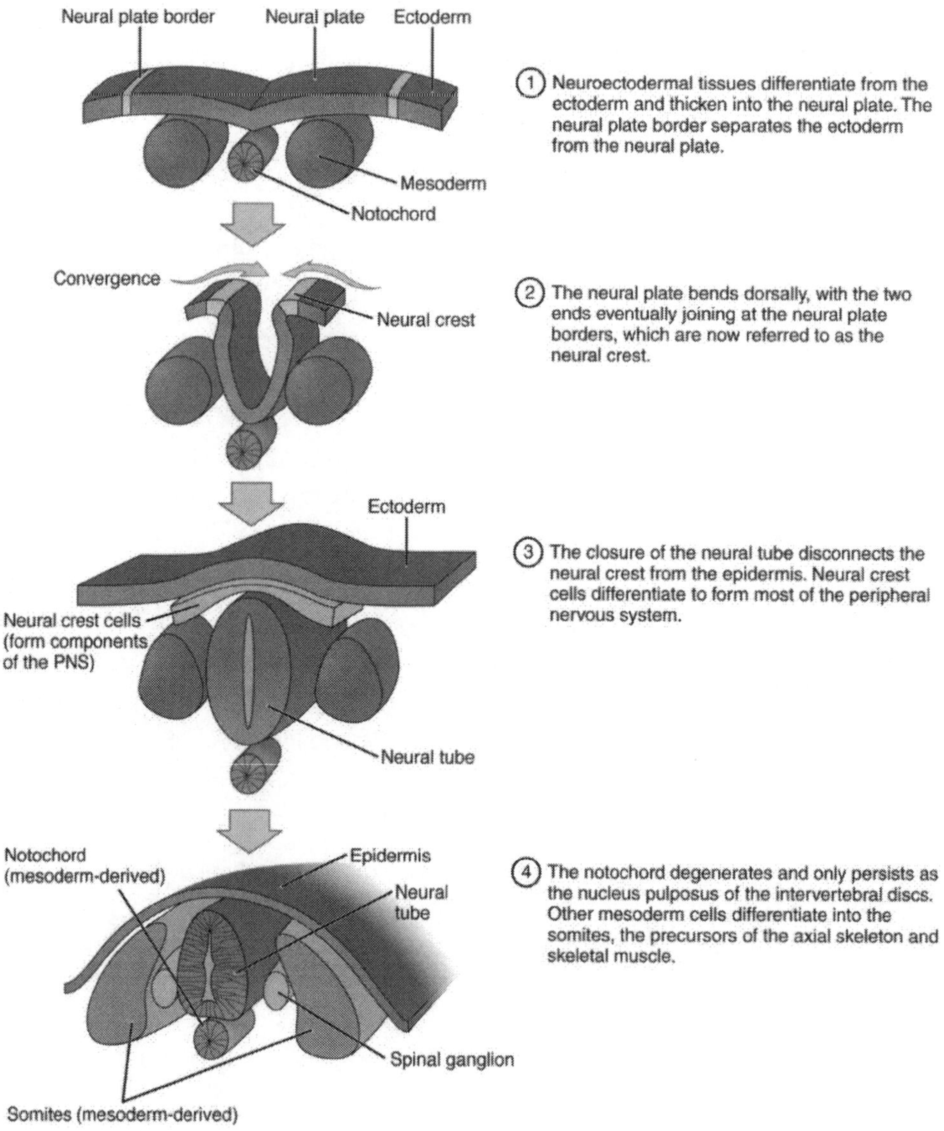

Neural plate border
Neural plate
Ectoderm
Mesoderm
Notochord
① Neuroectodermal tissues differentiate from the ectoderm and thicken into the neural plate. The neural plate border separates the ectoderm from the neural plate.
Convergence
Neural crest
② The neural plate bends dorsally, with the two ends eventually joining at the neural plate borders, which are now referred to as the neural crest.
Ectoderm
Neural crest cells (form components of the PNS)
Neural tube
③ The closure of the neural tube disconnects the neural crest from the epidermis. Neural crest cells differentiate to form most of the peripheral nervous system.
Notochord (mesoderm-derived)
Epidermis
Neural tube
Spinal ganglion
Somites (mesoderm-derived)
④ The notochord degenerates and only persists as the nucleus pulposus of the intervertebral discs. Other mesoderm cells differentiate into the somites, the precursors of the axial skeleton and skeletal muscle.

Fig. 1.3 – Illustration of neurulation, as the ectoderm thickens to form the plate, which folds into the crest which eventually yields the nervous system

Image Courtesy of OpenStax College CC by 3.0 via Wikimedia Commons

SOMITOGENESIS

The extra embryonic mesoderm helps provide nutrition to the fetus by way of the epithelium and villi of the amnion and yolk sac. It is also involved in developing fetal blood and in forming the connecting stalk that is the primordium of the umbilical cord. (Medical Embryology website, Drexel University College of Medicine; Anatomy Website, University of Michigan Medical School) A unique oscillation, often referred to as a 'clock wavefront' pattern, is set in motion around day 20. The paraxial mesoderm induces somitogenesis, which is responsible for the axial skeleton, along with muscles of the back and ribs. (Hester et al, 2011) Keeping with the theme of employing practical therapeutic applications related to embryological relationships, consider releasing the paraspinal muscles using the ribs. It is very effective!

Other studies have shown that transcription signaling is a significant part of what sets this relational process in motion. Transcription factors are DNA binding proteins that regulate the expression of genes. For example, developmental pathways Wnt/β-catenin, BMP, Notch, and FGF-8 are all involved in these timed, clock wavefront oscillations. (Robert Resnik, MD, 2019) Pairs of somites begin to form cephalo-caudally every 90 minutes at the rate of 3-4 pairs per day until they reach 44 pairs. ("Derivatives of Mesoderm - Embryonic Period," howmed.net) Since Wolpert first offered an explanation in 1969, numerous biologists have attempted to propose formulas for this incredibly mysterious and almost poetic orchestration of cellular positioning. Wolpert states:

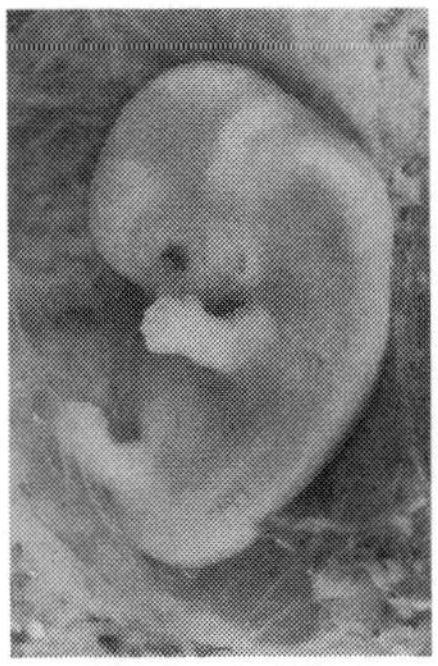

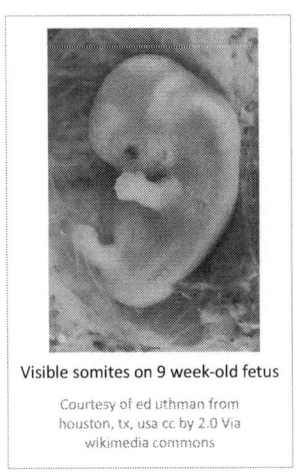

Visible somites on 9 week-old fetus

Courtesy of ed uthman from houston, tx, usa cc by 2.0 Via wikimedia commons

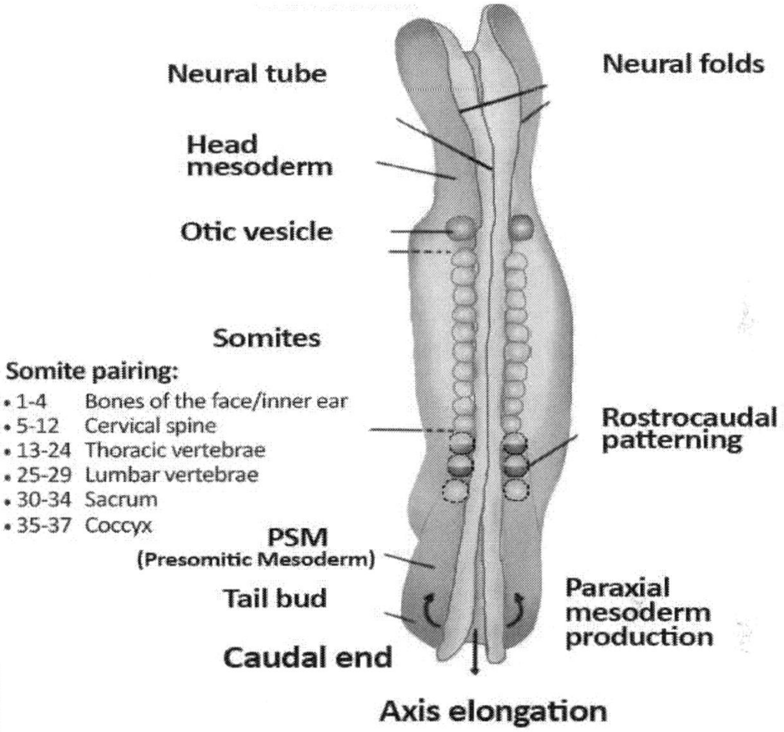

At about one month, 44 - 45 pairs of somites regress into 37 pairs. (Adapted from Larsen, 1993 by NeuPsy Key) The somites of the paraxial mesoderm also gives rise to the rib cage, voluntary muscles,dermis of the neck and trunk,some tendons and endothelial cells.(Shoishiro Tani,et al.,Experimental and Molecular Medicine, 2020).

Fig. 1.4 – Somitogenesis fate map of segmentation clock starting day 20

(Ágnes Nemeskéri, "Development of vertebral column and trunk," 2017, Melanie I. Stefan, Biomodels, April 2009; Larsen's Human Biology, 5th Edition, 2009 & 2015);

"The basis of this is a mechanism whereby the cells in a developing system may have their position specified with respect to one or more points in the system. Cells which have their positional information specified with respect to the same set of points constitute a field. Positional information largely determines, with respect to the cells' genome and developmental history, the nature of its molecular differentiation. [9](L. Wolpert, October, 1969).

At about one month, 44-45 pairs of somites regress into 37 pairs, as the most caudal pairs fall away. (Fig. 1.4) (Adapted from Larsen, 1993 by NeuPsy Key, and Nemeskéri, 2017) The somites of the paraxial mesoderm also give rise to the rib cage, voluntary muscles, dermis of the neck and trunk, and some tendons and endothelial cells. [10](Shoichiro Tani, 2020) Professor James Glazier at the Indiana University

Department of Physics mentions that the segmentation process isn't always perfect, and that some people are born with 13 sets of ribs, additional cervical vertebrae, and other mishaps that could produce scoliosis or other uncomfortable conditions. [11](Glazier, October 2011)

The ventral region of the maturing somitomere grows into the mesenchymal cells of the sclerotome that become the axial skeleton. [23](D Šošić et al, 1997) Mesenchymal stem cells continuously replicate themselves, based upon signaling from the ectoderm, "while a portion becomes committed to mesenchymal cell lineages such as bone, cartilage, tendon, ligament, and muscle," states Bruder. [24](Bruder, Fink, and Kaplan, 1994) These researchers go on to say that, "*Progression from one state to the next depends on the presence of specific bioactive factors, nutrients, and other environmental cues, whose exquisitely controlled contributions orchestrate the entire differentiation phenomenon*."

More attention has been given to these areas of research in the last decade in the hopes of increasing the effectiveness of stem cell therapy. Haibin Xi quoted Murray and Keller from 2008 as, "*To fully harness their power, it is imperative to design robust and effective protocols to differentiate hPSC's (human pluripotent stem cells) toward desired lineages, which often involves following cues seen during development of the tissue or organ systems of interest.*" [12](Haibin Xi. 2017) We will later explore some of the maternal and paternal influences that could interfere with this delicate developmental stage. Prevention is a worthy investment of time and resources, equal to investments in future treatment options for developmental anomalies.

CARDIOGENESIS

The fetal heart begins as a cardiogenic plate at the cranial end of the trilaminar disc lateral to the neural plate. It seems plausible that this proximity could explain why heart cells also contain nerve cells. The plate is derived from a few areas: the splanchnopleuric mesoderm which contains cardiogenic precursor cells, proepicardium, and cardiac neural crest cells. [13](Thomas Brade et al., 2013)

Brade explains that a variety of cell types make up what we later come to call the 4-chambered heart that most consider to be a muscle as well as an organ. He lists them as, "*atrial and ventricular cardiomyocytes, endocardial cells, valvular components, connective tissues, conduction system cells, as well as smooth muscle and endothelial cells of the coronary arteries and veins*." Also during the third week, blood islets coalesce at the cranial end of the embryo, arising out of the intra-embryonic mesoderm. [14](J-Marc Schleich, 2002)

Around day 17 to 18, the cardiogenic cells form the first and second heart field. A crescent or arc shape arises, which becomes enveloped by the second heart field. The first heart field forms into the right and left endocardial tubes that fuse at the midline. (Fig. 1.5) Both are just caudal to the head field that is unfolding simultaneously. The cells that form the crescent develop into the first beating linear tube. This tube begins looping to the right. As the primitive heart tube elongates, it begins to fold within the pericardium, eventually forming an S shape, which places the chamber and major vessels into an alignment similar to the adult heart.

Lindsay M. Biga et al., from Oregon State University describe the process like this: “Originally, it consists of a pair of strands called cardiogenic cords that quickly form a hollow lumen and are referred to as endocardial tubes. These tubes then form into a single heart tube. The five regions of the primitive heart tube develop into recognizable structures in a fully developed heart. The truncus arteriosus will eventually divide and give rise to the ascending aorta and pulmonary trunk. The bulbus cordis develops into the right ventricle. The primitive ventricle forms the left ventricle.”

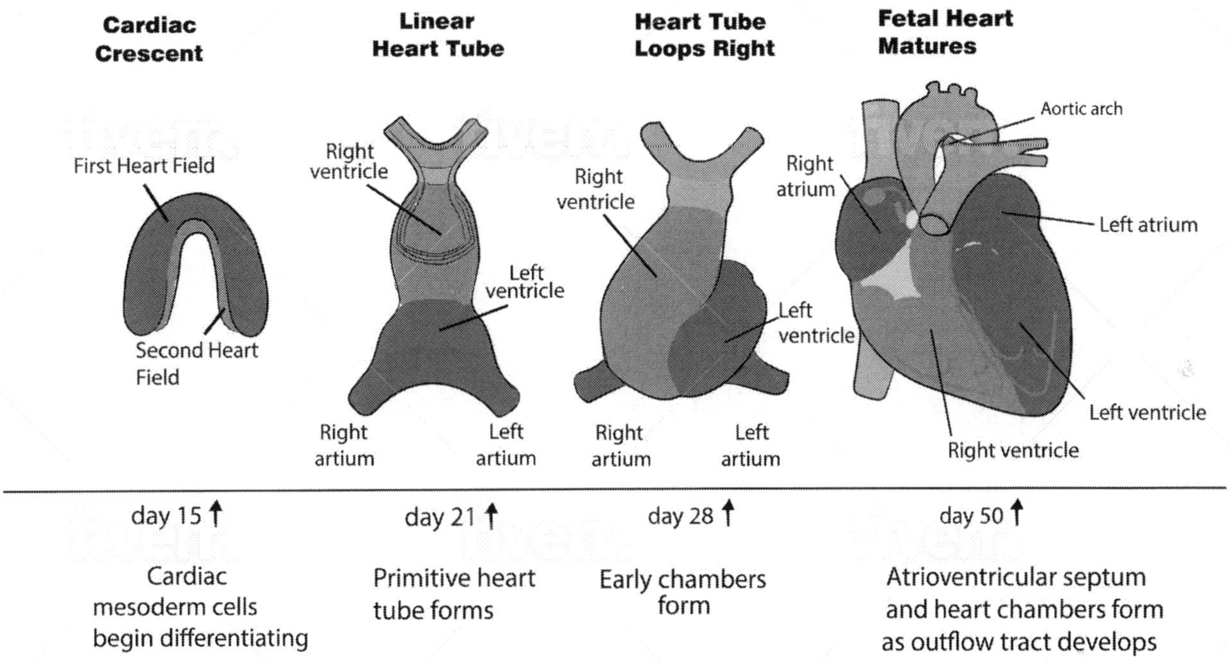

Fig. 1.5 Development of the primitive heart over 50 days, described by Dr. John A. Mc Nulty, Professor of Cell Biology, Neurobiology and Anatomy, Loyola University Medical Center

The circulatory system is the first functional unit in the developing embryo, and the heart is the first functional organ to nourish the embryo. [15](S.F. Gilbert, 2000) Initially, the umbilical vein brings oxygenated blood from the placenta, travels to the aorta, then to the right atrium of the heart. The blood leaving the heart through the right ventricle bypasses the lungs, which are not developed enough yet to process blood. (Fig.1.6) It uses the ductus arteriosus for the bypass, which sends the blood to the lower body before it leaves using the umbilical arteries. (American Heart Association, 2022)

The signaling and gene transcription processes are what’s still in debate. Andrew J. Lilly et al. proposed that for cardiac, vascular, and lymphatic systems, the SOXF factors, *“appear to have an indirect role in regulating cardiac mesoderm specification and differentiation. Understanding how SOXF factors are regulated, as well as their downstream transcriptional target genes, will be important for unraveling their roles in cardiovascular development and related diseases.”* [16](Lilly et al., 2017)

It is during these earliest stages that a congenital heart defect can occur. So there is keen interest to more fully understand the intracellular communication factors so that therapeutic interventions can be found. Congenital heart disease is the most common birth defect among congenital abnormalities due to disruptions during that phase of cardiogenesis. Familial chromosomal mutations contribute to the rising number of cases the last decade or so, along with mutations in transcription factors and signaling molecules such as NOTCH1, and JAG1.

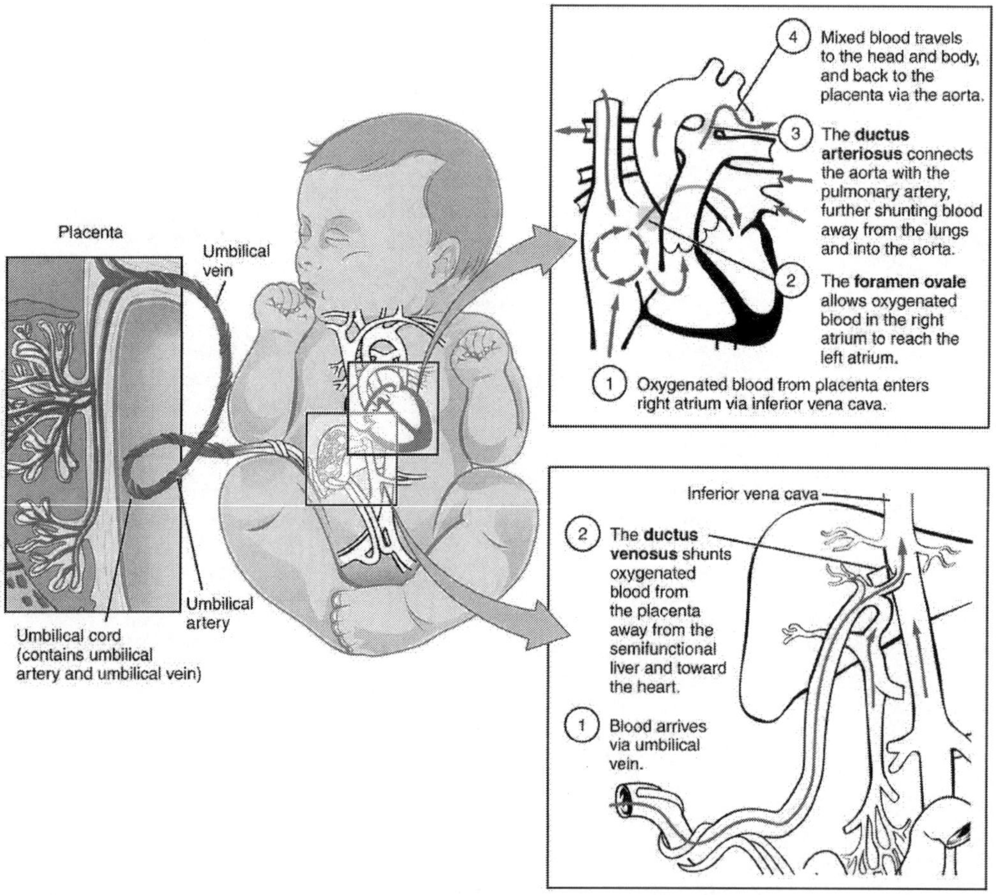

Fig. 1.6 – In the fetus, oxygenated blood arrives through the umbilical vein, but initially bypasses the immature lungs and liver using the ductus arteriosus before it leaves the body through the umbilical artery.

OpenStax College CC BY 3.0 via Wikimedia Commons

Although a large percentage of heart defects still remain a mystery, certain factors are becoming clear as causation. It is clear so far that maternal infections, certain drugs, diseases, stress, and maternal nutrition are directly related to some defects. The factors are being considered both from the perspective of the damaging impacts, as well as what could happen from the lack of protection the fetus would have had under optimal conditions. [17](Radha O. Joshi et al, 2021) Madhumita Basu and Vidu Garg report that,

"Maternal diabetes mellitus is a well-established and increasingly prevalent environmental risk factor for congenital heart disease." (Basu and Garg, 2018)

These researchers listed numerous transcription factors, ligands, and pathways that are involved in 'disease genes', along with several modifications in gene encoding for histone modifying enzymes.

Key areas of study regarding congenital heart disease include DNA methylation that's regulated by several enzymes and ncRNAs (non-coding) or micro RNA activity that mediate post-transcriptional gene silencing. RNA activity regulates gene expression during mesoderm formation and differentiation. Histones — important regulatory proteins — grossly influence RNA expression, along with the downstream expression of transcription factors. Transgenerational epigenetics is a current area of study as it becomes more obvious that ancestral phenotypes can be transmitted through more than one generation. The same holds true for patterns of trauma and inadequate nutrition. Exposure to toxins that alter any of the above factors is also an important growing field of study.

There is already evidence that dietary fat and maternal obesity affect gene expression in the fetal heart. It dysregulates NKX2-5 controlled transcription factors during cardiogenesis, and it "programs progressive heart dysfunction in adult offspring of mice." [18](Abdalla Ahmed, et al, 2021) Both mouse and human studies have discovered a connection between maternal blood sugar levels and fat intake on the developing fetus, showing implications for health later in life. Metabolism is a key feature in many aspects of fetal growth and development, because cellular energy and cellular communication are dysregulated when metabolism is dysregulated.

Keating and El-Osta reported that, *"Several components of the epigenetic machinery require intermediates of cellular metabolism for enzymatic function. Furthermore, changes to intracellular metabolism can alter the expression of specific histone methyltransferases and acetyltransferases, conferring widespread variations in epigenetic modification patterns. Specific epigenetic influences of dietary glucose and lipid consumption, as well as undernutrition, are observed across numerous organs and pathways associated with metabolism."* [19](Samuel T. Keating, 2015)

A normal heart as well as a defective heart can have electrical issues. The actual beating of the heart is set in motion by an electrical impulse through the sinoatrial node in the right atrium. The current passes through the heart, one conducting cell at a time, in a coordinated fashion, facilitating the contraction created by the muscle cells. The signal travels from the right and left atria causing them to contract and pump blood into the left and right ventricles. [20](Rakesh K. Pai, MD, 2021) An irregular heartbeat, whether too fast (tachycardia) or too slow (bradycardia) can happen in a fetus, but it isn't common. At 16 weeks the fetal heart is fully formed and beats at 110 – 160 bpm.

According to Texas Children's Hospital's Pediatric Cardiology Department, possible causes for a dysrhythmia include an electrolyte imbalance, inflammation, genetic defect, or medication. There is evidence that the father's preconception habits can influence the fetal heart. Sons of fathers who drank alcohol regularly had a higher incidence of irregular electrical activity in the heart as well as cognitive and behavior issues. In a 2022 longitudinal review of over 1200 births in Shanghai, preconception paternal alcohol increased incidences of neurodevelopmental and behavioral issues in their children, who still expressed sleep, anxiety/depression, acting-out and cognitive issues at 6 years-old. This team suggested that changes in ncRNA of the sperm could be part of the cause of these and other birth defects. (Min Luan, et al., Scientific Reports, 2022) A review of 55 studies in 2020 showed a 44% increase in the risk of congenital heart disorders if the father drank 3 months prior to conception. (Julia Riles, Healthline, 2021)

Both preconception and post-conception smoking also have potential birth defect impacts on the fetus. A study of over 566,000 couples in China showed that preconception smoking by the father may be associated with congenital heart disease, neural tube defects and limb malformation. (Q. Zhou et al., 2020) In a review of 125 studies involving 8.8 million parents from around the world, a father who smoked while the mother was pregnant increased the risk of heart defects by 74%, compared to 25% when the mother smoked while pregnant. [21](Ankur Banerjee, 2019) Second-hand smoke is quite harmful! There is a likelihood that planned pregnancies can take these findings into account and avoid the risks to the child, which later might otherwise be interpreted to be arising 'out of nowhere.'

Osteogenesis

Osteogenesis begins at this same embryonic stage, but the growth, remodeling, and ossification process continue for several years after birth. During the fourth week, as part of somitogenesis, the multipotent somitomeres begin to form an epithelial layer to distinguish themselves from other somites while the specialization process is set in motion. The cells that form the kidney — or mesonephros — arise out of the same portion of the lateral mesoderm that gives rise to the skeletal bones. A disruption in this process that might lead to a spinal defect could also create kidney problems. [22](Corinne DeRuiter, 2010)

There is also evidence that bone marrow cells participate in the formation of several types of kidney cells. (Yoko et al., 2008) The cells transition from the pronephros in the 3rd week, to the mesonephros by the 4th or 5th week, which serves as the excretory organ for the fetus. (Alan Partin, MD, PHD, 2021) Partin explains that a few mesonophros cells become efferent ducts of the testes in males, and the muscular portion of the vaginal walls and broad ligament of the uterus in females. We go into great detail about the relationship between bones and kidneys in a later chapter.

Bone formation also begins in the third week as the divisions of the mesoderm differentiate and migrate. The axial (thorax) skeleton forms out of the sclerotome division of the paraxial mesoderm, and the limbs (appendicular skeleton) develop out of the somatic division of the lateral mesoderm. (Fig.1.2) The axial skeleton consists of the skull including the facial bones, laryngeal skeleton (hyoid bone and voice box), the spine including the sacrum and tail bone, and the rib cage including the sternum and manubrium.

In practice, it can be observed that compression or malalignment in one area of the lateral mesoderm directly affects another. For example, alterations in rib or sternum alignment can adversely impact the skull. Conversely, in practice, it can be a valuable tool to employ the ribs, sternum, and sacrum to help rebalance and remove pressures on the skull, as is common in Biodynamic Cranial Sacral therapy and Cranial Osteopathy.

According to Grant Breeland, between the 6th and 7th week of development, two types of ossification begin: 1.) **intramembranous**, which converts mesenchymal tissue into the flat bones of the skull, clavicle, and most cranial bones; and 2.) **endochondral** ossification that converts mesenchymal tissue into cartilage that becomes long bones and the rest of the axial skeleton. Intramembranous mesenchymal cells are derived from neural crest cells of the trilaminar disc. Because they are directly connected to the nervous system, all flat bones may be implicated in pain patterns related to concussions. The process apparently can continue until 25 years of age.

Bones in different parts of the body grow at different rates, and in general are growing more in length than in width which makes them vulnerable to fractures. In fact, there is a high fracture rate in childhood and adolescence averaging 40-45% for active children. Nonetheless, it is advisable to maintain physical activity that stresses (high impact) and therefore strengthens the bones during this time, as it also sets the stage for healthy bones throughout life. (Gordon, 2020; Elkaheem, PhD et al., 2019, Tan et al., 2014)

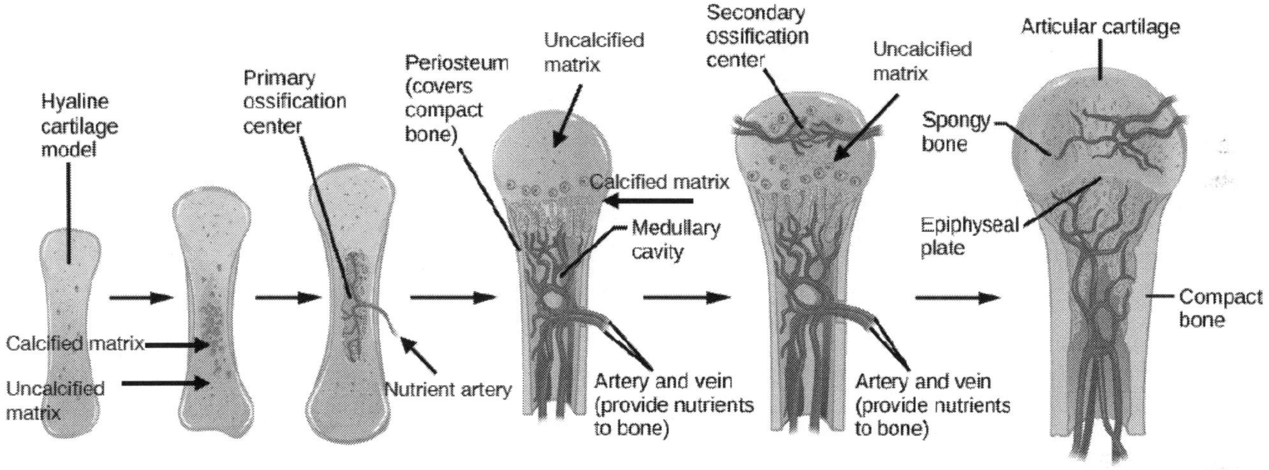

Fig. 1.7 -Stages in the ossification process of long bones

"As they (mesenchymal cells) gather in the cartilage, the cells form an ossification center where osteoblasts differentiate and spawn osteoids. Osteoids consist of an unmineralized collagen proteoglycan matrix that can bind calcium resulting in the hardening or mineralization of the matrix and entrapment of osteoblasts." (Breeland, 2021)

Image courtey of CNX OpenStax CC BY 4.0 via Wikimedia Commons

As they gather in the cartilage, the intramembranous mesenchymal cells become osteoblasts and form an ossification center — or template — where osteoblasts differentiate to form osteoids. (Fig. 1.7) Osteoids consist of an unmineralized collagen proteoglycan matrix that can bind calcium, resulting in the hardening or mineralization of the matrix and entrapment of osteoblasts. [25] (Breeland, et al., May 2021) Breeland continues the description of transformation in this way, *"The calcification of the extracellular matrix prevents nutrients from reaching the chondrocytes and causes them to undergo apoptosis. The resulting cell death creates voids in the cartilage template and allows blood vessels to invade.(Fig. 1.8) Blood vessels further enlarge the spaces, which eventually combine and become the medullary cavity (or spongy bone)."*

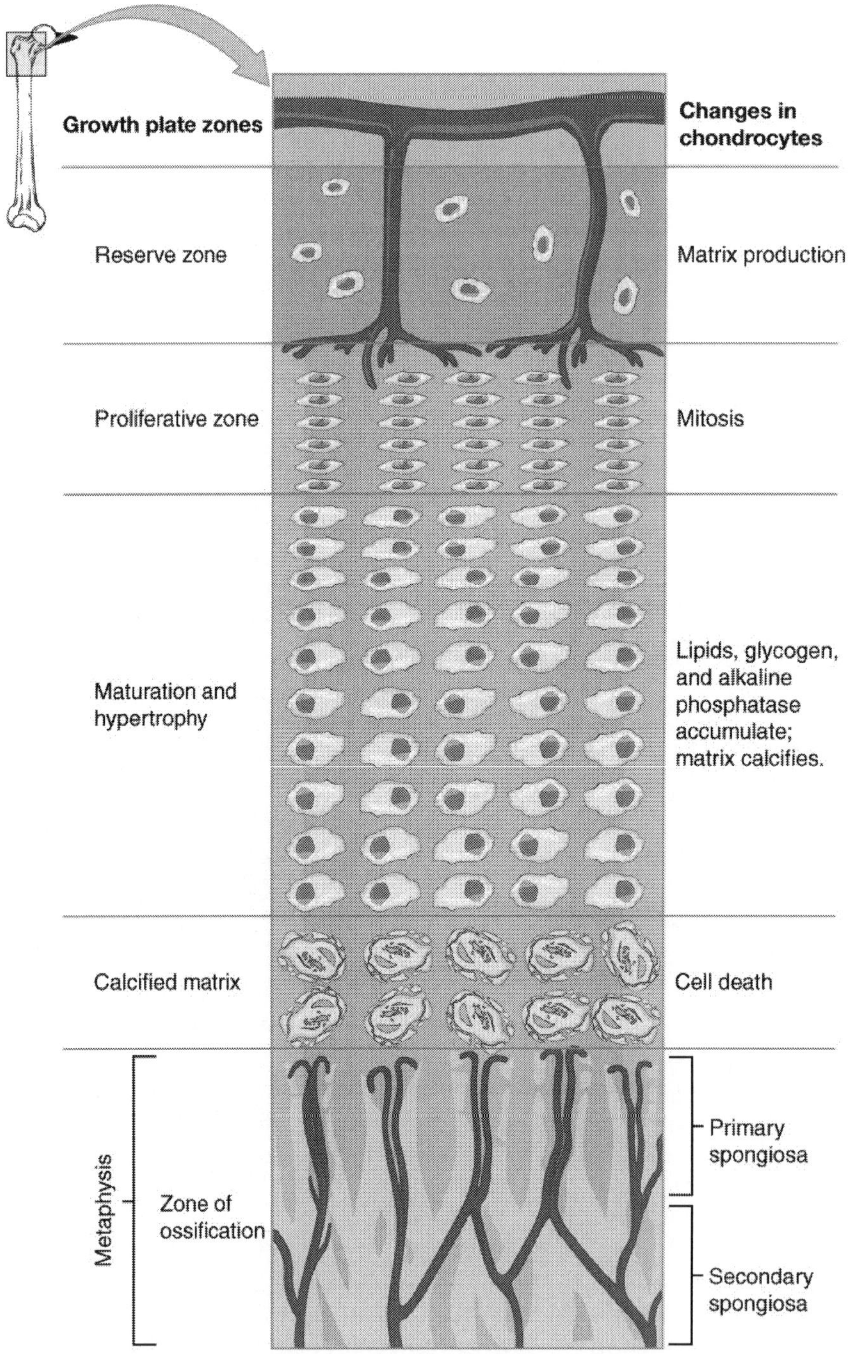

Fig. 1.8 – Long bones continue to grow in length and in width throughout adolescence. Each section plays a role in the continuation of the process. The reserve zone contains chondrocytes that secure the epiphyseal plate to the epiphysis. Mitosis happens in the proliferation zone where new cells are being produced. The substances in the maturation zone help to enlarge the cells and calcify the matrix, while the vascularized metaphysis deposits new bone cells on top of the newly formed matrix. (LibreTexts, UC Davis, 2020)

Image courtesy of OpenStax College CC BY 3.0 via Wikimedia Commons

The dense tissue of the periosteum is also formed during this stage, which serves as an entheses - the attachment site for tendons and ligaments. A secondary ossification center develops as the signaling from the notochord stimulates chondrogenesis. Then the notochord dissolves. Fusion of these areas in the spine concludes between the 5th and 8th year after birth at the epiphysis of the long bones, where ongoing growth of the bone happens (at the epiphyseal plate). The hyaline cartilage that remains becomes the articular surface of the bone. (Fig.1.7) Ossification centers are especially relevant, and along with related transcription factors, have been studied more often because these centers support bone repair during fracture healing.

Particularly for the spine, the timing of the release of these repair 'instructions' is critical. Kevin Kaplan, MD, explains that, *"Development of the spine is a complex event involving genes, signaling pathways, and numerous metabolic processes. Various abnormalities are associated with errors in this process."* [26] (Kaplan, et al, 2005) In 2020, Yūcel Ağirdil described the complexity of the process this way: *"There are many pathways, signals, receptors, mediators, agonists, and antagonists that interact with considerable mixing and matching, making it possbile for bone tissue to develop within the cartilaginous template... This complex system is vulnerable to a wide variety of genetic abnormalities, and to date nearly 500 genetic skeletal disorders have been described."[27]* It might be useful to note that bone begins as cartilage during this phase, and that later in life, errors in cartilage repair can generate osteoarthritis, or the inaccurate depositing of bone in a joint.

The vertebral arch alone has three ossification centers; one in the center and one on each side. In 1998, Persaud Moore described 5 secondary ossification centers for the vertebrae: one for the tip of transverse processes, one for the tip of the spinous process, and one for both the upper and lower aspects of the vertebral body. This endochondral ossification process utilizes signaling from hormones, such as estrogen and parathyroid hormone. It also uses transcription factors, growth factors, and cytokines. [27] (Yūcel Ağirdil, 2020) In manual medicine, there are contact points on the vertebrae that signal reorganization, repositioning, and cross-talk with other vertebrae and connective tissue. Additional research in this area could be very helpful for fracture repair as well as for rebalancing.

A greater understanding of these centers also becomes an exciting source for the potential reversal of osteoporosis later in life. Although the original formative stimuli were biochemical in nature, it has been shown that mechanical forces can also initiate biochemical responses. Aikiko Mammoto expressed in 2012 that, *"In the past, most work has focused on how transcriptional regulation results from the complex interplay between chemical cues, adhesion signals, transcription factors, and their co-regulators during development.*

Accumulated evidence indicates that mechanical cues, which include physical forces (tension, compression, shear stress), alterations in extracellular matrix mechanics, and changes in cell shape, are transmitted to the nucleus directly or indirectly to orchestrate transcriptional activities that are crucial for embryogenesis and organogenesis." [28](Mammoto and Ingber, 2012)

The matrix mechanics are the aspect of signaling that empowers us to have an effect on our own bones as well as on our organs. For as remarkable and sturdy the bones and other forms of connective tissue are that provide the tensegrity necessary for communication to flow, they are also fragile and prone to dysregulation. This makes our conscious participation in its powers of adaptation and resetting even more important, as it holds the key to the epigenetic potential. You will find as you read through this text, that countless researchers have affirmed over the years that how we relate to our bodies and the cells therein as we lead our lives acts as a form of communication that reaches the nucleus of each cell.

The ways in which we are active and inactive on a regular basis contribute to the framework of our very existence. How we can self-regulate by understanding the process is possibly the most exciting part of realizing how many other systems our bones influence. Bones will come up again and again throughout the book as their multiple roles and areas of influence - even at the level of transcription factors - will be discussed. In the meantime, let's take a look at the many ways these developmental stages can be compromised, most of which are avoidable, fortunately.

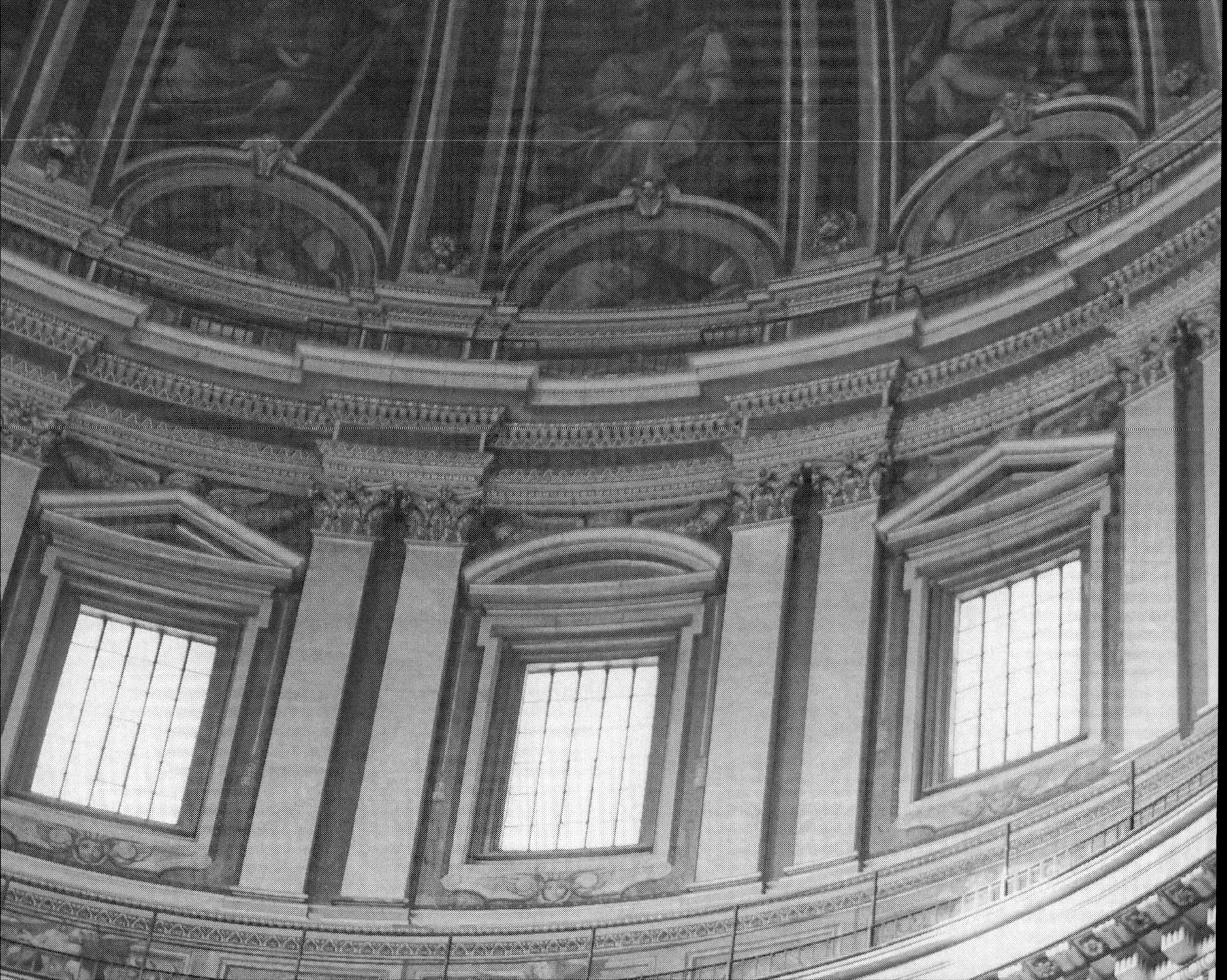

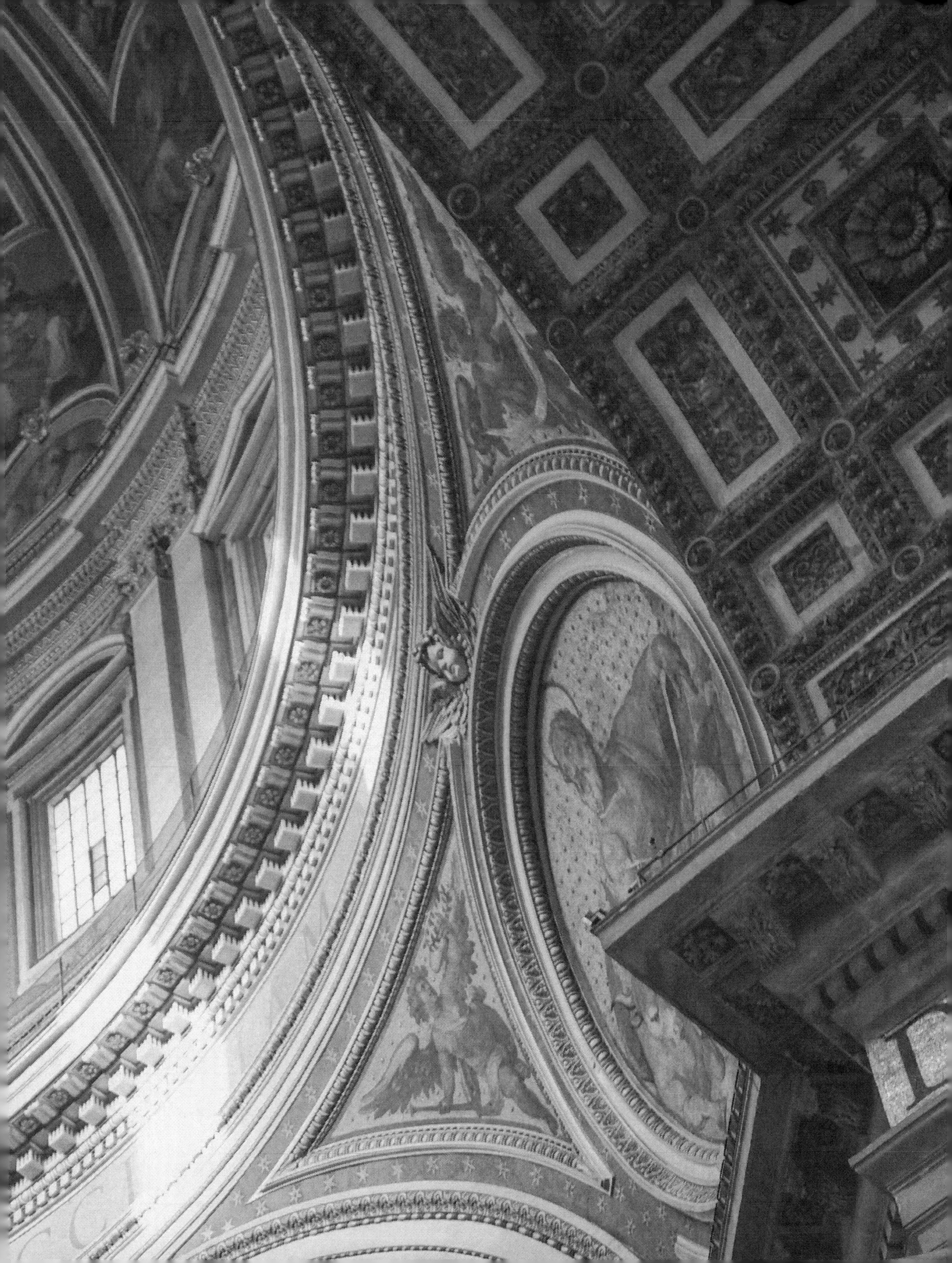

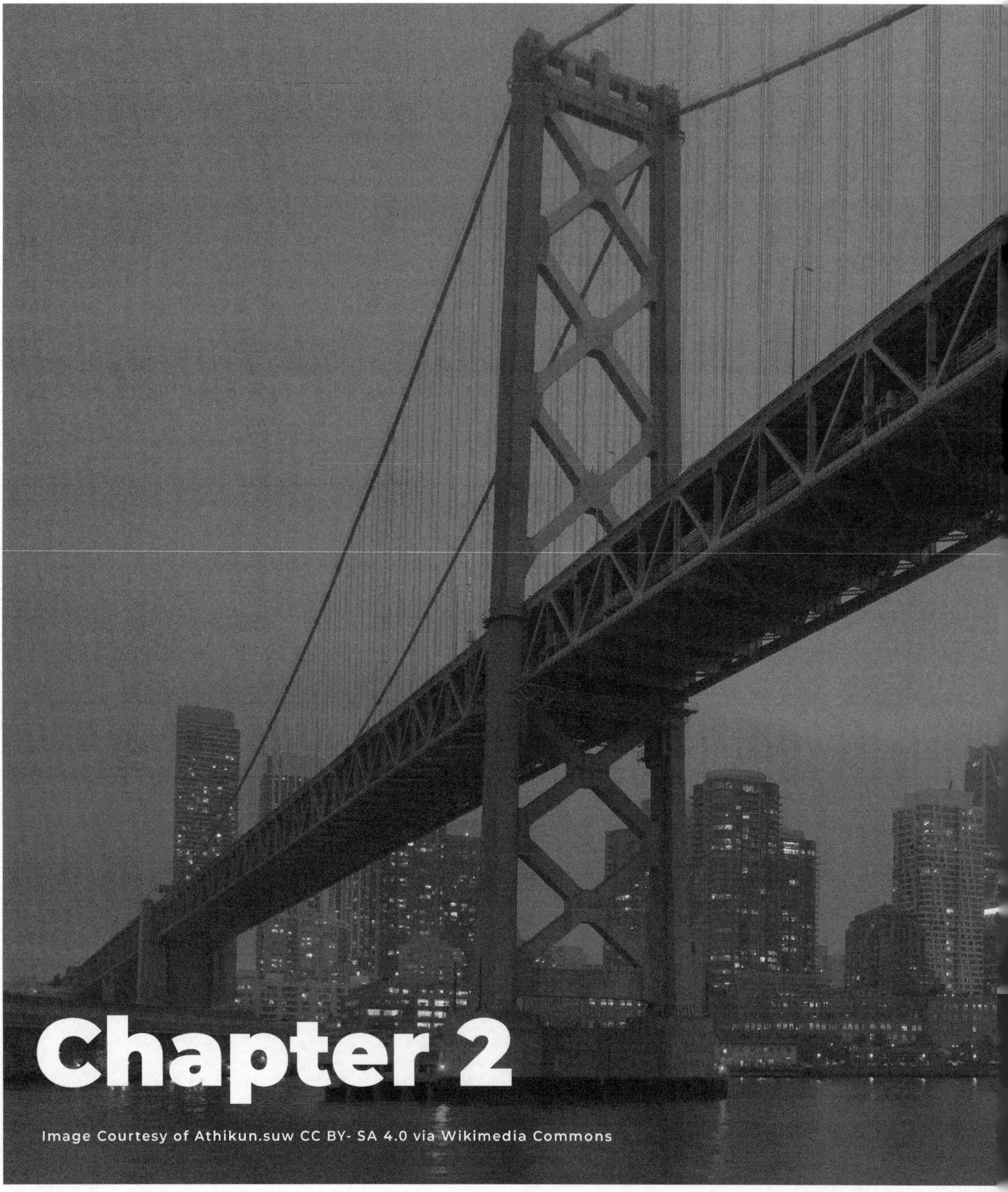

Chapter 2

Preconception Risks for the Fetus

Our bodies are the laboratories and manufacturing plants where new humans are being conceived and built. Everything about the status of these facilities matters. The preconception behaviors of both parents impact the health, cognitive capacity, and personality of the infant. Preconception health is defined as the health of both men and women throughout their lives until they conceive. It might be difficult to consider the fact that everything affecting your well-being can impact the child you haven't produced yet, but it's been proven.

Moss and Harris conclude that:

> *"The benefits of good preconception health include improved pregnancy and birth outcomes, including birth weights and gestational ages in the normal range, which produce reduced risk for adverse health conditions throughout the lifetime, including cardiovascular disease, metabolic diseases, and cancer."*

Health factors being studied during preconception for their effects on the child later in life included: diabetes, high blood pressure, alcohol and fast food consumption, and depression. [29] (Jennifer L. Moss, Kathleen Mullan Harris, 2015)

In 2017, a group of researchers focused on childhood neurological impacts from preconception and prenatal conditions that were based upon malnutrition, stress, and inflammation. Betty Vohr stated that, *"Fetal growth restriction in both term and pre-term infants is associated with neonatal morbidities and a wide variety of behavioral and psychological diagnoses within childhood and adolescence, including attention-deficit/hyperactivity disorder (ADHD), anxiety, depression, internalizing and thought problems, poor social skills, and autism spectrum disorder."* [30](Betty R. Vohr et al., 2017)

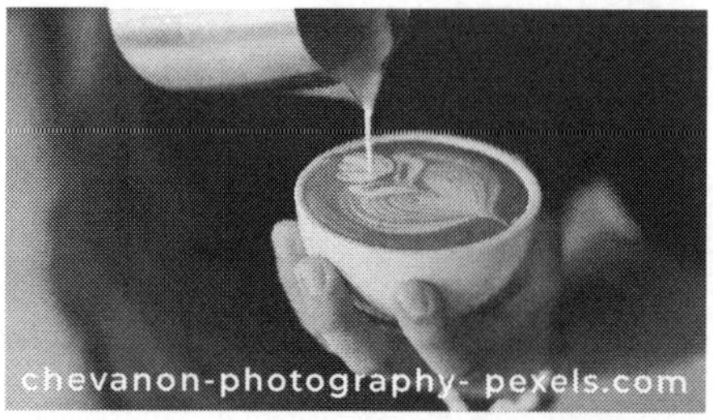

Zohra Lassie found that preconception lifestyle factors weigh heavily on fetal development, and that the harm can impact two generations. For example, their study revealed that drinking over 300 mg. (3 cups) of **caffeine**/day preconception increased miscarriages by over 30%. Smoking before conceiving can triple the risk of congenital heart defects. [31](Zohra S. Lassi et al., 2014) Maternal exposure to radiation while working prior to conception can lead to increased rates of miscarriage, which has also been shown in cases of exposure to **non-ionizing radiation** from wi-fi, smart meters, computers, and the like.

Segal and Guidice reported in 2019 that, "*There is a growing consensus that preconception exposure to* environmental toxins *can adversely affect fertility, pregnancy, and fetal development, which may persist into the neonatal and adult periods and potentially have* multigenerational *effects*." [32](Thalia R. Segal and Linda C. Guidice, 2019) Segal and other researchers are recommending consultations with doctors before conceiving to assist parents in optimizing health outcomes for the family.

Risks during Early Stages of Pregnancy

Since McBride established the relationship between pregnant women taking the drug thalidomide and infants born with phocomelia — or limb reduction formation — a large number of drugs and supplements have warning labels on the bottle regarding their safety during pregnancy. [33](Hill & Kleinberg, 1984) Unfortunately, most women are unaware that they're pregnant during this critical first month while the blueprints for the organization of the body are being established, and up to half of pregnancies are unplanned. A study by Shizhao Li, et al. in 2019 found that both health and disease later in life can be directly related to circumstances in the first month of pregnancy.

They report that:

> *"Exposure to environmental facts such as nutrition, climate, stress, pathogens, toxins, and even social behavior during gametogenesis and embryogenesis has been shown to influence disease susceptibility in the offspring.*

From atmospheric pollution, endocrine-disrupting chemicals to heavy metals, research increasingly suggests that environmental pollutants have already produced significant consequences on human health. Moreover, mounting evidence now links such pollution to relevant modification in the epigenome. The epigenetics diet, referring to a class of bioactive dietary compounds such as isothiocyanates in broccoli, genistein in soybeans, resveratrol in grapes, epigallocatechin-e-gallate in green tea, and ascorbic acid in fruits, has been shown to modify the epigenome leading to beneficial health outcomes." [34](Li et al., 2019)

ENVIRONMENTAL EXPOSURES

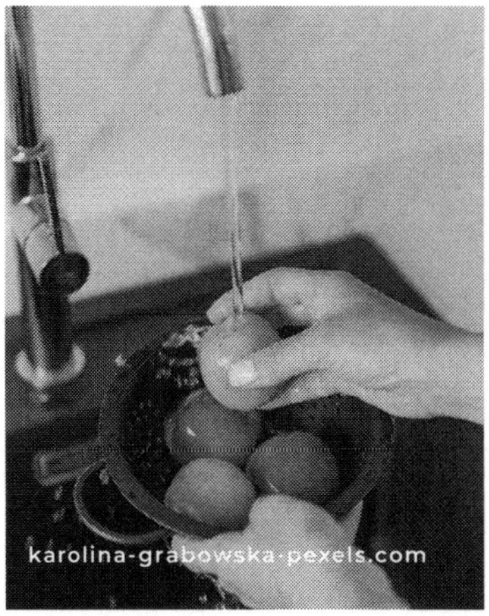

It has been shown in a 5-year study that air pollution above a certain particulate level (2.5ppm) can produce gestational diabetes in women whether exposed before or during pregnancy. [35](Amal Rammah et al, 2020) Baccarelli and Bollati report that, *"In environmental health, the recognition that exposures could produce DNA mutations represented a major landmark for risk assessment and prevention. Consequently, chemical agents have been categorized according to their capability to alter the DNA sequence (In vitro). Several classes of environmental chemicals have been identified that modify epigenetic marks, including metals: cadmium, arsenic nickel, chromium, methylmercury; peroxisome proliferators, air pollutants, and endocrine-disrupting toxicants like BPA (in many plastic bottles) and dioxin (used in herbicides and winds up in food. [36](Andrea Baccarelli and Valentina Bollati,* 2008)

PRENATAL STRESS

Although the cause may not be realized when symptoms develop years later, stress, anxiety, or depression in the mother while pregnant can have a lasting effect on the child. In 2015, Phelan and colleagues found during a study of 3000 women that, *"Maternal prenatal stress is associated with increased reporting of infant illness as well as increased frequency of both urgent care visits and emergency department visits."* In fact, they found that high prenatal stress was a significant predictor of maternal reporting of infant gastrointestinal and respiratory illness along with urgent care visits. The women reporting highest levels of stress were unmarried, younger minority women without college degrees on public insurance. [37] (A.J. Phelan, et al., 2015).

LaPlante observed in a smaller 'distress–related-to-temperament' study of 121 infants — half male, half female — that both maternal stress and illness can predict temperament at 6 months old. LaPlante states that *"There is a growing body of literature linking measures of maternal stress during pregnancy and adverse infant/child outcomes. For example, higher levels of prenatal maternal stress are associated with poorer intellectual, linguistic, and behavioral outcomes."* He goes on to state that *"Human research indicates that maternal infection during pregnancy is associated with higher rates of schizophrenia and autism among offspring."* [38](David P. LaPlante et al., 2016)

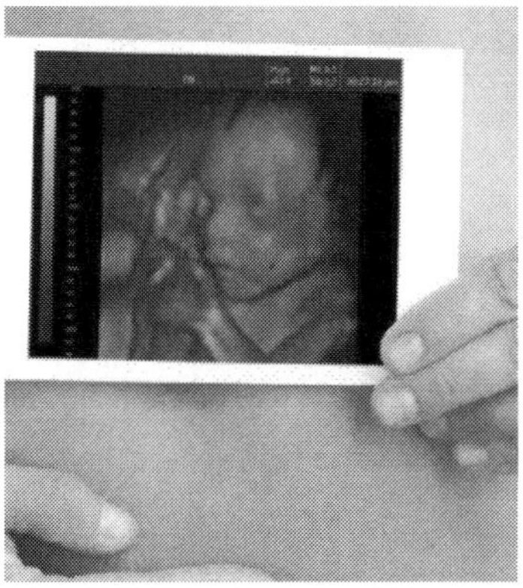

Recent findings show that the sex of the child can be influenced by maternal stress, and since the male fetus is more vulnerable, it's also more likely to miscarry. The male fetus was more affected by psychological rather than the physical stressors of the mother, and pregnant women who had higher levels of social support have increased odds of male versus female births. The study by Walsh and colleagues also showed that anxiety and depression in pregnant women doubled the likelihood of having offspring with neurological issues, such as ADHD or anxiety. [39](Kate Walsh et al., 2019)

Perhaps pregnant women could be made aware of classes that prepare young mothers to navigate the emotional waters that may become turbulent during or after birth. There have been programs offered in hospital settings that curbed maternal stress by a large margin when the mothers knew what to expect, and had some guidance on how to handle the new situations with infant care, and with care for their own bodies.

ANTIBIOTICS

Professor David Burgner from the Murdoch Children's Research Institute ran a study from 1997 to 2009 in Denmark that included 750,000 pregnancies and found that,

> *"Children born to mothers who were prescribed antibiotics during pregnancy may have up to a 20% higher risk of being hospitalized with infection."*

He went on to say that the increased risk persisted throughout childhood. The likelihood becomes greater the closer to delivery, and if the antibiotics were prescribed more than once. [40](Sophie Scott, 2018) There is no recommendation to not take antibiotics if the mother contracts an infection, but to be aware of the dangers, and to consider that the impacts on the microbiome of the mother influences the microbiome and immune system of the fetus in ways that are not yet fully understood.

FEVER

A change in temperature in the developing fetus, such as having a fever during the process of neurulation, can create defects in the neural tube which could lead to spina bifida, anencephaly and encephalocele, when the ends of the tube don't close properly. It has been shown that women taking 400 mg of folic acid in the earliest stages of pregnancy did not produce these birth defects even though they had a fever at that stage. (Slone Epidemiology Center at Boston University in collaboration with the CDC) More serious stress, trauma, illness, infection or fever during the first couple of weeks before implantation may more often result in the termination of the pregnancy.

ALCOHOL

In 2007, Kapil Sayal and his team chose to look at long-term impacts of moderate alcohol consumption rather than the heavier usage that can lead to fetal alcohol syndrome. They found that just one drink per week during the first trimester was *"associated with clinically significant mental health problems"* in 4-year-old girls, which continued to be noticed two years later. [41](Kapil Sayal et al., 2007) In 2011, Erica O'Neil discussed various defects that can occur based upon which structures are differentiating and developing during that critical third week in her article, *"Developmental Timeline of Alcohol-Induced Birth Defects."* She listed neurological deficits, physical deformities, heart valve issues leading to heart disease, vision issues, and so on, as the signaling from each germ layer becomes compromised.

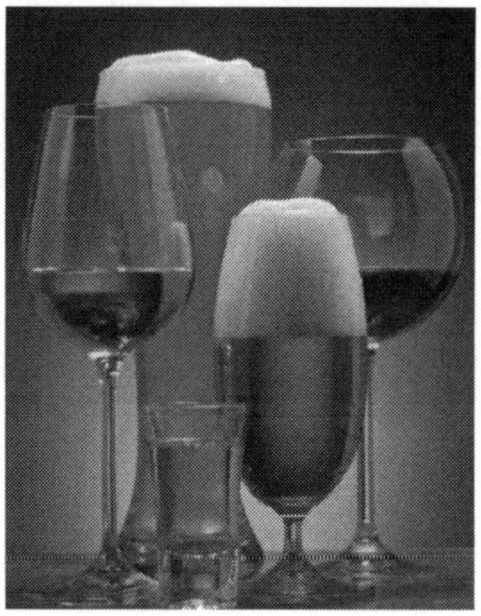

Giorgia Sebastiani and her researchers found in 2018 that restricted micronutrients due to impaired absorption by the addicted mother contributed to physical and neurological impairments similar to the disruptive effects of ethanol. The March of Dimes went as far as to say that no amount of alcohol is safe for pregnant women. Theodore Cisero, PhD discovered in the 1980s that regular consumption of alcohol by the father can create excessive or abnormal electrical activity in their sons which can lead to behavioral or cognitive disorders. In addition, twin studies in the late 1980s showed that even when raised by a non-alcoholic father, both twins with an alcoholic biological father demonstrated a much greater risk of becoming alcoholics themselves. (Cloninger, 1989; Pickens, 1991)

Several researchers are mentioning the need to increase the current limited research on gender variations in susceptibility. The area most needed involves how paternal alcohol intake contributes to fetal alcohol syndrome and adult onset glucose intolerance. [42](Chang et al., 2019) Chang and his team also discovered an increased incidence of growth restriction, fibrotic livers, and metabolic dysfunction in male and female offspring of preconception paternal drinking, along with "long-term immune signaling alterations, and an abundance of inflammatory cytokines in the liver, pancreas, and plasma".

A new paradigm is opening up in the field of addictions. Neurobiology is acknowledging the changes in brain anatomy, chemistry, and cellular communication, but is also acknowledging neuroplasticity as a viable option; the ability of the neurons to form new pathways. Altering pathways result in altering mental, emotional, and physical states, but also means that brain changes would be a reflection of those states, not just the cause. The shift in paradigm from viewing addictions as a disease to viewing it as a reaction to trauma suggests that the system is using it as a coping mechanism. Coping mechanisms can be unlearned when given new coping mechanisms.

Coping better can lead to lowered sympathetic drive in the nervous system so that it can be open to new options. Perhaps then the trauma would be open to a safe way to be acknowledged and gently reframed. The felt sense of safety in the body would make it easier to be released from tissue memory, paving the way for new cells that have a 'clean slate' to be cycled in. Viewing the condition as dysregulated functioning changes the way treatment is approached, leaving the option open for healing. Gaining a skill set that can shift an automatic, unconscious behavior to a conscious, intentional one is beneficial in every circumstance. I've even heard from a client who was on a bike when she was hit by a car, that she was aware of herself flying through the air and did all she could to make conscious choices about how to land.

Neurologist, Antonello Bonci, from the National Institute on Drug Abuse states that,

> *"If addictions (such as sugar, alcohol, gambling, heroin, sex) are learned, then recovery can be 'learned' as well.*

However, creating new "recovery" neural pathways cannot be rewired and reassigned through healing the underlying trauma and core issues alone. The brain must be rewired through a specific set of evidence-based therapeutic protocols that help create new neural networks for recovery such as, but certainly not limited to: mindfulness techniques, HearthMath biofeedback, EMDR, brain supplement protocols, and energy medicine."

Author, Maia Szalavitz, once an addict herself, calls addiction a learning disability that happens 90% of the time in one's youth, if it happens. She echoes that it comes as a coping mechanism to trauma at a time when cognitive skills are still forming and perceiving outcomes to risk-taking behavior is not developed. Szalavitz reports that the majority of addictions in Europe, except smoking, resolve themselves by age 30. At that age, those executive function areas of the brain are more fully developed and conscious choices can override reactive patterns. [43](Szalavitz, 2022) Nonetheless, creating awareness and developing programs for children that include outlets for overwhelming emotions could be very helpful and preventative. There is already evidence of this being true as mindfulness programs enter the curriculum in some schools.

DIETARY CONSIDERATIONS

In general, but particularly for pregnant women, certain dietary options should be avoided. Large fish, such as swordfish, shark, king mackerel, tuna, marlin, and orange roughy, tend to eat smaller fish and accumulate more mercury. Raw fish, which is popular in some types of sushi, can contain parasites or be overrun with bacteria like Salmonella or even norovirus. The same holds true for eggs and meat that are undercooked, rare, or medium rare. Adda recommends also avoiding processed meats, raw sprouts, unpasteurized milk, cheese, and fruit juice, unwashed produce, processed junk food and alcohol. [44] (Adda Bjarnadóttir, MS, 2020)

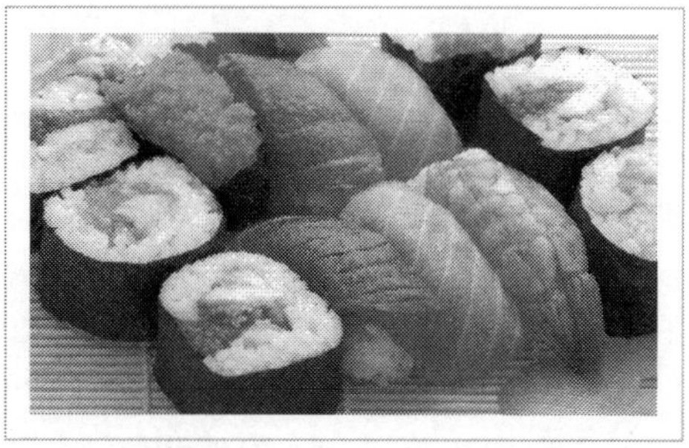

The American Pregnancy Association adds smoked seafood to the 'avoid' list, along with deli meat, pre-prepared chicken or tuna salad from a market, and fish from local lakes or streams that may contain PCBs (industrial solvents), such as striped bass, bluefish, pike, trout, salmon, and walleye. They also discourage the consumption of soft cheeses like Brie, Camembert, Roquefort, Feta, and Gorgonzola that may contain listeria bacteria, unless they're made from pasteurized milk. Paté that needs to be refrigerated is also risky according to this organization.

Food is information, carrying and transmitting over 26,000 biochemicals that our system decodes and uploads on a regular basis. (Barabási, 2020) Everything we put in our bodies or experience through our senses becomes a type of information that is digested by our system, and while pregnant, it includes the system of the baby. Thoughts, behaviors, feelings, and emotions are all a type of input that can be leaving impressions upon the unborn fetus whose consciousness is ripe for messaging and imprinting. It can take a while before those impressions can become conscious.

The first month is critical, when much of the cellular communication is in high gear while building the foundation of the form and their functions. This continues through the rest of the first trimester. Although the fetus is not quite as vulnerable during the second trimester, according to Johns Hopkins University, it is still recommended to avoid alcohol, smoking, excessive caffeine, undercooked meat, hot tubs or sauna, and cleaning the litter box to prevent exposure to some infectious bacteria. ("The Second Trimester," Health Magazine)

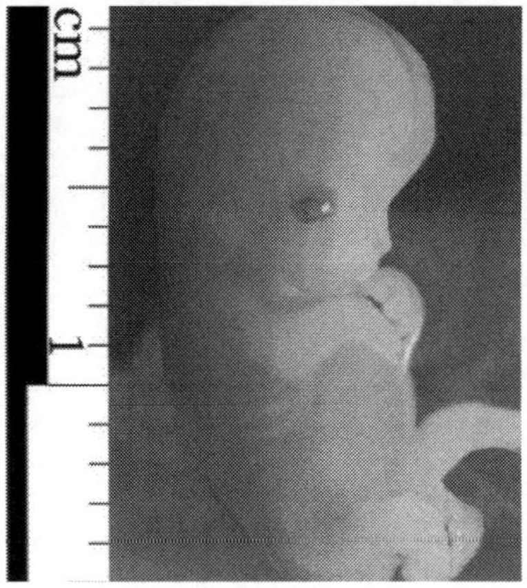

7 week-old fetus

GoldenBear at German Wikipedia, CC BY-SA 3.0 via Wikimedia Commons

The third trimester is mainly a time for growth of the fetus, as it gains weight, gets stronger, moves more, grows hair, opens its eyes, develops bone marrow, and practices breathing. ("Pregnancy week by week," Healthy Lifestyle, Mayo Clinic) Everything the mother ingests should still be considered carefully, as complications can arise even though the body of the infant is largely fully formed. Some systems, such as the brain, lungs, and bones are still maturing.

RADIATION AND EMFS

Due to an ever-increasing exposure to electronics in the digital world we now live in, and the fact that no safety measures have been instituted before the technology was released, the health hazards are increasing. Non-ionizing radiation is emitted from the magnetic fields generated within common household and work environments. Appliances, power lines, smart meters, computers, Wi-Fi routers, microwave ovens, cell phones, and more can produce emissions that are capable of penetrating walls. Young children, the elderly, and pregnant women are the most vulnerable and the most at risk of receiving harm. In fact, pregnant women who are exposed to this type of radiation are almost 3 times more likely to miscarry. (Ronnie Cohen, Reuters, 2017)

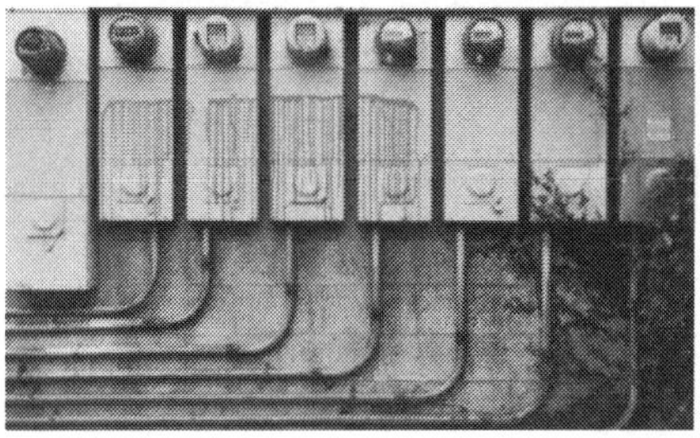

In addition, a multi-year project conducted by the National Toxicology Program "has revealed an increased risk of cancer associated with MF (magnetic field) non-ionizing radiation exposure." Although the risk was higher if the women were exposed on a daily basis, the source of the MF didn't make a difference in the outcomes. One study found an increased risk of embryonic bud (arm and leg) growth and cell death with higher exposures. [45](De-Kun Li, et al., 2017) These researchers state that The International Agency for Research on Cancer has classified magetic fields as a possible carcinogen.

Nida Ahmed writes in a 2020 article covering a Kaiser Permanente 20-year study of 2600 pregnant women that,

> *"Recent human studies have suggested that maternal exposure to MF non-ionizing radiation in pregnancy is linked with an increased risk of various childhood illnesses including asthma, obesity, and neurological conditions such as ADHD."* She goes on to say that over 6 million children in the U.S. have been diagnosed or are receiving treatment for ADHD. *[46](Nida Ahmed, 2020)*

There is evidence that Wi-Fi exposure impacts the body's cellular signaling via voltage-gated channels within seconds. One study showed that calcium channels could be blocked by pulsed, low-intensity magnetic fields emitted by Wi-Fi, and that chloride, potassium and sodium channels were also gated. The researchers interpreted the findings to indicate that the plasma membrane was affected. They went on the say, "*Moreover, different biological manifestations occurred within the exposure time frame, including calcium overload, raised steroid hormone levels, lower male and female fertility, neurological impairment, oxidative stress, cell damage and cell death*."[47](Martin L. Pall, 2018)

"Excessive Wi-Fi exposure can also lead to reduced melatonin, which interrupts sleep patterns as well as causing increased norepinephrine," reports Dr. Sanchari Sinha Dutta. Increased oxidative stress and free radical damage are responsible for damage to cellular macromolecules like proteins, lipids, and DNA, Dutta reports, along with "chromosomal mutations, which is one of the causes of spontaneous abortion of the fetus." [48](Sanchari Dutta, PhD, 2020)

There are energetic, frequency, chemical, electrical, neurological, and mechanical sources of communication that happen constantly in the body. Maintaining balance and health at any age is dependent upon these avenues of communication being able to happen efficiently and accurately. Some alterations can take years to show damage, but others can happen immediately. Those that occur during pregnancy and the first few years of a child's life can have long lasting impacts on many different systems, and some alterations affect the health of future generations. These biological systems overlap and interact in ways that aren't readily apparent when conceiving of them as individual entities.

They began as, and still are collections of cells with certain predetermined functions that continue to regulate cell behavior throughout our lives. There is inherent cellular common ground, as all cells arose from the primitive ectoderm and still experience shared signaling pathways. From this perspective, whatever you expose yourself to has the potential of impacting many different layers of functioning. That may be why the source of some conditions is hard to track when looking at the symptoms. It may not be as difficult when looking at the signaling. In fact, much research has already made the connections between most manifestations of disease and faulty signaling.

Something that begins as a mechanical force from repetitive strain, or a sudden fall could develop into tissue disorganization that produces biochemical changes which alters signaling systems. Optimally, as manual or movement practitioners, we can facilitate the restoration of balance in the systems' communication processes, either by helping the system to discharge and balance tension, or by using approaches that stimulate the system's capacity to self-correct. In this case, it may reveal itself as a chicken or egg situation where either one facilitates the other.

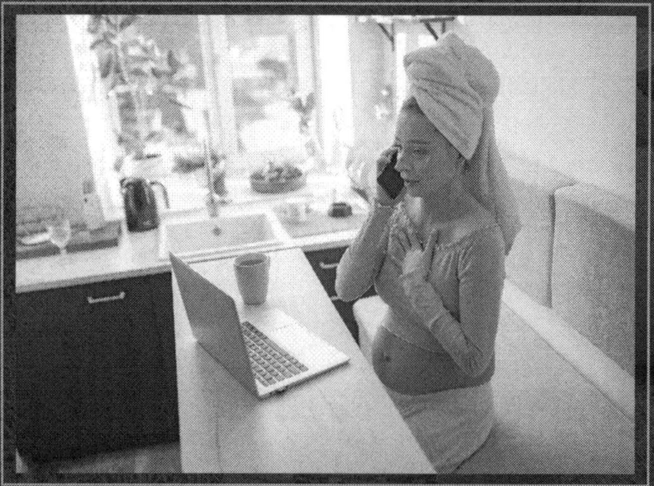

As individuals, a paradigm shift into every experience becoming a potential regulator for our cells' behavior can be very empowering. Realizing that whatever we eat, and how or if we move in certain ways can determine whether or not we acquire a major health issue is liberating. Knowing how to offer tactile, kinesthetic, or even dietary input into a system that can catalyze a reset across many layers of communication is both exciting and motivating. Opening the embryological avenues of interaction for reexamination as a catalyst for a profound somatic reset is the aim of this text.

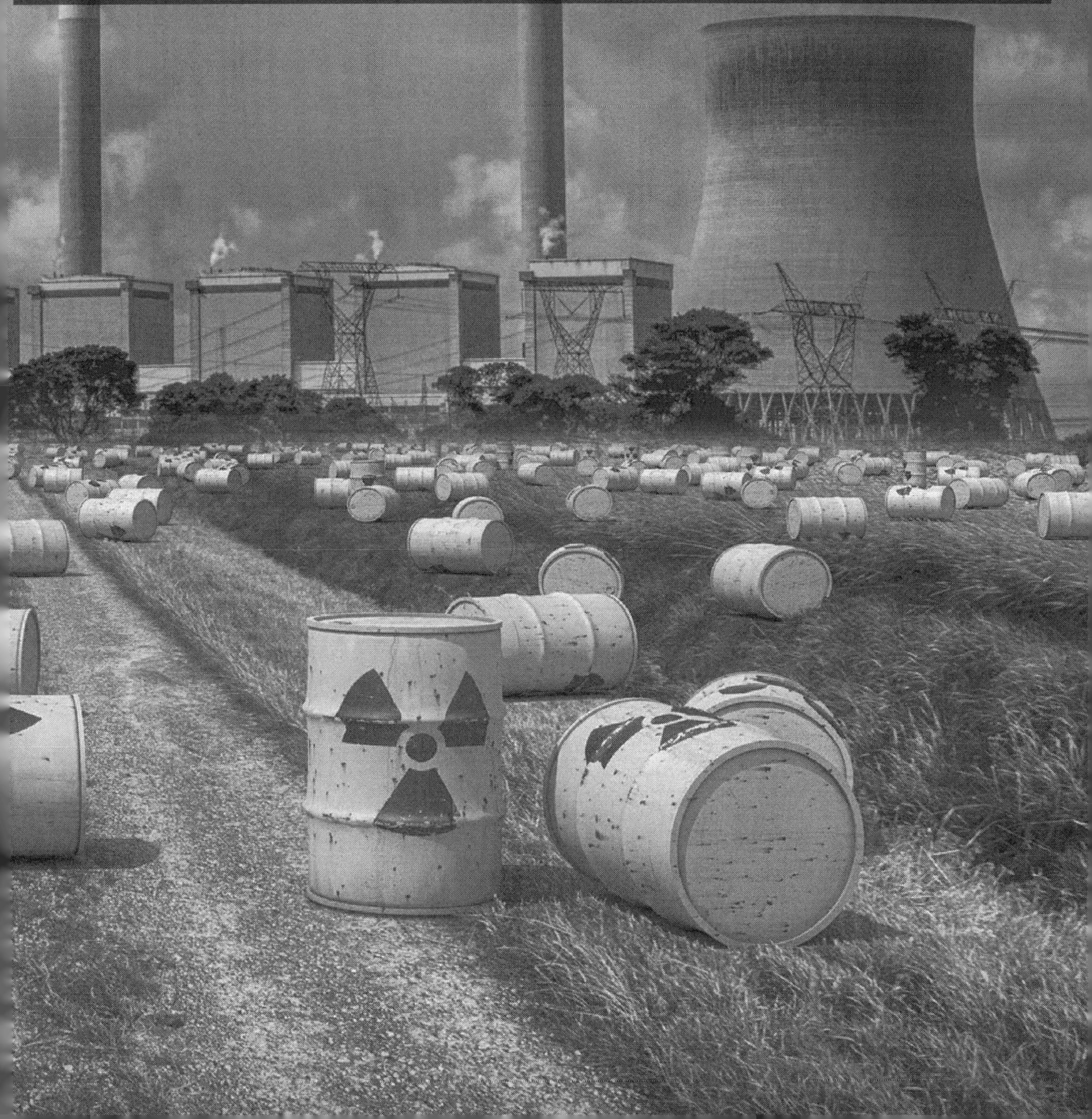

Chapter 3

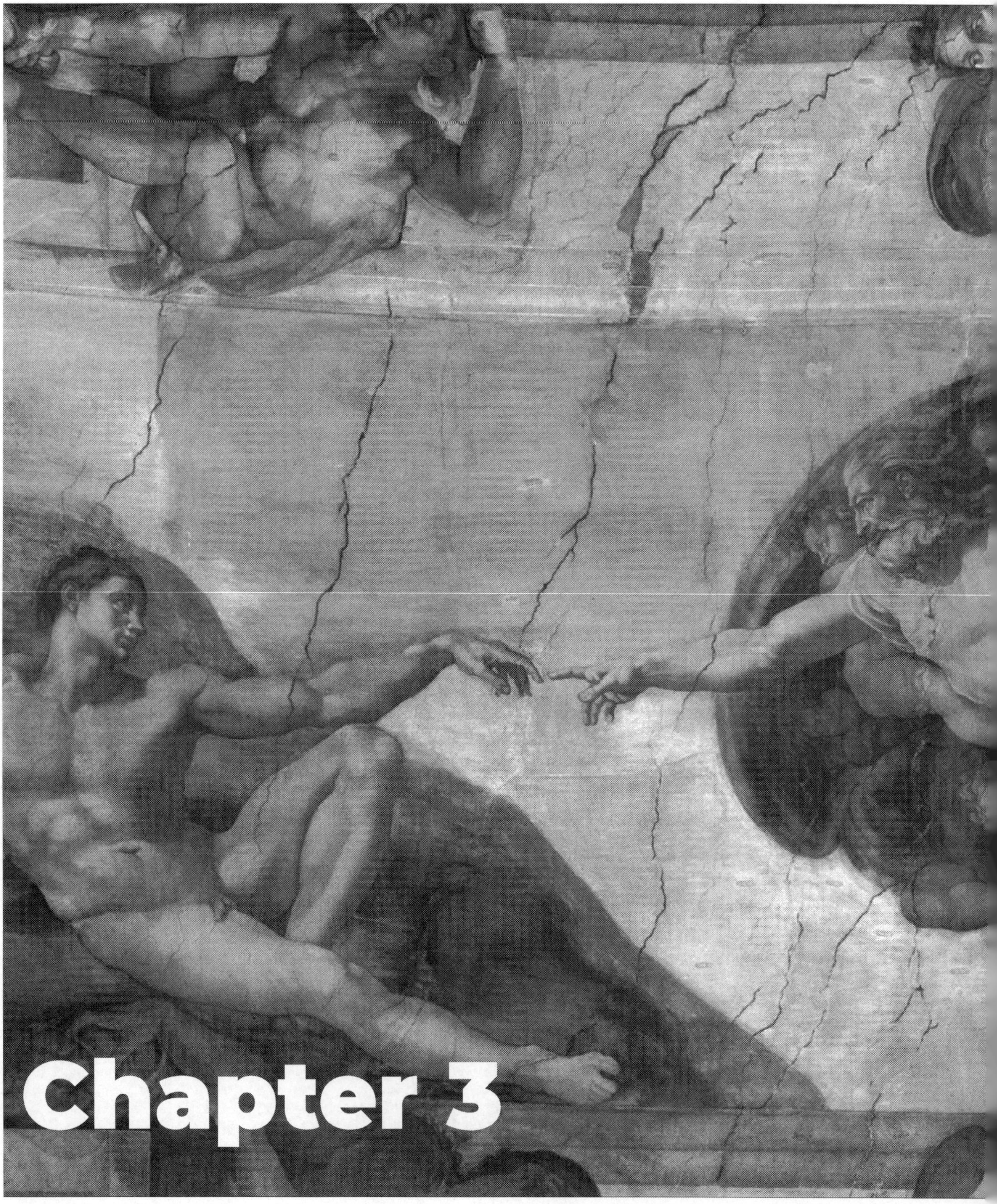

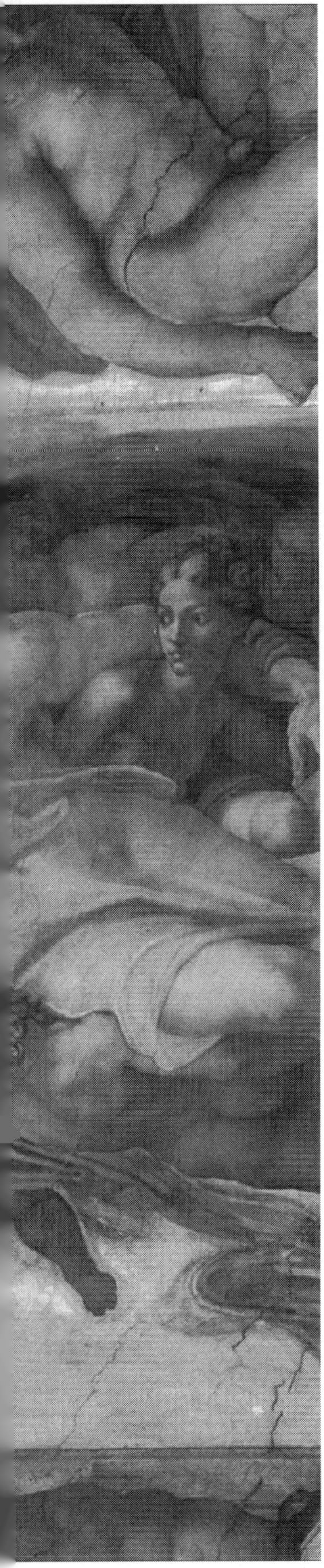

Communication and Connection

Our bodies are responding to something within itself or something in its outer environment every millisecond. Ideally, these processes would be efficient and effective. For many people, for many years they are effective. Since our bodies are built to function in response to inter- and intra-cellular communication, it makes sense that becoming a part of those conversations could help retain or regain balance. Food is also information and is a huge part of what the body listens to, as well as various herbs, nutraceuticals, homeopathic approaches, thoughts, emotions, frequencies, and movement.

Pharmaceutical companies are studying active components of countless herbs, roots, leaves, and other natural substances to create patentable drugs that can manage or minimize symptoms. Some of the ways that those types of research are being utilized in relation to cellular communication will be discussed, along with a few break-throughs in the imitation of form and function at the molecular level. A wider variety of communication methods was covered in earlier Somatic Intelligence volumes, so for this text, we'll focus on the cellular level of interactions. Touch and movement can bring about a cascade of cellular responses, so this will be the direction each discussion on the subject is headed in.

THE BODY'S METHODS OF CELLULAR COMMUNICATION

Four Basic Types

There are four basic types of cellular communication**: paracrine, autocrine, endocrine, and direct (juxtacrine) contact,** using either short or long forms of sending the signal. (Fig.2.1) When there is a chemical messenger (ligand) moving a short distance between cells and binding to a receptor on the receiving cell, it's called **paracrine** signaling. In the case of synaptic or **electrical** signaling, there are both electrical (depolarization) and chemical (neurotransmitter) signals traveling both short and long distances. (Fig.2.5) The initial electrical charge has to be converted into a chemical signal for the messengers to become activated. It is not included in the four basic types but it is very common as it involves the nervous system.

AUTOCRINE

When a cell gives itself a message by using a ligand that binds to its own membrane and activates a change within the cell, it's called an **autocrine** process. Examples of this type of cellular activity involve homeostasis of the cell, and immune responses. For example, the binding of IL-1 on a macrophage that triggers the release of additional cytokines is an autocrine signaling process. (King, 2007) Autocrine messaging is also found in pathological conditions whereby a tumor will signal itself to increase in size. There are instances whereby a cell can use multiple methods, such as the pituitary gland which uses endocrine, paracrine, and autocrine means of signaling.

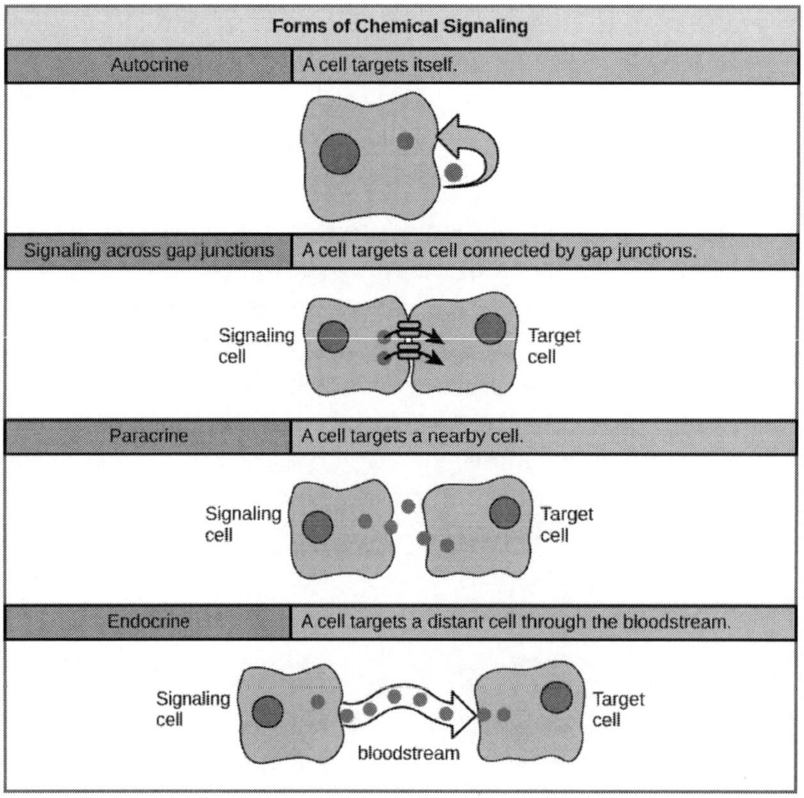

Forms of Chemical Signaling
Autocrine
A cell targets itself.
Signaling across gap junctions
A cell targets a cell connected by gap junctions.
Signaling cell
Target cell
Paracrine
A cell targets a nearby cell.
Signaling cell
Target cell
Endocrine
A cell targets a distant cell through the bloodstream.
Signaling cell
bloodstream
Target cell

Fig. 2.1 – Illustration of Autocrine, Juxtacrine, Paracrine, and Endocrine signaling

Illustration Courtesy of CNS OpenStax CC BY 4.0 via Wikimedia Commons

ENDOCRINE

Endocrine signaling generally happens over a distance by endocrine gland cells using fluid transport systems, such as hormones traveling through the bloodstream, which is slower. (Fig.2.2) The most plentiful signal detectors on the endocrine target cell membrane or receptor are called G protein-coupled receptors or GPCRs. These receptors are often a subject of research because they have been seen to be mutated in a variety of endocrine diseases. [49](Lap Han Tse and Yung Hou Wong, 2019)

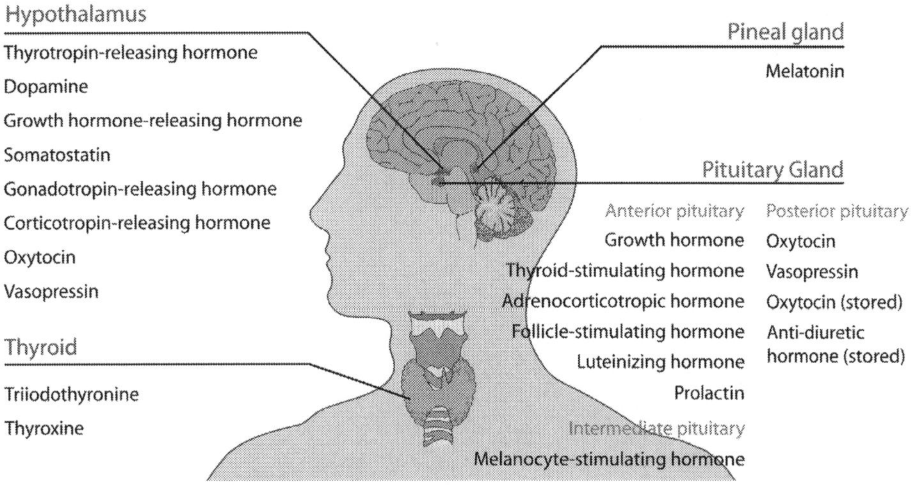

Fig. 2.2 - Examples of endocrine signaling via hormones

Image courtesy of CNX OpenStax CC BY 4.0 via Wikimedia Commons

These researchers make the point that, *"It is now firmly established that the endocrine glands are regulated by a plethora of internal and external signals via blood circulation, and that these input signals can further trigger the release of autocrine/paracrine messengers. Various autocrine/paracrine factors are known to contribute to the communications and intricate feedbacks between different types of cells within an endocrine gland, resulting in a coordinated hormonal output and the corresponding physiological outcome. Remarkably, the same chemical molecules can be used in multiple contexts of endocrine, paracrine or autocrine signaling, or even in synaptic signaling."*

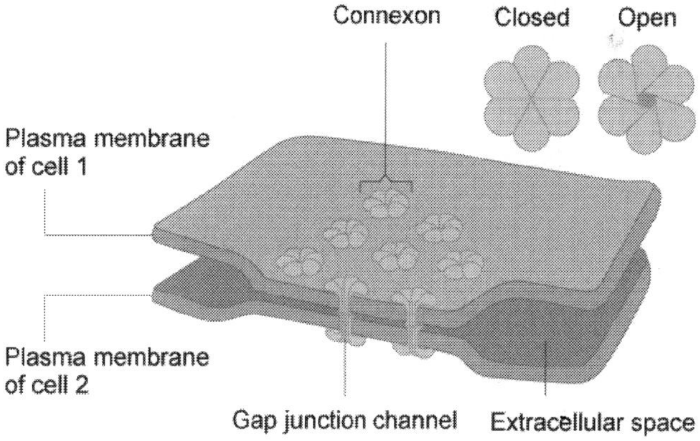

Fig. 2.3 - Gap junction juxtacrine signaling with connexons example

Courtesy of Kassidy Veasaw, CC BY-SA 4.0 via Wikimedia Commons

JUXTACRINE

Juxtacrine, or direct-contact signaling can happen in a few different ways: (1) a protein on one cell binds to its receptor on the adjacent cell, (2) a receptor on one cell binds to its own ligand on the extracellular matrix secreted by another cell or, (3) a signal transmitted from the cytoplasm of one cell passes through conduits (gap junctions) into the cytoplasm of an adjacent cell. There are a group of proteins called '**connexons**' (Fig. 2.3) that act as a bridge or gap junction between the neighboring cells, allowing the passage of ions, amino acids, and small molecules to be transported directly.

The extracellular matrix option is particularly critical in developmental stages for mammals. Gilbert states that, "*Cell adhesion, cell migration, and the formation of epithelial sheets and tubes all depend on the ability of cells to form attachments to extracellular matrices.*" [50](Gilbert and Sunderland, 2000) They describe this matrix as being comprised of collagen, proteoglycans, and a variety of specialized glycoprotein molecules like fibronectin, which serves both as an adhesive to link molecules, and as a network upon which the cells can migrate. (Fig. 2.4)

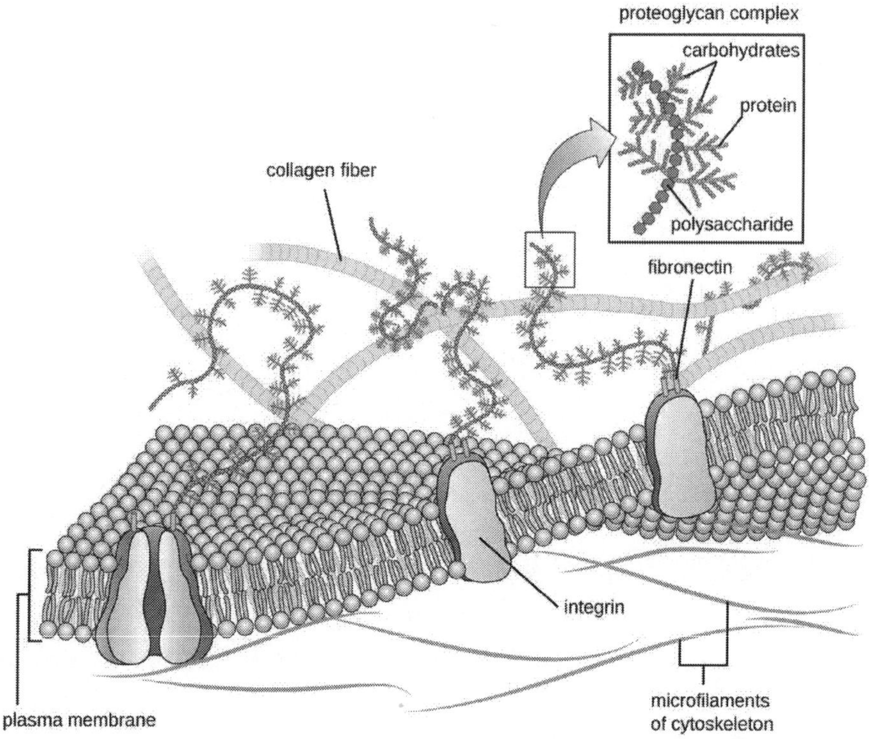

Fig. 2.4 - Example of fibronectin and integrin bridging the ECM to the cell membrane

Courtesy of CNX OpenStax CC BY 4.0 via Wikimedia Commons

Fibronectin receptors serve as a bridge between the fibronectin matrixes outside of the cell to the intracellular scaffolds. They also act as an anchorage site for the actin microfilaments that move the cell. In this function they are labeled as **'integrins'** because they integrate extracellular and intracellular scaffolds. Laminin, and collagen type IV are also part of the ECM, or basal lamina. "*Laminin helps to assemble the ECM by promoting cell adhesion and growth, changing cell shape, and permitting cell migration.*" (Hakamori, 1984)

ELECTRICAL SIGNALING

Electrical signaling between neurons is a type of juxtacrine communication, even though it sends signals over long distances. (Fig.2.5) Dominick Purpura from the Department of Neuroscience in Einstein's College of Medicine in New York, reports that, "*The most hotly debated question in neuroscience in the 20th century was whether synaptic transmission, which is the currency of the brain, is mediated electrically or chemically.*" In more recent years, it has been more widely accepted that communication between neurons is an electrochemical process.

There are two ways that electrical transmission happens: (1) using a pathway of low resistance between neurons known as a gap junction, and (2) as a consequence of extracellular electric fields generated by neuronal activity. [51](Faber and Pereda, 2018) The channels along the cell membrane that facilitate the flow of positive or negatively charged ions across the membrane from the outside to the inside of the

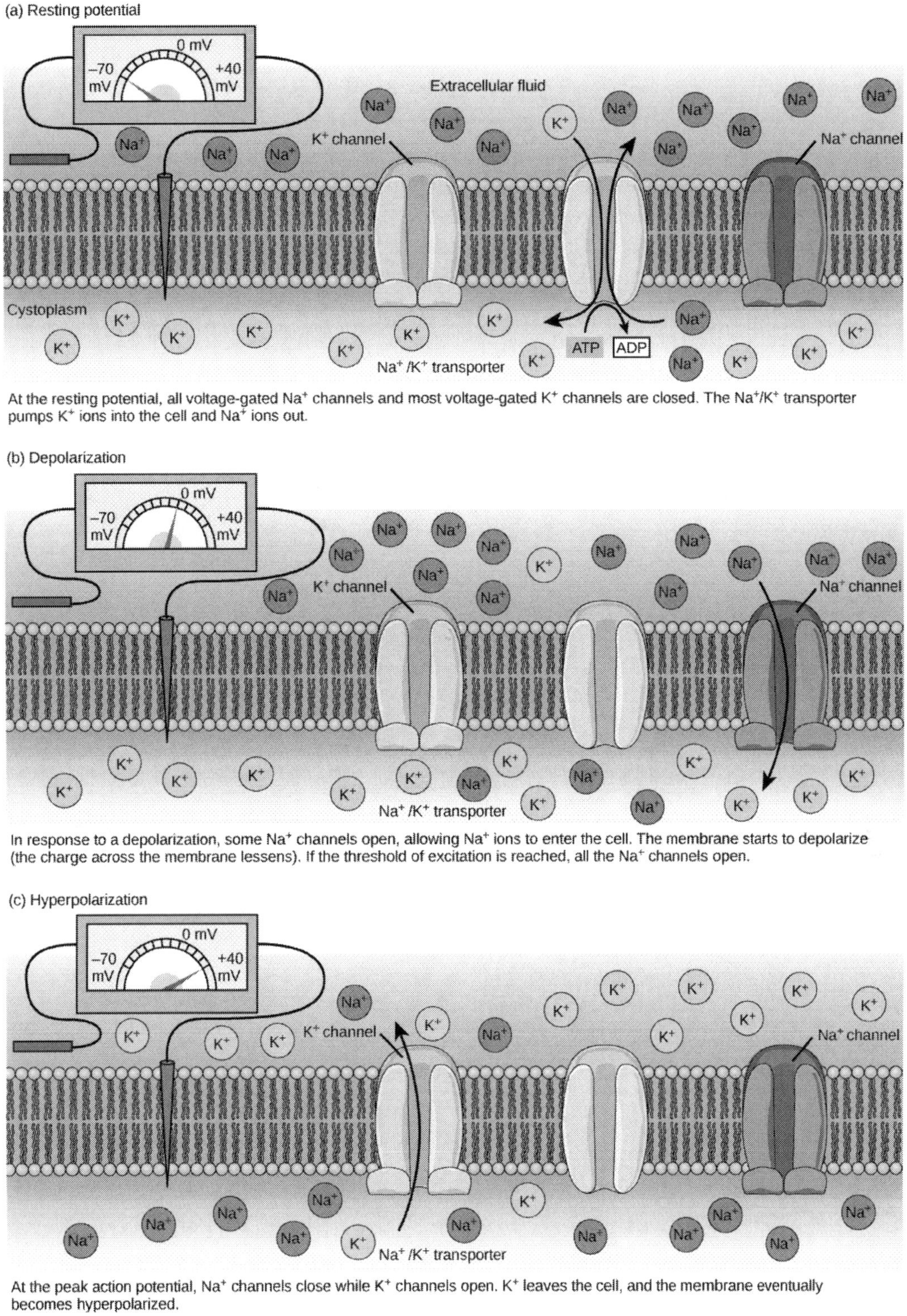
(a) Resting potential
0 mV
–70 mV
+40 mV
Extracellular fluid
K^+ channel
Na^+ channel
Cystoplasm
ATP
ADP
Na^+/K^+ transporter
At the resting potential, all voltage-gated Na^+ channels and most voltage-gated K^+ channels are closed. The Na^+/K^+ transporter pumps K^+ ions into the cell and Na^+ ions out.
(b) Depolarization
0 mV
–70 mV
+40 mV
K^+ channel
Na^+ channel
Na^+/K^+ transporter
In response to a depolarization, some Na^+ channels open, allowing Na^+ ions to enter the cell. The membrane starts to depolarize (the charge across the membrane lessens). If the threshold of excitation is reached, all the Na^+ channels open.
(c) Hyperpolarization
0 mV
–70 mV
+40 mV
K^+ channel
Na^+ channel
Na^+/K^+ transporter
At the peak action potential, Na^+ channels close while K^+ channels open. K^+ leaves the cell, and the membrane eventually becomes hyperpolarized.

Fig. 2.6 – Example of action potential from resting phase to depolarization and hyperpolarization after potassium leaves the cell, which prevents a signal from traveling in the opposite direction

cell can build up to what is called an **'action potential'.** The action potential then stimulates a chemical (neuro-transmitter) response that either excites or inhibits the neuron.

Normally the inside of the cell carries a more negative charge with a resting potential of around -70mV, but it does fluctuate slightly. (Fig. 2.6) When the input signal causes the membrane to reach -50mV it is said to have reached its 'threshold'. The spike that is produced by the change in potential sends a neurotransmitter into the synaptic cleft where the electrical signal briefly becomes a chemical one until it binds onto the postsynaptic receptor. At that point, it again becomes an electrical signal that flows down the axon. (University of Queens-land, Queensland Brain Institute)

The neuron has three main components: (1) the dendrites, thin fibers that extend from the cell in branched tendrils to receive information from other neurons; (2) the cell body, which carries out most of the neuron's basic cellular functioning; and (3) the axon, a long, thin fiber that carries nerve impulses to other neurons. (Fig.2.5)Two mechanisms have evolved to transmit nerve signals. First, within cells, electrical signals are conveyed along the cell membrane, which is essentially an autocrine type of signaling. Second, for the paracrine communication between cells, the electrical signals generally are converted into chemical signals conveyed by small messenger molecules called neurotransmitters. (Alcohol Health and Research World, 1997)

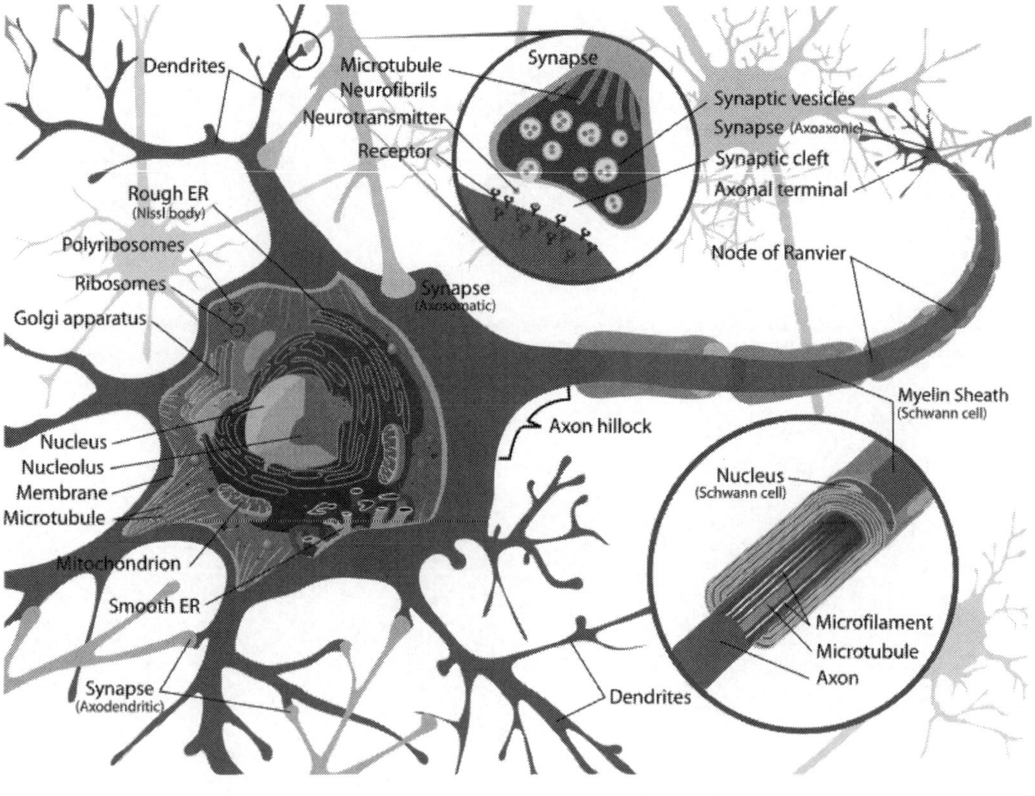

Fig. 2.5 – Example of electrical signaling with components of a nerve cell

Image courtesy of LadyofHats, Public Domain via WikiMedia Commons

PAIN PERCEPTION

Pain reactions are not set in stone. Pain perception uses its own nociceptors, transmitting sensation using both free nerve endings and touch perception pathways. While there are protective, reflexive responses built into the nervous system at the spinal cord before the signal reaches the brain, there is some evidence of subconscious and conscious adaptation to pain as well as thresholds that can vary from person to person. Reactions can vary greatly from one individual to the next, often based upon past experiences and trauma.

Emotions, depression, or anxiety can also intensify the body's perception of and response to a painful event or condition, whereas adaptation in the brain and nervous system can often reduce the amount of pain perceived or heighten the threshold. The American Pain Foundation reports that 30% of adults aged 45-64 experience pain lasting more than 24 hours, but only 21% of adults over 65. (WebMD, *"What's Your Pain Tolerance*?," March 31, 2014) That is a very curious finding since cumulative imbalances and degenerative issues seem like they would be greater later in life, but it could also be that retirement and the reduction of stress contributes to pain relief.

Somatic Pioneers and the CNS

IRVIN KORR AND THE FACILITATED SEGMENT

Irvin Korr, who received his PhD in Cellular Physiology from Princeton in 1935, mentioned the concept of the 'facilitated segment' as early as 1947. He theorized that an area of the spine, as a result of ongoing pain signals, could become hypersensitive and develop a habituated or learned pathway, which could in time spread to other segments. It is most likely that this type of progression confuses the system's ability to reset. The over-stimulation of the spine could also elicit neurovascular or neurovisceral changes, along with hyperarousal of the immune system. Lateral or adjacent hyper-sensitization was discussed by Sherrington in 1906, Eccles in the 1950s, and subsequently several others who verified the interrelationships between afferents and efferents up and down rhe spinal cord. [53](E. Lederman, 2000)

Korr, in his paper on, "The Neural Basis of the Osteopathic Lesion," lists the imbalances that can arise from joint 'derangements' and subsequent tissues and organs effected via the anterior and lateral horn cells as:

- Hyperesthesia (increased sensitivity) especially of the muscles and vertebrae
- Hyperirritability, reflected in altered muscular activity and altered states of muscle contraction
- Altered visceral and other autonomic functions
- Changes in tissue texture of the muscle, connective tissue, and skin
- Changes in local circulation and in the exchange between blood and tissues

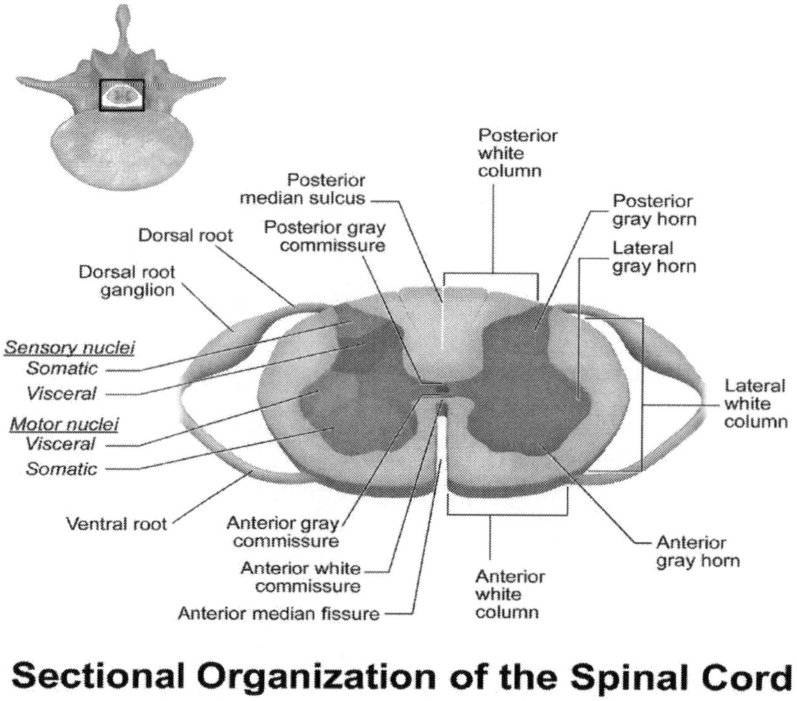

Fig. 2.7 – Anterior, lateral, and dorsal horn of the spinal cord

Image courtesy of OpenStax CC by 4.0 via Wikimedia Commons

Korr states that the principles of reciprocity and convergence facilitate the potential of spinal imbalances to have far-reaching impacts. He describes the process being, "*Each anterior horn cell receives impulses from a large number of sources through the presynaptic fibers which converge upon and synapse with it. The proprioceptors, stretch, and tension receptors situated in the tendons and in the muscles themselves are a steady and continuous source of impulses. (Fig.2.7)*

> *It is indeed, most important to keep in mind that the efferent neurons do represent final commom paths shared by a host of impulse sources, in addition to those associaed with joint and supporting tissues. In fact, every afferent nerve fiber, whether it mediates touch, pain, pressure, temperature, sight, or any other sense modality, exerts influence upon the final common path represented by the motor nerve."*

In recognition of the fact that fluctuating internal or external environments amidst daily activities create a vulnerability to reinforcement and facilitation, Korr states that, "Pathology results when the balance is shifted too far in one direction or the other (excitation or inhibition) for too long" which can have physical, psychological and physiological outcomes. Because midline structures were the first to become specified, out of which all other structures came into being, reinforces that they serve a primary function. It makes sense to look to the spine as a major organizing center or fulcrum and source of communication that helps to regulate other systems. In my opinion, the ectoderm is a powerful source as well.

SIR CHARLES SCOTT SHERRINGTON

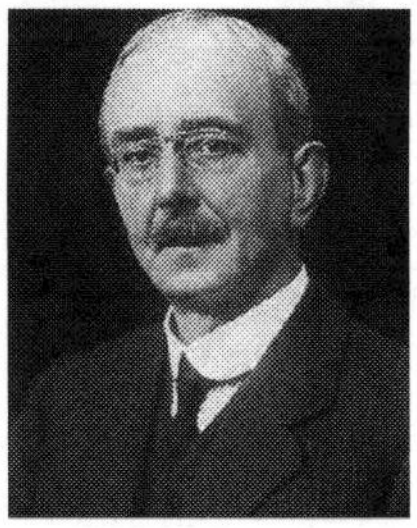

Sir Charles Sherrington

Sir Charles Scott Sherrington won the Nobel Prize in 1932 in 'Physiology or Medicine', and was bestowed honorary doctorates from 20 universities around the world. He forever changed the way that the central nervous system has been viewed since he published the book, "The Integrative Action of the Nervous System" in 1906, covering two decades of his work. He continued to elucidate the functions of reflexes, spinal nerves, muscle action, movement, and proprioception. (Proske and Gandevia, 2012)

Sherrington identified the structure and function of muscle spindles and golgi tendons organs and coined the term, 'proprioception'. (Fig 2.8) He identified it as the process by which the spindles and GTOs send information to the brain as sensory feedback from 'one's own body' regarding stretch, tension, position, muscle tone, and posture. [54]*(S. Finger,* 2022)

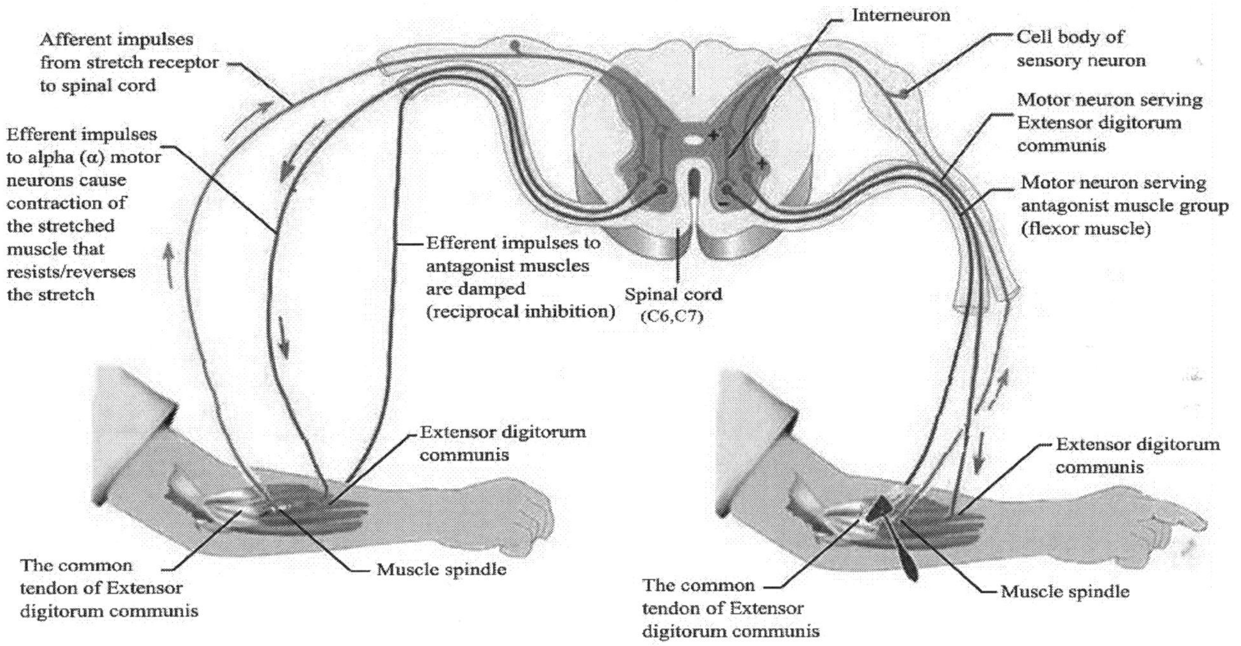

Fig. 2.8 – Illustration of muscle spindle cells (proprioceptors) sending sensory information about limb position or motor activity to the cord via afferent pathways, then using a direct route to trigger a fast, reflexive reaction

Image courtesy of Zhang, MJ, Zhu, CZ, Duan, ZM, Niu X. Department of Cardiology, Second Affiliate Hospital, School of Medicine, Xi'an Jiao Tong University, China CC BY-SA 4.0 via Wikimedia Commons

DR. F. M. POTTENGER

Another pioneer in viscerosomatic relationships was Dr. F. M. Pottenger, who noticed that certain post-surgical complaints after the removal of an organ created changes in the curvature of the spine. He reports that,

"The segmental relationship which exists between an afferent visceral neuron and an efferent somatic neuron probably also exists between an afferent and an efferent visceral neuron," leading to "a continuous flow of stimuli from the surface of the body inward to the visceral, and from the visceral outward to the skeletal tissues." (Fig. 2.9)

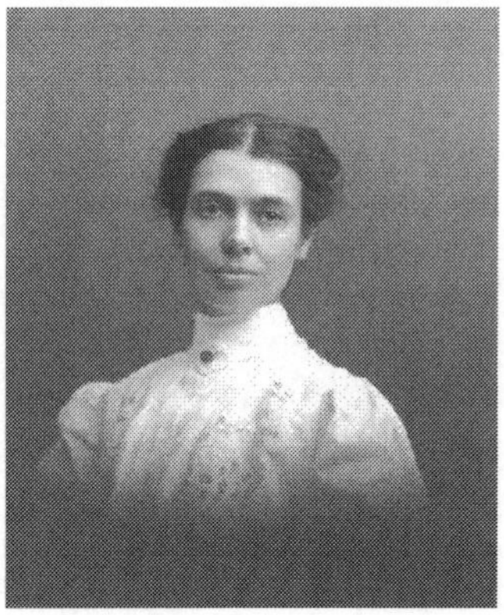

Louisa Burns, DO

LOUISA BURNS

Louisa Burns studied at the Pacific College of Osteopathy and began teaching there in 1906. She became the head of the A.T. Still Research Institute in 1914 after she was healed from spinal meningitis with osteopathy, and remained in that position for 22 years. She later created her own research center, called the Louisa Burns Osteopathic Research Laboratory, to study the 'osteopathic lesion' and wrote 5 books and numerous articles before she retired. She was able to validate somatovisceral and viscerosomatic reflexes or referral pathways using numerous experiments on animals.

DR. NEVILLE T. USHER

Dr. Neville T. Usher wrote an article in 1933 called, "Spinal Curvatures – Visceral Disturbances in Relation Thereto," in which he described a few case studies where the following symptoms arose solely from visceral irritation caused by a spinal curvature: fatigue, intercostal pain and neuritis, nausea and vomiting, gas, gastric distress, constipation, abdominal cramping, backache, sciatica, coughing and difficulty breathing, constant urination, and heaviness in the legs. All symptoms were relieved by balancing the curvature and subsequent pelvic distortion.

Some clinical practitioners or instructors may experience a preponderence of evidence from the viscerosomatic direction. They focus on freeing and mobilizing organs directly from connective tissue restrictions, which could liberate musculoskeletal issues along with the visceral symptoms. From the perspective of underlying interdependence due to communication pathways, it seems wise to incorporate movement patterns that help to decompress, align, and mobilize the spine as well as to include manual therapy methods that can facilitate finer, more specific releases in both the visceral and nervous systems.

These findings are reflective of the developmental processes whereby the ectoderm begets the endoderm, and either can be utilized to help balance the mesoderm. Because it functions as a type of connective tissue that still transmits volumes of information throughout the system, maintaining the health of the ectoderm layer could be very important. We'll go into much greater detail on incorporating the skin as a therapeutic powerhouse later in the text.

In a separate article, Korr emphasizes the extent of the nerves' ability to influence health at the level of cellular function. He declares, *"Among the neural phenomena important to musculoskeletal problems are the transport and exchange of macromolecular materials...Research supports the view that the trophic influence of nerves on target organs depends largely on delivery of specific neuronal proteins by means of axonal transport and junctional transfer. There is also retrograde transport from nerve endings to cell bodies."*

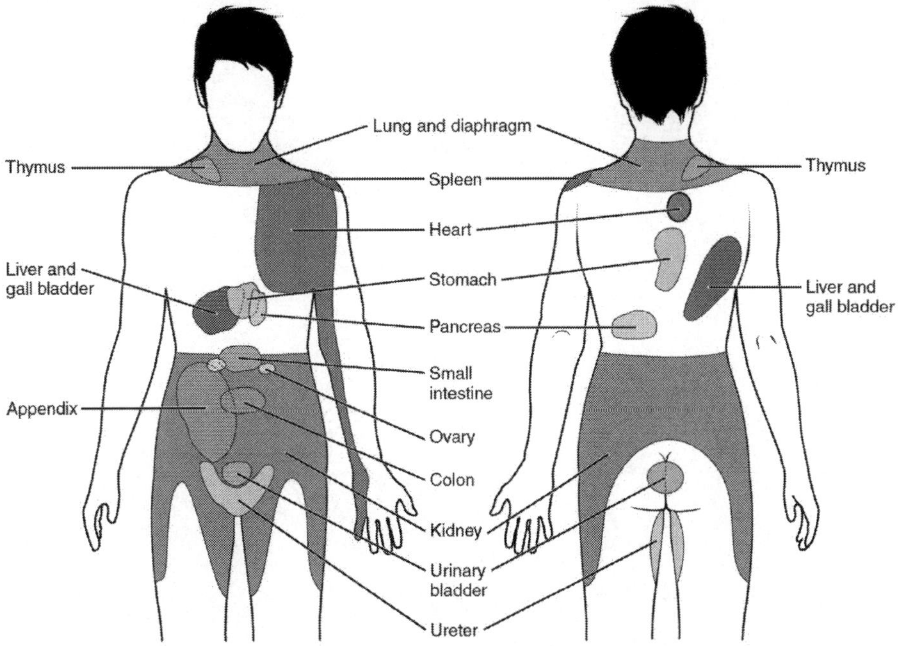

Fig. 2.9 - Potential Referred Pain Areas from organs and glands into soft tissue areas
Image courtesy of OpenStax CC by 3.0 via Wikimedia Commons

Trophic Nerves

Trophic nerves are believed to govern nutrition, differentiation, and regeneration of tissues, including nerve cells. Lorne Mendell in 2002 stated, "*There is considerable evidence that sensory neurons compete for a trophic substance in the periphery, and those that fail to obtain adequate levels of such a substance are the ones that do not survive*." In 2009, Neary and Zimmerman reported that trauma and injury including ischemia have been connected to the "release of extracellular nucleotides by damaged and dying cells, and in the development of neuropathic and inflammatory pain." This indicates that the structures meant to be a source of healing become part of the problem when the damage reaches a certain state. They listed the physiological outcomes of the release of nucleotides in response to nervous system injury as including neurogenesis, neuronal differentiation, glial proliferation, migration, growth arrest, and apoptosis. [55] (Joseph T. Neary and Herbert Zimmerman, 2009)

DR. JOHN DENSLOW

Dr. John Denslow was also a physiologist who did research at the Kirksville College of Osteopathy in Missouri along with Dr. Korr. Part of what they discovered was that the trophic function of the nervous system became a potential source of pathology for many other systems by way of their connections to soft tissue and vascular sites when the nerve became irritated, injured, or dysfunctional. An article in the Journal of Atrial Fibrillation in 2020 explained the role of the cardiovascular branch of the autonomic nervous system that regulates heart rate, blood pressure, and maintaining homeostatis during exercise.

In that vein, Ross Hauser MD describes the possibility that chest pain, racing heartbeat, panic attacks, fainting and near-fainting, anxiety, palpitations, tremors, tachycardia, and other symptoms could be related to cervical instability. This location of instability of the spine could interfere with communication between the brain and the heart and blood vessels and produce a myriad of disturbing and possibly life-threatening symptoms. The condition is called Postural Orthostatic Tachycardia Syndrome (POTS). [57] (Ross Hauser, MD, 2021)

Heart disease is the leading cause of death (one every 36 seconds) among men and women of most ethnic groups in the United States as of September 2021. Italian researchers, Rosa Bruno, et al., expressed that it's becoming increasingly clear that the sympathetic neural control is involved in vasomotor control of both small resistance arteries as well as the modulation of large artery function. They also mention that increased sympathetic activity is linked to decreased endothelial function and increased stiffiness. [56] (Rosa M. Bruno, et al., 2012) Recent research is showing promise in deepening the understanding of the roles BDNF plays in cardiac myocytes. However, it appears that patients with coronary artherosclerosis have lost much BDNF signaling. (Zierold et al., 2021)

DR. WILLIS HAYCOCK

A few decades ago, Dr. Willis Haycock, in his book entitled, "Osteopathy, Principles & Practice" Volume 2, agreed with his colleague on the importance of correcting spinal lesions in order to restore health, and stated,

> *"This research powerfully presents the concept of the role of the nervous system in the development of all disease processes, and should, I submit, be studied deeply by every osteopath."*

It seems that all manual and movement therapists would benefit from becoming more familiar with methods that help to regulate the nervous and vascular systems directly. Methods that palpably facilitate more ease and calm in the connective tissue of the surround as well as within the structures themselves can only further enhance cellular messaging.

JOHN MARTIN LITTLEJOHN

John Martin Littlejohn was a Scot, who after earning degrees in Divinity and Law, came to America to visit for a few months. Littlejohn became ill and found his way to A. T. Still's clinic in Kirksville where he was able to recover. Curious about how and why the methods worked, he became a student and professor of Osteopathy in Kirksville, then studied physiology for 10 years in Chicago to understand more fully the physiology behind the structural techniques. He founded The Littlejohn College of Osteopathy and Hospital in 1900 where he taught and worked until 1913.

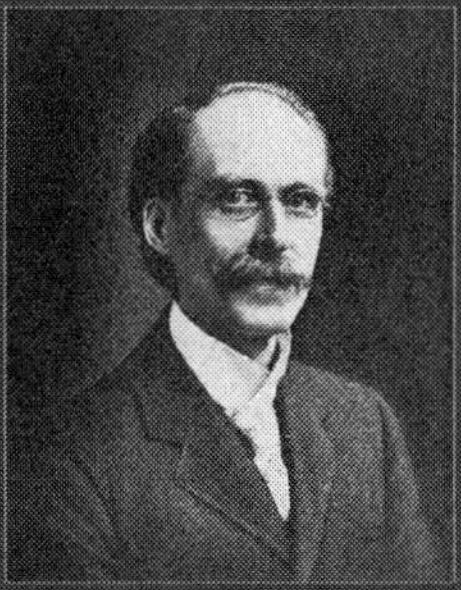

His theories included a form of 'vitalsim' as it was called in those days, whereby he wanted to discover the biochemical underpinnings of a healthy life force. He saw this as the true source of fully aligned structure and efficient organ functioning. His approach to treating the nervous system was in order to return the body's vital force to full function. He stated that, *"All treatment is, or ought to be, directed to the vital force through the property of the irritability of tissue, of which nerve tissue is the most highly irritable."* It seems that he's pointing to disease or dysfunction as a reflection of restricted vital force, similar to chi in Chinese Medicine. He went on to say that,

> *"The curative work is corrective of irritability; the curative work appeals more to the motor or efferent side of the nervous system."*

ANDREW TAYLOR STILL

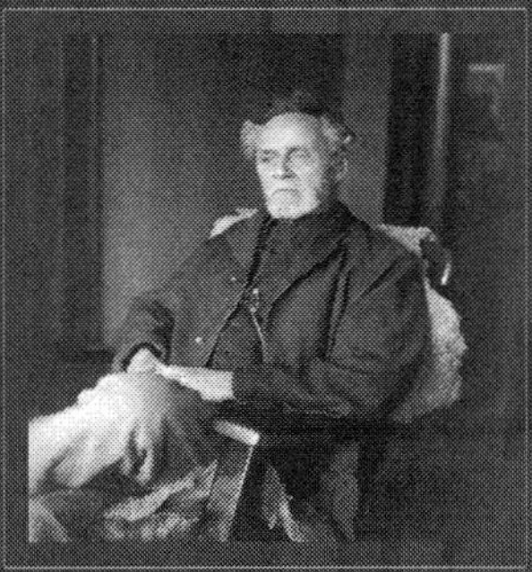

Andrew Taylor Still, thought by most to be the father and founder of Osteopathy, considered any change in the size, shape, texture, structure, or position to constitute an osteopathic lesion or somatic dysfunction. (Torsten Liem, 2016) According to Liem, the lesion or dysfunction also interrupted the flow of life force. Emmanuel Swedenborg took this concept a step further by theorizing that the soul was distributed throughout the body by way of its fluids, which are restricted during dysfunction or disease. Littlejohn said during one of his early lectures, *"The blood is life; it is bearer of the substances upon which vitality depends."* These doctors went beyond structure and function to what they intuited to be the true source of inherent health, yet also flows through the body to maintain homeostasis through its various systems.

As Biodynamic Cranial approaches began, made popular by **Dr. William G. Sutherland,** inherent health and the fluid body began being seen as the organizing principles that contained the information and power to reset the system. It is probably the branch of the osteopathic umbrella that has the most spiritual underpinnings. Minimal contact is made, and maximum allowance is given to the soma itself to cognize the imbalances and create the necessary shifts.

Using the tidal forces, vital energies (Breath of Life) and nutrients are liberated and transported by the fluid systems, and by way of the Primary Respiration system that gains amplitude as the nervous system settles. Universal rhythms, including the midline potency, find their way home. This approach allows the inherent intelligence to locate the lesion or fulcrum around which a certain amount of tension is organized and release it. French osteopath, Jean-Pierre Barral says, "The body 'hugs' the lesion." It most certainly does point to it without fail, although there can be changes when the system is in 'freeze' mode.

DR. ERICH BLECHSCHMIDT

Dr. Erich Blechschmidt was an embryologist who believed that the 'generative forces of the developing embryo' are identical to the regenerative forces used for healing in all of us. The dynamism of embryogenesis that sets cascades of metabolic and informational activity in motion, creating shifts in structure moment-by-moment, remains with the body to a lesser degree as the 'cellular foundation of life.' These dynamic, self-aware, self-regulating forces can be palpated and followed by the practitioner, usually with awe as it moves from lesion to lesion, gracefully unwinding restrictive imbalances and bringing them back into the fold in a simultaneous 3 if not 4 dimensional inclusivity.

I think it's safe to say that most forms of touch with a therapeutic intention, whether directed at the viscera, soft tissue, bone, the nervous, vascular, or fluid systems, will elicit a response at the cellular, biochemical, and energetic levels. The extent to which manual therapy and movement reeducation have an effect at the level of transcription factors is something that would be fascinating to study. There's not a whole lot of data available on the subject right now, but in the coming chapters I will present what I found and how I believe it's relevant and applicable to both manual and movement medicine. In general, the takeaway from science so far is that the majority of how genes express themselves can be modified, which is pretty exciting.

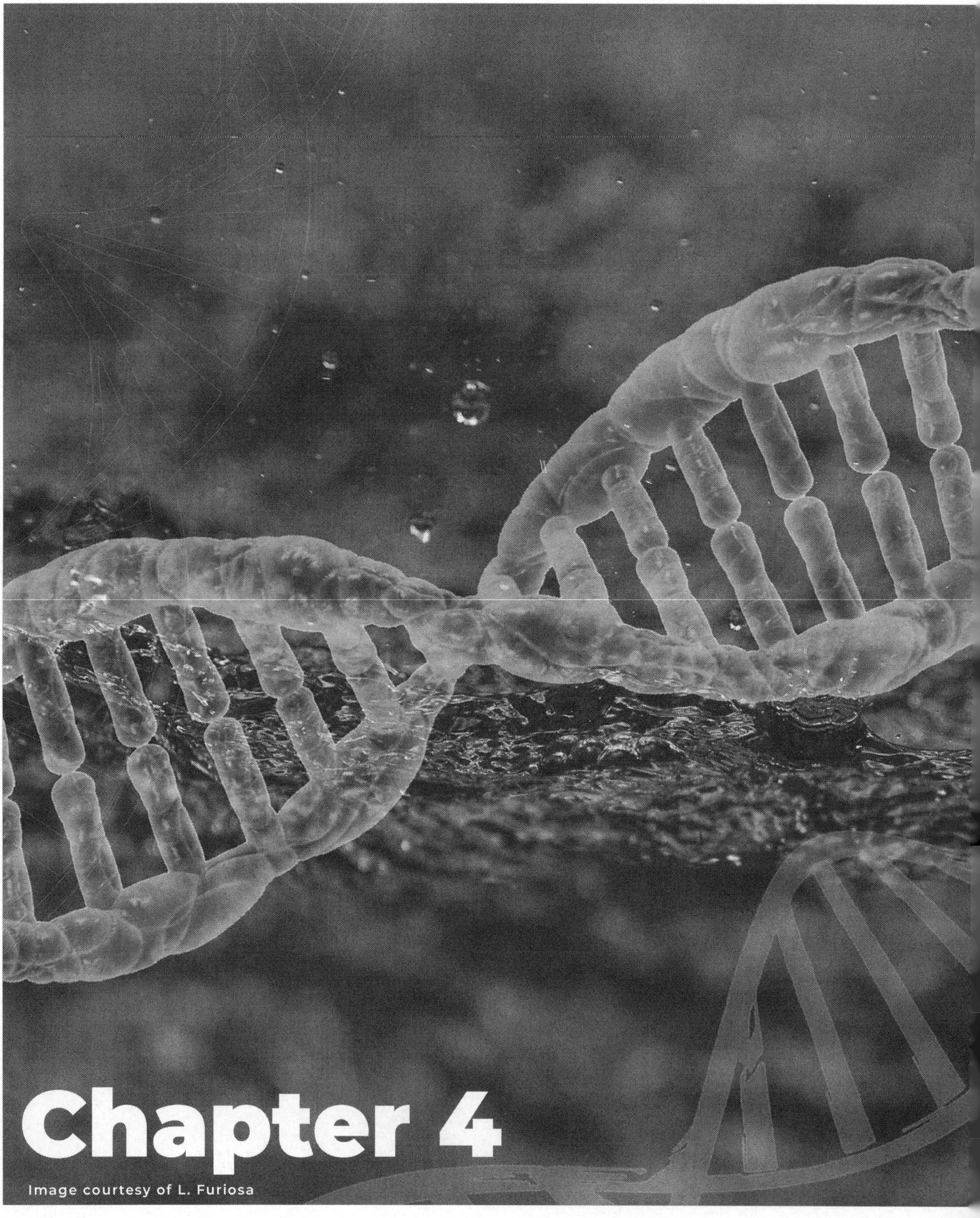

Chapter 4

Image courtesy of L. Furiosa

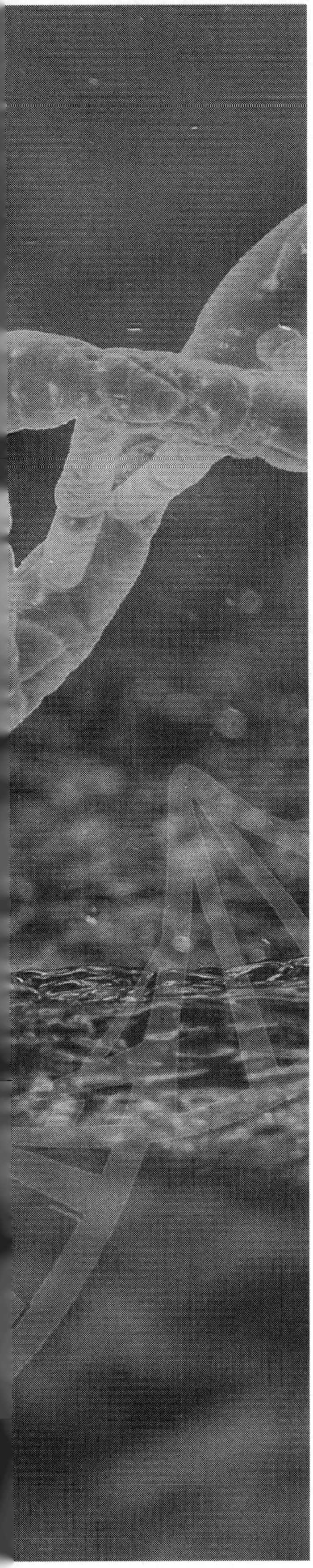

How Does our DNA Perceive our Lives?

Although abbreviated in this text, the process by which our bodies come into being is thoroughly and profoundly programmed. It is inherently and almost overwhemingly complex and specific. It needs to be so to help oversee, regulate, and hold steady the foundation while responding instantly to current input. Each system has its own discreet role which is interlaced and interdependent with other systems and their roles. They cannot compartmentalize even though we can do so in our minds. Unprocessed input remains in waiting in some form or other systemically. A cascade of energetic and biochemical responses happens with each type of information that our senses perceive. There are structures that enable the system to perceive the environment inside and outside of the cell, each of which considers the 20% pre-programmed, and 80% epigenetic options. The good news, is that we are able to influence those epigenetic options, and this chapter summarizes how and why.

Role of the cell membrane

Signaling issues at the cell membrane may be similar to cars on the freeway who come upon a roadblock due to a huge, fiery accident piled up on the road. The cars and people in them with their travel plans don't leave because the traffic stops. If they have to sit there too long without food, water, or resolution of the stagnation in the flow of traffic, many types of trouble will eventually erupt. An ambulance and police will come at some point to help those injured. Some people waiting behind the pile up may get out and walk or try to find other forms of transport to their intended destination, but the car and roadblock are still there. Immune cells and internal cell messengers respond to help extinguish the fire, get the injured cells out of play, deliver nutritive factors and begin a repair process. But signaling is still interrupted for a while, and the road may have sustained damage as well.

INTEGRINS AS RECEPTORS

Stephanie Hehlgans explains that, "Integrins are heterodimeric cell-surface molecules that on one side, link the actin cytoskeleton to the cell membrane, and on the other side mediate cell-matrix interactions. In addition to their structural functions, integrins mediate signalling from the extracellular space into the cell through integrin-associated signaling and adaptor molecules such as FAK (focal adhesion kinase) ILK (integrin-linked kinase), PINCH, Nck2... and others. (Fig.4.1) Via these molecules, integrin signalling cooperatively interacts with receptor tyrosine kinase signalling to regulate survival, proliferation, cell shape, as well as polarity, cell adhesion, migration, and differentiation." [58](Hehlgans, 2007)

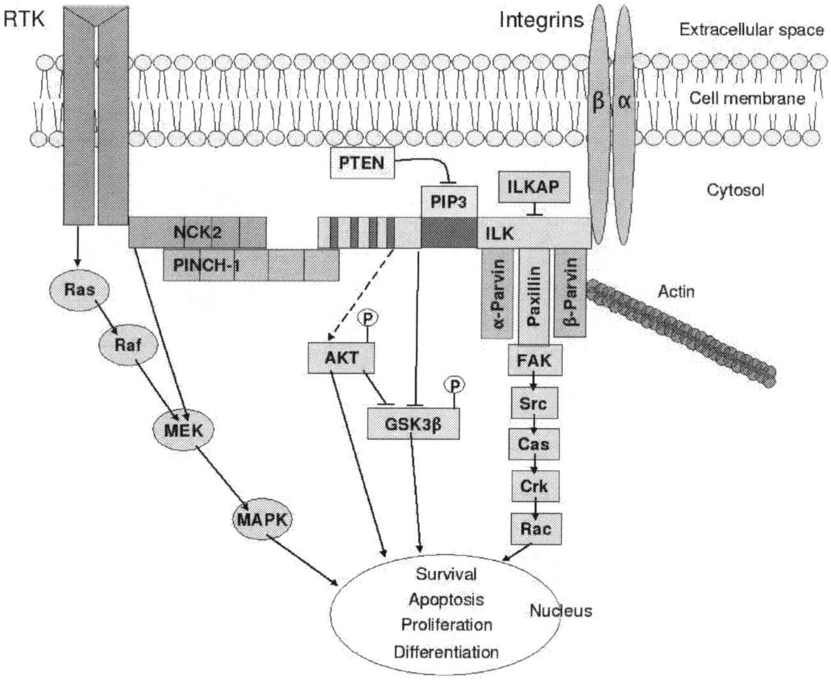

Fig. 4.1 Example of cellular signaling using integrins

Courtesy of K.murphy at English Wikipedia, Public domain

Hehlgans' researchers go on to report that disruptions in this process have been associated with various types of cancer. The cell membrane can be seen as a major intersection — if not a brain — in coordinating the traffic that has to pass through it. Integrins have been defined as a superfamily of receptors that bind ligands at the cell surface in both health and disease. They have affinities with certain ligands from the extracellular matrix related to tissue repair, inflammation, infection, and agiogenesis (creating blood vessels). [59](Mezu-Ndubuisi and Maheswari, 2021) Integrins are landmarks to us related to manual or movement medicine, because they support intracellular communication.

Mezu-Ndubuisi lists the four categories of alpha and beta subunits of integrins according to which type of ligands they bind. Integrin αβ heterodimers types are: leukocyte-binding, 2.) collagen-binding, 3.) Arg-Gly-Asp(RGD)-binding, and 4.) laminin-binding. The first type involves inflammatory cytokines used during injury or cell damage. The second involves amino acids that mediate the adhesion of molecules and collagen for organization of the cytoskeleton and repair. The laminin-binding subunit is the most ancient, as its role is to secure the cell to the basement membrane (BM).

It is currently presumed that this tissue bears and corrects changes in shape due to mechanical forces, in addition to regulating how cells perceive biochemical signaling. [60](Khalilgharibi N. and Mao Y., 2021) These researchers comment that the BM (Fig.4.3) is a dynamic participant in tissue development, integrin

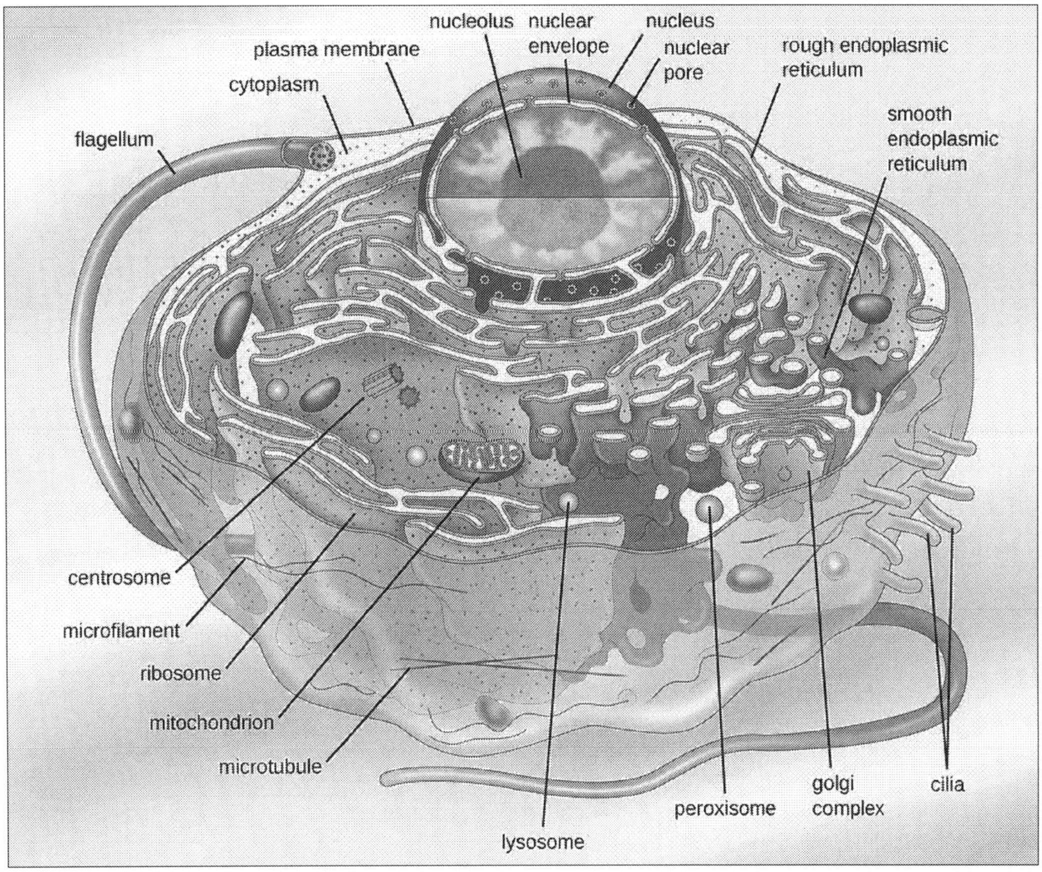

Fig 4.2 – Components of a basic eukaryotic (contains a nucleus) cell

Courtesy of CNX OpenStax CC BY 4.0, via Wikimedia Commons

signaling, and ligand availability. A ligand is a chemical messenger. And, like nearly all other aspects of cell functions, it can also become dysregulated and contribute to disease.

BASEMENT MEMBRANE FUNCTION

The **basement membrane** is a vitally important, specialized type of extracellular matrix (ECM) made of collagen type IV and laminin. It is a very thin, yet very dense tissue that is present in all organized cells (Fig.4.2). It underlies epithelial and endothelial cells, and surrounds muscle, fat, and Schwann cells, providing a structural barrier, elasticity, growth, and shape. [61](Sekiguchi and Yamada, 2018) The BM also provides an adhesive substrate and signaling platform for migration, polarization, and differentiation. Loss of epithelial polarity is often observed in cancer, with the most aggressive cases correlating to the extent of the loss. Certain types of aneurysms and retinopathies are related to the BM losing its structural integrity, along with perforated tissues in the lungs, kidneys, and small intestine, causing other pathologies.

Integrins respond to biochemical changes and can mediate both outside-in and inside-out cross-talk through the cell membrane. *(Sino Biological, 2021)*

This functon would become activated during infection, injury, or trauma. Additional cascades of signaling and messenger transport happens in the presence of inflammation, tissue damage, and cell death, as well as to attempt to prevent the death of an injured or dysfunctional cell. (Fig.4.4) Biomechanical irregularities are just as significant for our health as biochemical ones. That is what makes repatterning using movement and touch such a potent therapeutic tool.

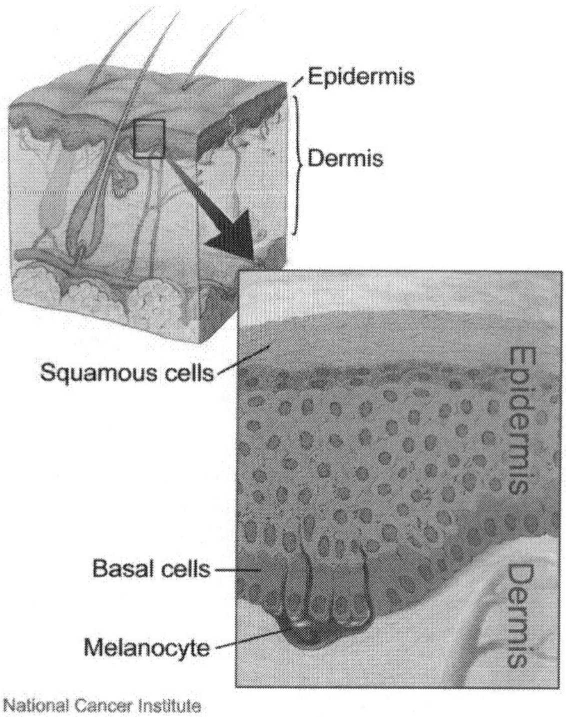

Fig. 4.3 – Illustration of the basement membrane beneath epidermis

Courtesy of Don Bliss (Illustrator) Public Domain via Wikimedia Commons

Molecular responses to trauma

Chaudry and Bland reported in 2009 that, "Protracted reduction in tissue perfusion after major trauma in an individual produces profound effects on tissue metabolism, structure, and function. This is apparent at cellular, organ, and systemic levels. Major changes after trauma occur in the micro-circulation, cell membrane transport and function, energy metabolism, and the function of mitochondrial, immunological and cardiovascular systems... T and B cell functions are also depressed after trauma." [62](I.H. Chaurdy and K.I. Bland, 2009)

SURGERY AND EMOTIONAL TRAUMA

Surgery is included in many reports as a type of trauma, as are cases of PTSD where there is emotional trauma. Part of the issue in slow recovery is the restriction of energy at the mitochondrial level — like ATP — which is needed to moblilize the necessary resources, such as growth factors for tissue repair. A recent therapeutic intervention called photobiomodulation seeks to overcome that issue by stimulating the mitochondria and the production of ATP and the downstream release of growth factors. Using low level laser radiation as well as specific near and far infrared frequencies have been shown to help stimulate the mitochondria, promote the blood flow in otherwise ischemic tissue, and accelerate wound closure.

Leyanne describes the cellular responde to trauma this way: "*The binding of growth factors to cell surface receptors induces signalling pathways that transmit signals to the nucleus for the transcription of genes for increased cellular proliferation, viability, and migration in numerous cell types, including stem cells and fibroblasts.*" [63](Thobekile S. Leyane, et al., 2021)

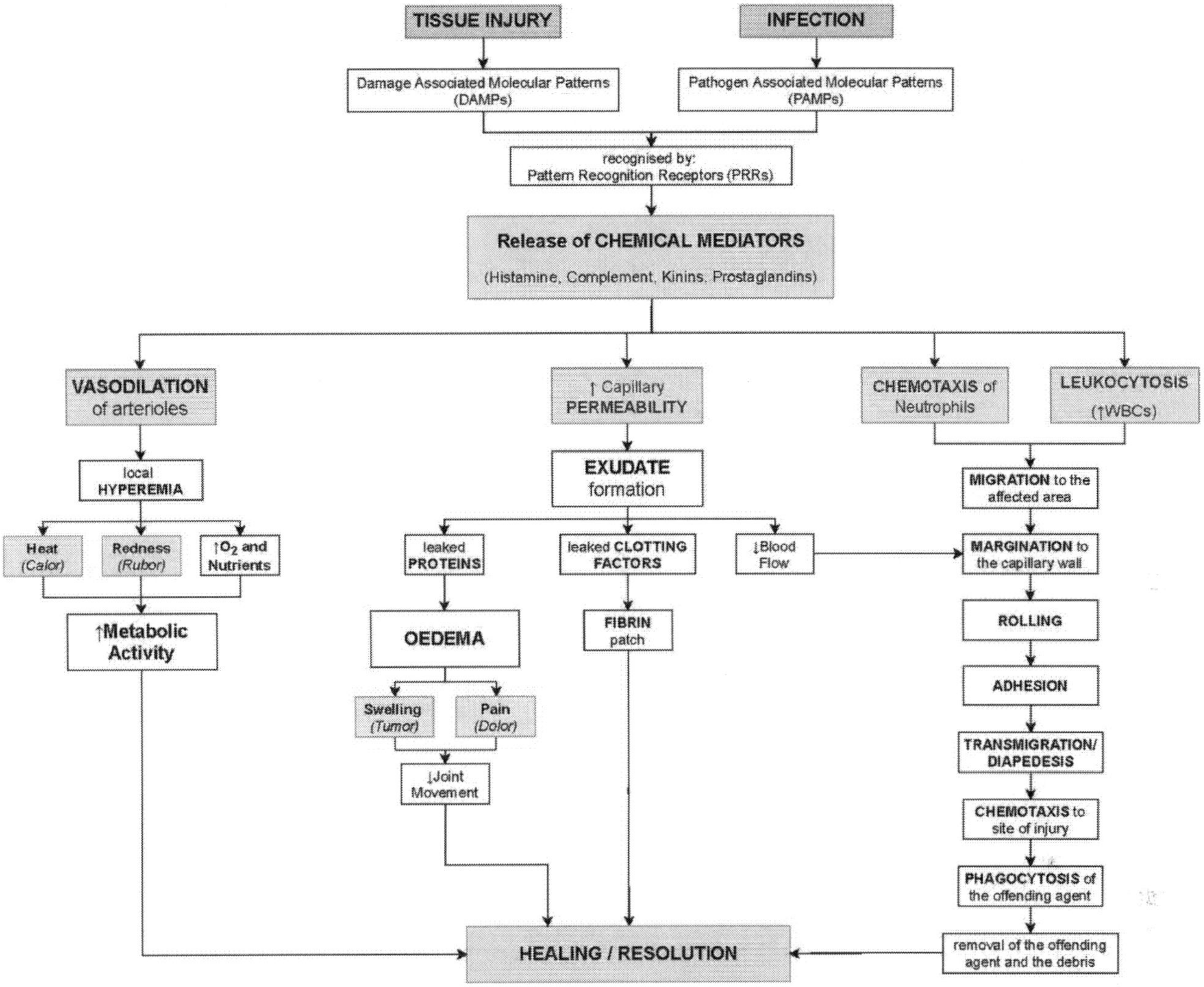

Fig. 4.4 – Illustration of cellular changes during trauma, injury, or infection

Courtesy of Creative Commons Attribution – Share Alike 4.0 International

INJURY-INDUCED CASCADE

Calcium 2+ (Ca2+) or calcium cation is a large ion that can bypass some of the initial transcription-dependent pathways and initiate keratinocyte and fibroblast activities along with cellular binding proteins that can quickly get the wound healed. Elevated Ca2+ levels are triggered when an injured cell releases ATP into the extracellular matrix, which affects various signalling pathways, including the MAPK (mitogen activated protein kinases). MAPK was originally called ERK (extracellular-related signal kinases) pathway, which is active during viruses, cancer, cardiovascular diseases, inflammation, and physical tissue injury.

On the other hand, some traumas can also cause dysfunction in the up-regulation of Ca2+ and often stimulate even greater injury due to the toxic levels of influx. (Blazek, 2015; [64]Mohammed M. Sayeed, PhD, 2000) Epidermal growth factor (EGF) stimulates the proliferation of various cell types, but mainly fibroblasts and epithelial cells. It's receptor, EGFR, is particularly active in the CNS and plays a significant role in neurogenesis. (Wong, 2004) There are obviously several steps along the way after the initial signal that crosses the cell membrane by the growth factor (EGF).

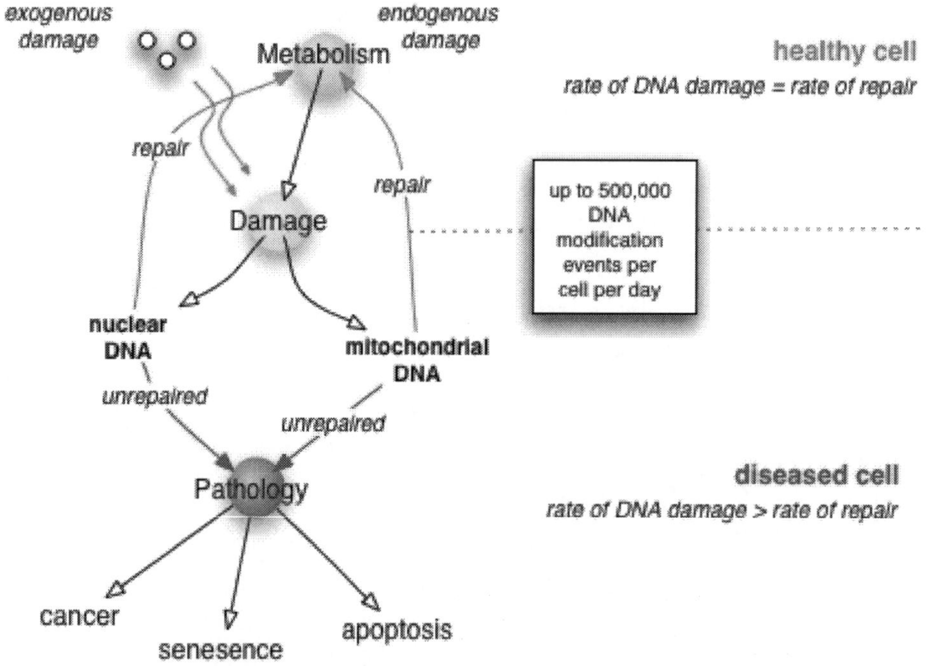

Fig. 4.5 – UV light, environmental toxins, heavy metals, tobacco smoke, among others, can cause countless lesions daily to DNA and its ability to replicate properly or be repaired. (Stephen P. Jackson and Jiri Bartek, 2009)

Image courtesy of Harold Brenner via Wikimedia Commons

BIOCHEMICAL RESPONSES

Enzymes enhance the signal, provide feedback, activate, regulate, and energize other proteins downstream that determine the switching on or off of genes that could repair or regulate the cycle of the damaged cells. If the genes get stuck 'on' while reaching the nucleus and the feedback loop becomes compromised, the stage is set for the damaged cells to become cancer cells (Fig 4.5) The potential for a breakdown in communication creating confusion, hyperactivity, inhibited activity, or mutation is great. There are starts and stops along the way that need to be well coordinated for healthy outcomes. One current way of thinking about it, is that damage to the cell membrane where the transfer or transport of information happens, can be a central cause of the issues. Later in the text I'll point out several studies that describe how tactile and kinesthetic inputs communicate to the cell nucleus and have the potential to restore homeostasis. The fact that Elsa Gindler cured herself of tuberculosis using sensory awareness and A.T. Still facilitated the healing of the black cholera using manual therapy, establishes the precedents for reversal of major cellular dysfunction using conscious movement and manual therapy.

I'd like to think that the potential to reset and rebalance is just as great as the potential for imbalance and dysfunction, elucidating the science of which, is the purpose of this text. The other aim is to make it clear why incorporating signaling pathways from embryological regulatory perspectives during movement and manual therapy practices make sense. These intricate signaling processes suggest that approaching an imbalance from a few different perspectives may be wise and more effective in the long-term experience of well-being.

Multiple systems-signaling approach to homeostasis

EPIGENETIC POTENIALS OF MOTHER NATURE

A case in point for the complexities involved in healing, using my own example, happened when dealing with an onset of eczema. It seemed to come out of nowhere after an exposure to a stick (not poison oak) in the garden. I began a four-year journey that was truly eye-opening. Although it was given the term 'contact dermatitis', that diagnosis didn't hold up over time. Finding out why some systemic reactivity traveled to the skin was arduous, but rewarding.

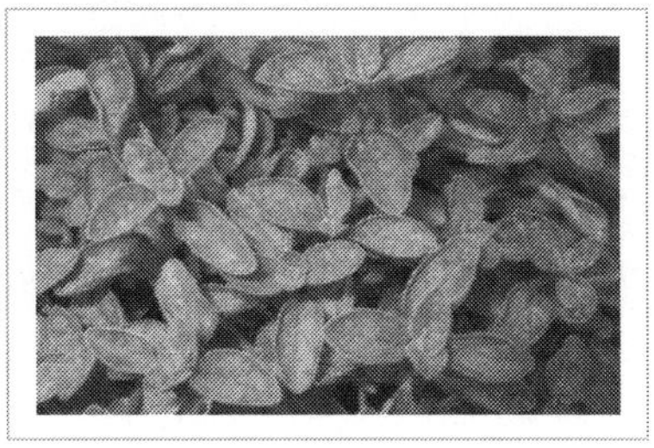

It wasn't necessarily true that the 'cause' was the stick, or something coming into direct contact with it. Remember that the ectoderm is the beginning of embryogenesis and invaginated into the endoderm, and then the mesoderm. According to the early pioneers in osteopathy, any irritation in the system could build into a response that travels through the nervous system and reveals itself in the skin, an organ, or vice-versa. This is also a case in point for 'terrain theory' as opposed to 'germ theory'.

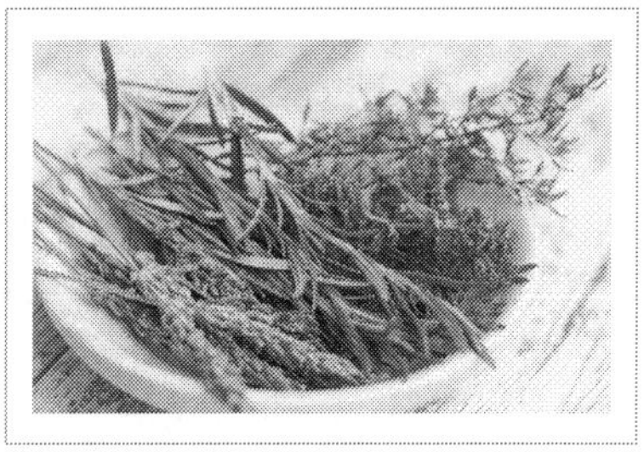

The initial treatment recommended by the dermatologist was to apply a mild steroidal cream, which I did, but it kept coming back and the cream was wearing my skin thin. I began trying a myriad of products from the health food store that claimed to help eczema but they had very little to no effect. I researched creams and oils on my own and began making my own remedies. They stopped the itching and in some cases made the patches (on my ankles) smaller, but didn't heal them. What did eventually work, was using several approaches that involved – you could say – several different signaling pathways with varying functions. It must have changed the gene expression which broke the cycle.

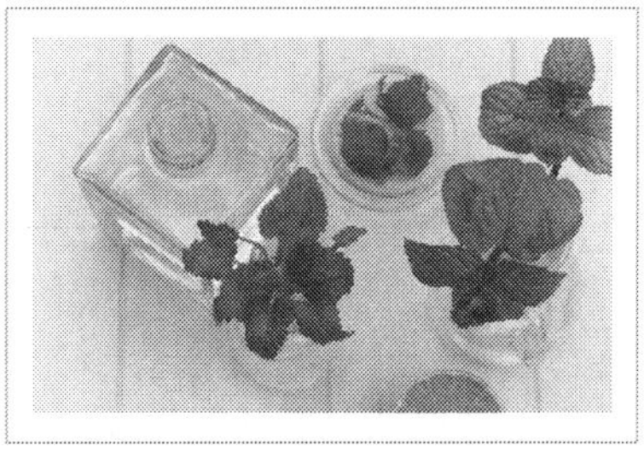

The most potent approach involved rotating a cellular detox blend (of rainforest butters and essential oils), with a blend for skin tags, and an anti-proliferation formula for 'rogue' or mutating cells. Unhealthy cells may have had layers of issues needing to be dealt with, including certain types of bacteria, fungi, or oxidation – an abundance of senescent cells — particularly if they were clumped together and not getting enough oxygen, nutrition, or able to remove waste properly. There's a good chance that this situation in my ankles was partly due to adhesions after spraining them seven times. After those adhesions were addressed the scarred skin healed more fully. Adhesions can alter or restrict cellular communication.

I'd always included a blend to nourish, repair and rejuvenate skin cells, along with oils to combat inflammation and boost immune response. Essential oils are ripe with volatile organic compounds that have countless medicinal properties. The compounds/chemical constituents within them are also specific, and have been researched to identify which species of an oil has the most of the active compounds. For example, with cancer, studies identify which type of cancer they're effective for, if it blocks the pathway, stimulates apoptosis, prevents cancer cells from attaching, or outright kills them.

For example, **carvacrol**, a phenolic monoterpene found in **oregano** and **thyme**, has anti-microbial properties for viruses, fungus, and bacteria, is an anti-oxidant, and stimulates apoptosis in cancer cells. (Medhi Sharif–Rad, et al, 2018) There are at least 60 compounds in oregano, but its potency for a particular action depends upon the percentage of that compound, along with the co-activators that may be present, and where the compounds are in the plant.

According to some studies, the greatest anti-oxidant power or free radical scavenging activity was from essential oils using the leaf and flower parts of the plant, which is over 30% carvacrol. It also has over 18% thymol, which also has anti-microbial, anti-oxidant, and anti-tumor properties. Oregano has "multiple therapeutic actions against various cardiovascular, neurological, rheumatological, gastrointestinal, metabolic and malignant diseases at both biochemical and molecular levels." (Mohamed Meeran et al., 2017)

These plants are grown all over the world, and a certain region may have different growing or harvesting conditions that mean the compounds will be modified, and therefore become more potent or less potent. In addition, there can be different species within a single genus of a plant. When creating a blend that would help restore skin cells, I had to be sure to include Galangal, Frankincense Serrata and Frankincense Carterii in the non-proliferation blend. Boswelia Carterii and its boswelic acids have been shown to arrest cancer cell growth, suppress growth, and stimulate apoptosis in specific (J82) types of bladder cancer cells without damaging healthy cells or fragmenting DNA. (Mark Barton Frank, et al., 2009)

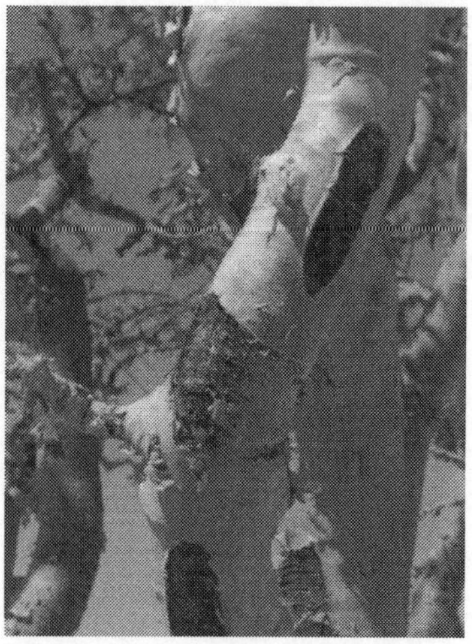
Frankincense tree

Boswellia Sacra has a similar effect on breast cancer cells (Mahmoud M. Suhail, et al., 2011) while Boswellia Serrata has been shown to be effective against colon, pancreatic, and prostate cancer, in addition to leukemia and brain tumors. (Neeta and Harish Dureja, 2014) The boswellic acids in frankincense may be so effective because they are very specific in how they communicate with cancer cells. Rafie Hamidpour and his team of researchers found that:

"Among boswellic acids, Acetyl-11-ket-β-boswellic acid (AKBA) has special inhibitory effects in prostate cancer by suppressing vascular endothelial growth factor receptor 2-mediated angiogenesis. Also,

tirucallic acids isolated from the oleogum resin of Boswellia carterii effect Akt inhibitors. Akt has been associated as a major factor in many types of cancer since it can block apoptosis and promote survival of the cell.

> *"The boswellic acid acetate seems to induce apoptosis in six human myeloid leukemia cell lines through a Caspace-mediated pathway which is activated by the induction of the death receptors 4 and 5 (DR4, DR5). The anticancer activity of AKBA is attributed to the inhibitory effect on the lipoxgenases leading to the inhibiton of cell proliferation and induction of apoptosis in tumor cells." [65](Rafie Hamidpour et al., 2016)*

Neeta Dureja is in full praise of Frankincense saying, "Boswellic acids are bioactive pentacyclic triterpenes derived from a natural plant source...and represents one of the most promising cancer agents (treatments)." (Neeta and Harish Dureja, 2014) It also has powerful anti-inflammatory actions which is the basis for many systemic imbalances and expressions of symptoms. Alpha pinene, another constituent of Frankincense essential oil, is able to reduce pro-inflammatory cytokines, enhance T-cell activity, and potentially modulate immune responses while reducing stress hormones.

> Xuesheng Han and his group of researchers analyzed the effect of Frankincense essential oil on 21,224 genes and found that it had "*a robust effect on regulating human genes, which many being upregulated and many being downregulated*."

Using an independent analysis company, they were able to establish that Frankincense 'affected many signaling pathways that are closely related to inflammation, immune response, and tissue remodeling.' [66](Xuesheng Han, 2017) This is most likely why it was so helpful for skin eruptions like eczema.

This is just one essential oil – and there are some with up to 300 organic compounds, each with its own function that may work in concert with the others in particular ways. It's helpful to be reminded that foods, herbs, oils, plants, flowers, seeds, roots – all have the potential of affecting our systems in a very fundamental and profound way – down to the DNA. Mother Nature is the most resourceful source of medicine, and I guess the *only* source of medicine and nourishment we have when you think about it.

Although it can be mind-boggling to see the list of active organic compounds in essential oils, the effectiveness of a particular quality of that oil may be more effective synergistically and in certain quantities. For example, linalool, the main compound that is calming and relaxing in oils like lavender contains around 35%, however, essential oils of coriander and Ho have 80-85% linalool. It communicates with the nervous system and has been shown to also exhibit anti-microbial, anti-inflammatory, antioxidant and anti-cancer properties. Perhaps enhancing the trophic effects of the CNS, combined with alpha-pinene, linalool and pinene influence multiple neurotransmitter, inflammatory and neurotrophic signals as well as behavior, demonstrating psychoactivity. (Green et al., 2021)

LIMITING ANTI-NUTRIENTS

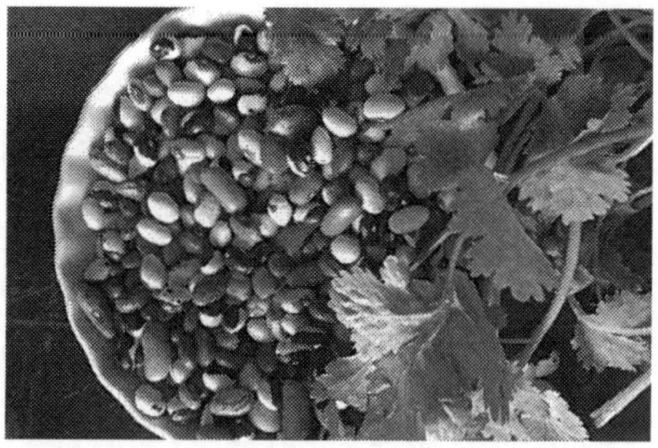

There likely have been numerous cellular changes happening in the cells that were involved in producing the eruption of eczema in my skin, yet the true source was deeper. The real surprise came when I read an article somewhere that **lectins**, including those in chicken and turkey, can create inflammation in the epithelial lining of cells, and during this breakout phase, (and since childhood) I'd had issues with veins bursting in my hands. After eliminating lectins – including beans, lentils, chicken, soy, grains, etc. from my diet, my skin cleared up and stayed that way. My veins stopped bursting. I knew the connection was real because when I tried to eat a bowl of dahl, the eczema began to return immediately. If I ate chicken more than once or twice a month, either the rash would begin or the veins in my hands began to pop again. Food is information and there may be numerous determing factors in why some people respond differently than others to the same stimulus, but with the introduction of so many toxins into our environment, things that our immune systems previously could easily have prevented or managed are now able to cause issues.

I took the investigation a little further. Apparently, some lectins are not fully digested and can bind to the cell membrane of the intestines and interfere with digestion, absorption, and metabolism. The dysregulation of the wall of the gut can interfere with its regeneration and allow substances to exit into the bloodstream creating inflammation, cramping, or nausea. They are more harmful if consumed raw, so much of the issue can be resolved with soaking or cooking for over 30 minutes for most people. There's more. Lectins also have an agglutinating (to stick together – as in rouleau in red blood cells) feature, which is present in the type found in chicken and turkey. The majority of plants have this type of lectin, and the effects are across all blood types.

Nadja Zubecevic describes it this way:

"Plant lectins are carbohydrate-binding proteins or phytohemagglutinins present in most plants, especially seeds and tubers, which include cereals, potatoes, and beans.

> *Lectins have great significance in the diet because of their involvement in gastrointestinal difficulties and erythrocyte agglutination....The concentration of plant lectins depends upon the part of the plant. Lectins from the seeds of certain plants cause the greatest percentage of erythrocyte agglutination, and the lowest agglutination was caused by plant bulbs and leaves." [67](Zubecevic et al., 2016)*

There is some evidence that the potential harm done by lectins can be offset by EDTA, (Tunis, 1965) a chelating agent that prevents it from binding to erythrocytes. They can also be made to be inactive by proteolytic enzymes such as papain, and by simple sugars. (Gorakshakar and Ghosh, 2016). Lectins are seen as communication molecules for plants and have been under study for the ways in which they can be of benefit in the treatment of disease as their functions become more clarified.

Lifelong experiences of trauma, accidents, and surgical procedures are likely to alter the accuracy of the information delivery systems, adaptability, and tolerance thresholds. They also alter the availability of the energy needed to accomplish the necessary information processing, which may be even more common in aging populations.

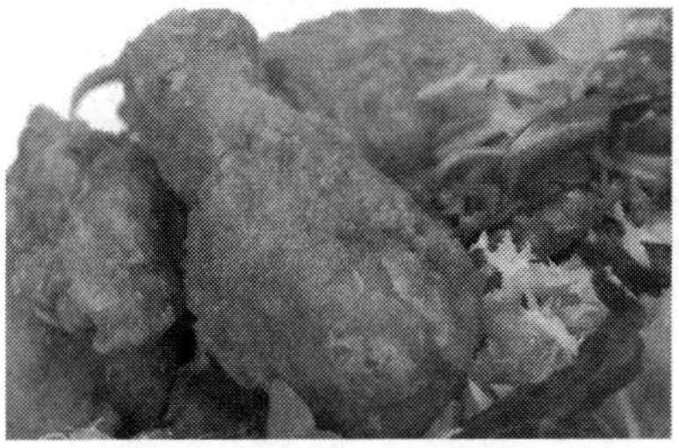

Chicken contains agglutinating lectins

Other anti-nutrients like oxylates, phytates, phytoestrogens, and histamines may create issues for those whose systems are already struggling with an auto-immune conditions or gastrointestinal issues.

If you have enough curiosity to check your symptoms against an elimination diet of those potential anti-nutrient triggers, there could be pleasant surprises waiting for you.

Nonetheless, even though a molecule may have many faces, there are ways to influence which face it wears. Lectins can be very harmful or very helpful, perhaps even within the same system. People have different tolerance thresholds, so something your system may not be agreeable with every week may be fine once in a while. Keep in mind that substances or activities your system was open to earlier in your life could change, particularly during those middle-age years.

The central point to adhere to, is that our systems rely on multiple, complex cascades of communication processes through several different pathways, biochemicals, receptors, and signaling processes for every event that the senses perceive. Developing our felt-sense to build upon a library of languges the body uses to communicate with us can make a tremendous difference in the duration, efficiency, and accuracy of the cascading molecules during a crisis, as well in the outcomes.

POTENTIAL SOURCES OF HARM FOR DNA

All natural and unnatural substances have the potential of communicating with us on a molecular level, right down to the DNA in the cell nucleus. That's why it's so vital to conceive of things this way and to realize that certain substances, reactions, or experiences can alter the cells' ability to communicate with themselves or with other cells. Some substances can even break one or more strands of DNA pairs, which may lead to mutations if not repaired.

One of the most common ways to damage DNA is through exposure to the sun, something we seldom avoid while growing up. Our body's photoreceptors in the skin are a perfect example of the preprogrammed specificity for acceptable frequencies. Light frequencies can be helpful or harmful, depending upon which range they're being transmitted in. We very much need the red frequencies of the sun, particularly between 600 and 850 nm (300 GHz-400 GHz) for the therapeutic benefits, and 100-600nm for low level light therapy. We need UVB rays for the production of vitamin D. The UVC frequency range has a powerful antimicrobial, santizing effect.

High noon is the best time to receive UVB rays to stimulate vitamin D synthesis, but high noon is also the easiest time to get sunburn and skin damage for certain types of skin. Apparently, DNA damage isn't unusual. Unfortunately, this common area of damage is nearly impossible to detect until it already has some mutated skin cells. Melanin, the substance that gives the skin its color, is protective against UV rays, but darker skin will still get damaged after about an hour, according the the researchers at the Institute for Quality and Efficiency in Health Care. (NIH, 2018)

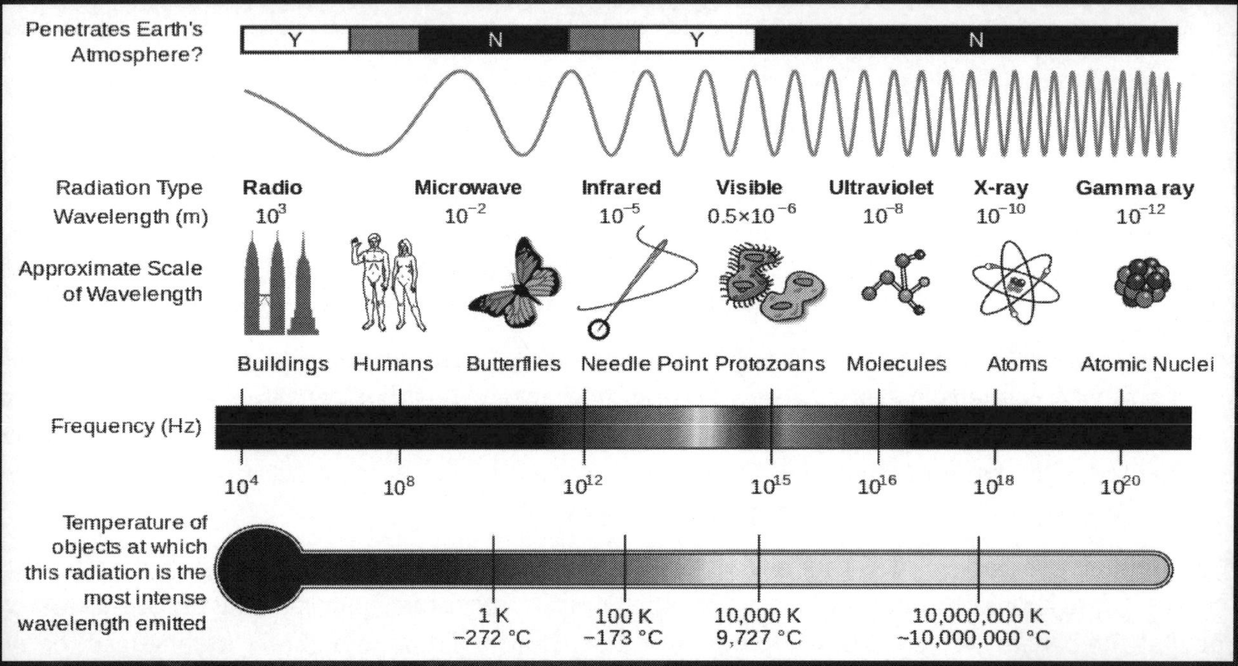

Fig. 4.6 – Spectrum of wavelengths; the sun emits rays from Infrared to Gamma

Image courtesy of Inductiveload, NASA, CC BY-SA 3.0 via Wikimedia Commons

That said, the amount of UVB rays received depends upon the color of one's skin and the distance from the equator. Darker-skinned people will need to spend a longer time in the sun to get an adequate amount, and those in the very northern part of the globe, like Norway or Canada may not get any at all in the winter months even if they're outside for long hours. (Rayan Raman, MS, 2018)

To put this issue in perspective, Tom Ellenberger, at the Washington University School of Medicine in St. Louis, explains it this way: *"DNA damage, due to environmental factors and normal metabolic processes inside the cell, occurs at the rate of 1,000 to 1,000,000 molecular lesions per cell per day. A special enzyme, DNA ligase, encircles the double helix to repair a broken strand of DNA. Without cells to mend such breaks, cells can malfunction, die, or become cancerous."*

Suzanne Clancy, PhD, emphasizes that the integrity and stability of DNA is of utmost importance because it is the repository of information that is essential to life. The most common examples Clancy mentions are the sun damage from UV light of the sun, tanning beds, and the damage to lung cells by tobacco smoke. [71] (Clancy, 2008) She describes a 'proofreading' enzyme that would normally catch and correct these errors in the cell, but some do slip through the cracks. Depending upon the rate of replication errors per cell, mutations will begin to accumulate and set the stage for a disease process.

When the bases become damaged by oxidation (free radicals) or metabolic issues, by alkylation or hydrolyzation, the system's mechanisms of repair come into play. Ionizing radiation, such as that from x-rays, gamma rays, microwaves, or heat and light from the sun, can kick the electrons out of an atom. That will create an ion, which can cause double-strand breaks in the DNA. Hydrolyzation happens when a water molecule splits a protein molecule, like with hydrolyzed collagen that is broken down in smaller particles like peptides or amino acids so the body can use it more readily. (Patrick Carroll, MD, 2019)

However, the bases of DNA are somewhat fragile, and water (hydrolysis) can separate purine from a base, a process called depurination, which happens daily to everyone. Amino groups on DNA bases can also be damaged by water, (Fig. 4.7) which is called deamination and also happens several times a day. Ideally, repair enzymes are set into motion and correct the damage before it becomes a problem. [68] (Toshinori Suzuki, 2006) Hydrolyzed protein as a food additive is more concerning as it is a precursor to MSG, according to Muthusamy Ramesh. Ramesh says that as it is being broken down to release glutamic acid, it combines with sodium to form monosodium glutamate. [69](Ramesh, 2018)

Alkylation damage is caused by drugs used for chemotherapy and autoimmune disorders, by some industrial chemicals, environmental contaminants, and various carcinogens, including food sources. There is some evidence to support the fact that orange juice and citric acid can reduce DNA damage from two types of alkylating agents. [70](Silvia Franke et al., 2005) Although some processed foods have been linked to mutations in cells, there is also evidence that dietary phytochemicals, or diets rich in fruits and vegetables can counteract those mutations and prevent cancers from forming.

For example, gallic acid, found in green tea, pomegranate, some berries, apples, walnuts, avocado, Boswellia daizielil, and more, is a phenolic acid that can block the mutagenic activity of alkylating factors. It also has powerful anti-inflammatory characteristics involving MAPK and NF-kB signaling pathways, weakening the release of inflammatory cytokines, chemokines, adhesion molecules, and cell infiltration. (Jinrong Bai et al., 2021)

Clancy explains that base excision repair (BER) is the most common form to handle spontaneous DNA damage from free radicals. This type of damage generally is cut out by DNA glycosylases that break the bonds and fill the gap with special polymerases, then sealed with ligase, also shown in Fig. 4.7. The double-strand breaks from ionizing radiation can lead to chromosomal rearrangement and interfere with transcription and replication. Double-strand helix breaks, according to Featherstone and Jackson, can be repaired using non-homologous end joining, and homologous recombination. Optimally, the cell's protective mechanisms wall off the cell and prevent it from replication while being repaired, and if repair efforts fail, signals for apoptosis may begin. [71] (Suzanne Clancy, PhD, 2008)

That said, food and environmental toxins aren't the only potential threat to cells being able to function efficiently. Lack of movement in a sedentary lifestyle is just as harmful if not more so. Sitting may well be the new 'smoking'!

> The surprising results of a study by researcher, Yin Cao, ScD, of 89,278 Americans declared that one additional hour of watching tv for those under 50 increases colorectal cancer risks by 12%.

The same may hold true for video games. The rate of risk rises to almost 70% if spending over two hours watching televison per day.

The outcomes were the most consistent for women with a family history of cancer, and all results were independent of exercise and body mass. Apparently, young-onset colorectal cancer has different molecular characteristics that make it more aggressive, so fewer survived. [72](Oxford Unversity Press USA, 2019) This study underscores how important biomechanical input is for the system to be able to sense itself and properly regulate its functions. Movement is medicine.

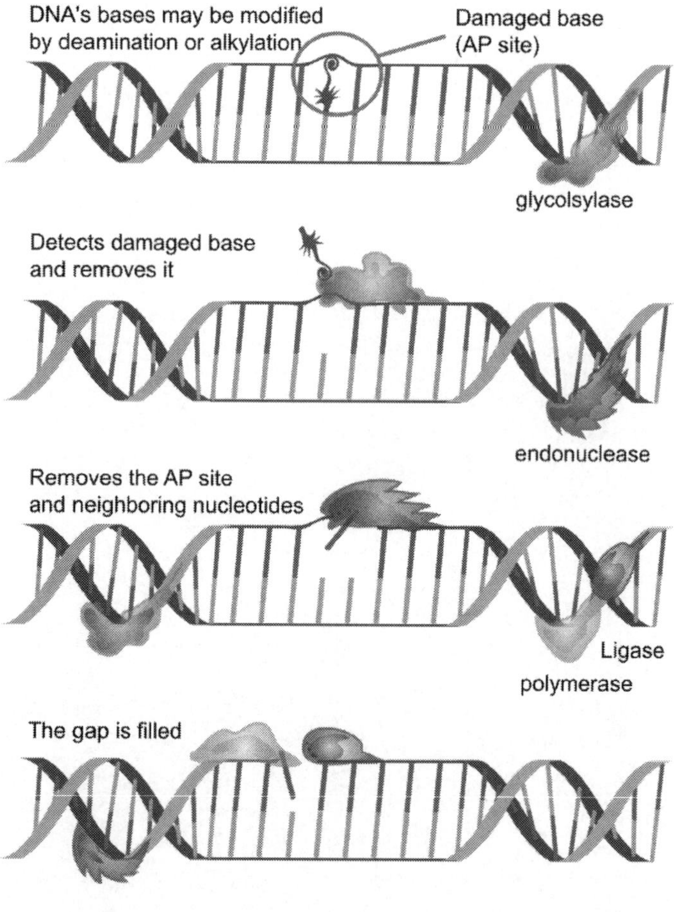

Fig. 4.7 Repairing DNA base damage with enzymes on the right: glycosylase, endonuclease, and polymerase, using the template on the other side of the double helix as a reference to copy from for the repair

Boumphreyfr CC BY SA-3.0 via Wikimedia Commons

POTENTIAL SOURCES OF BENEFIT FOR DNA

Micro-neurocurrent, a modality that was invented in the early 1900s by a Canadian Osteopath, disappeared for a while. It re-emerged when it was refined in the 1980s by Dr. Carolyn McMakin after it was proven to be a viable and reliable form of treatment for pain, inflammation, and wound healing. It has been shown to Increase levels of ATP by up to 500% and speed healing by modifying the intensity according to the needs of each patient. Individualized specificity acheives the best results. ATP (adenosine triphosphate), the form of energy that all cells use, has among its many functions the ability to signal the synthesis of RNA and DNA.

> Cellular signaling in general relies upon ATP, so whatever can support the production of this cellular requirement is supporting the overall health of the body. *(Jacob Dunn, 2022)*

Cells can absorb light, which in turn can signal other processes to occur. Tsai and Hamblin describe photobiomodulation (PBM) using the infrared frequency of light as being able to "*promote wound healing, help alleviate pain and inflammation, and stimulate tissue regeneration as well as immunomodulation*." These researchers also spoke about its ability to stimulate the production of ATP, metabolic processes, cytoskeleton organization, cell proliferation/differentiation, and homeostasis. [73](Shang-Ru Tsai, PhD and Michael R. Hamblin, PhD, 2017)

Even though the communication in our systems is inconceivably detailed and the opposite of random, most of the inherent programming is not set in stone; only a small percentage of it is. As more details emerge in recent research about how interlaced the soma is functionally, new discoveries are also happening on a structural level that allow those structures to be included on the self-regulatory playing field. For example, the perineural system was thought for decades to function as insulation for the nerves, but is now known to be responsible for complex trophic and repair activities. With that understanding, during injury, substances that stimulate the trophic secretions from glial cells can speed healing. (University of Zurich, 2018)

How DNA responds to self-care

MOVEMENT AND EPIGENETICS

Practitioners of Yoga, Somatics, and Chi Kung can also attest that more benefit will be derived in each according to the specificity of the position of each and every part of the body, how the breath and the mind are employed, and several other factors according to the level of practitioner or teacher. Manual therapy falls under the same principles, in that specificity in the touch and its intention elicits more specific responses from the body. A specific local intervention can have a global response, however. System-wide shifts can often be felt on several levels as the changes are being integrated, until they come to rest after the opening, softening and lengthening of the tissue fields.

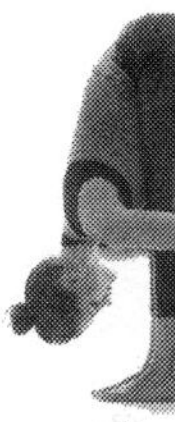

There is much to still be discovered in the field of epigenetics, as it is becoming increasingly clear that the majority of our programming is open for modification. In fact, countless forms of input, such as thoughts, emotions, diet, pollution, lifestyle choices, forms of exercise, and so on have the ability to determine whether certain genes are turned on or off. The placebo effect demonstrates consistently that we all have the ability to change how genes express themselves.

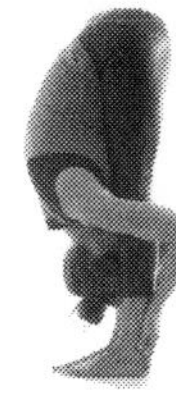

Biologist, Bruce Lipton, has expressed in different ways that the cells and their receptors change their shape and receptivity based upon our beliefs and perceptions. *(Criag Gustfson, 2017)*

A few minutes of exercise signals cellular responses almost immediately. Dr. Juleen Zierath explains it this way while she was being interviewed: "*We've studied the early, immediate changes at the level of the DNA, and how other proteins recognize it, and how they can regulate the production of specific proteins to support higher growth and the breakdown of sugar and fats with exercise.*" Zierath admits that low-level workouts have some benefits, but a workout for 35-minutes that is so intense you can't carry on a conversation is what's needed to *"support the production of these special proteins for glucose and lipid metabolism."* [74](Ira Flatow, 2012)

MOOD AND ATTITUDE

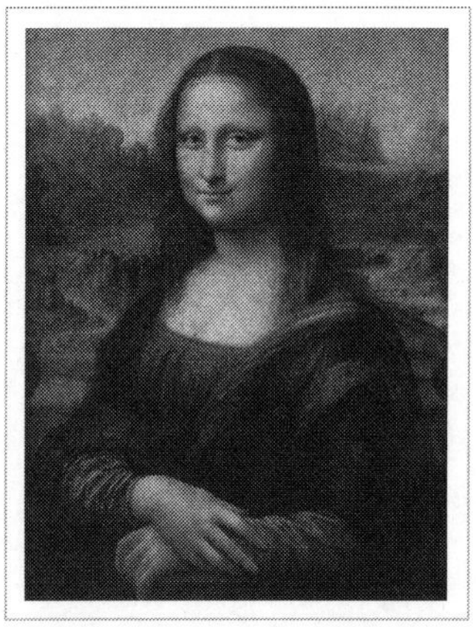

The research on how healthy cells function in happy, well-adjusted people is skimpy, as studies mostly focus on what's going wrong rather than on what's going right. One report distinguishes between how immune cells respond to the different types of happiness a person experiences. In a relatively small study, a team of researchers from the University of North Carolina found that those whose happiness was correlated with a sense of purpose in a cause larger than themselves had stronger anti-viral and lower inflammatory responses. [75] (Aditi Nerurkar, 2015)

Although the specifics weren't looked at on a molecular level, in a large study of 10,000 Australians, outcomes were measured based upon their general outlook on life. Overall, studies showed that happier people have more robust immune systems, lower inflammation, increased longevity, and dramatically reduced incidences of heart disease. Smiling and laughing have been shown to be relaxing, reduce stress (cortisol levels), release endorphins and neurotransmitters like dopamine, serotonin, lower your heart rate, and at times, reduce blood pressure and pain levels. [76](Mark Stibich, PhD, 2021)The most 'coveted' one, that has been associated with health and well-being years later, is the 'Duchenne smile', like the one borne by Mona Lisa in the famous painting.

Smiles have also been shown to be contagious, which feeds back even more good chemistry to the initiator of the chain reaction.

As far as the body's concerned, a certain response happens in the brain even if you fake the smile. Some psychologists have reported, however, that all smiles are not alike. French anatomist, Guillaume Duchenne, studied facial expressions using electrodes in the 1800s and expressed a theory on which muscles contract (obicularis oculi) during a smile coming from within, exposing the 'sweet emotions of the soul'. This type of 'low intensity' smile, Duchenne insists, connotes true enjoyment and real satisfaction. Happiness, he explained, has a higher intensity but is a more fleeting experience.

Psychologists bickered over this issue for 100 years, saying that the meaning of a facial expression couldn't be 'locked into a universal vault like that'. Then a facial expression coding system was developed. In 1970, Ekman and Freison from the University of San Francisco captured the muscular coordinates of 3000 facial expressions. They then ressurected the assertions of Duchenne, which according to their studies, activated the left anterior and parietal areas of the brain associated with positive emotions.

Predictive studies came in later on this issue, whereby longer marriages and longer lives could be associated with the type of smile a person had on their face decades earlier in photos. This is pretty fascinating, because the smile could even be fake and the body will take it at 'face value,' apparently, because it still

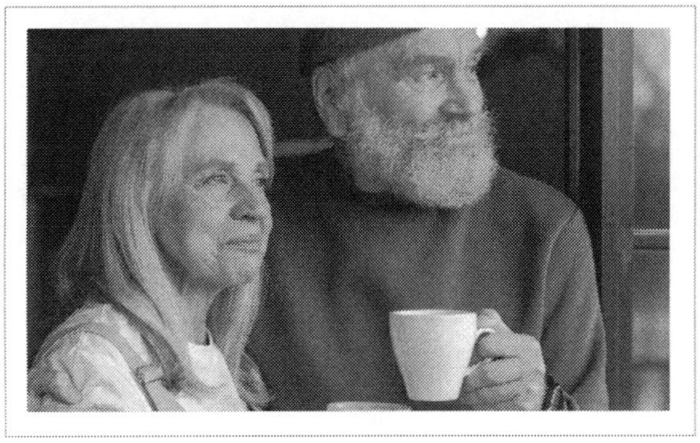

lights up brain regions. How we hold ourselves muscularly is being interpreted and responded to by our cells.

There is some evidence, however, that many facial expressions are inherited. Except for the more universal emotive changes that happen in joy and sadness, many other ways that emotions are expressed on the face come from the family you were born into. The results hold true even when the family members are blind. Evolutionary biologist, Eviatar Nevo, conducted a study in Israel labeled the phenomena 'family facial expression signature'. (Constance Holden, 2006) Most agree that emotions, facial expressions, and body language are wired into survival circuits so have a great deal of influence on how the body thinks we're doing.

Our facial expression and body positioning also communicates to us how we think we're doing. It's something worth exploring to see if we have expressions that have been unconscious, yet have been sending a steady stream of input to our cells that may be sending the wrong message. It could be that our inner state, which we can cultivate, along with the self-care we practice, can keep genetic switches operating in our favor; in the direction of balance and health. Knowing that numerous choices we make throughout the day can have an impact on every cell in our body, could be a key point in making decisions. In real time, choices in how we express ourselves have a molecular, biochemical equivalent.

HOW AGING AFFECTS GENE EXPRESSION

We covered the first three epigenetic mechanisms (listed top left corner on the image describing epigenetics) (Fig.4.8) related to the efficacy of cellular communication and gene expression. Those mechanisms concern environmental exposures, developmental and prenatal issues, pharmaceuticals, or alcohol and smoking. Maybe because of general upsurges in health consciousness, the last few decades have seen a growing body of research on what contributes to longevity. Healthy genes are certainly fundamental to healthy aging. A group of researchers began a study of 200 individuals in 2015 to determine if there were similarities in how specific tissues age, using at least 40 tissue samples from 9 tissue types. It was called the Genotype-Tissue Expression project (GTEx).

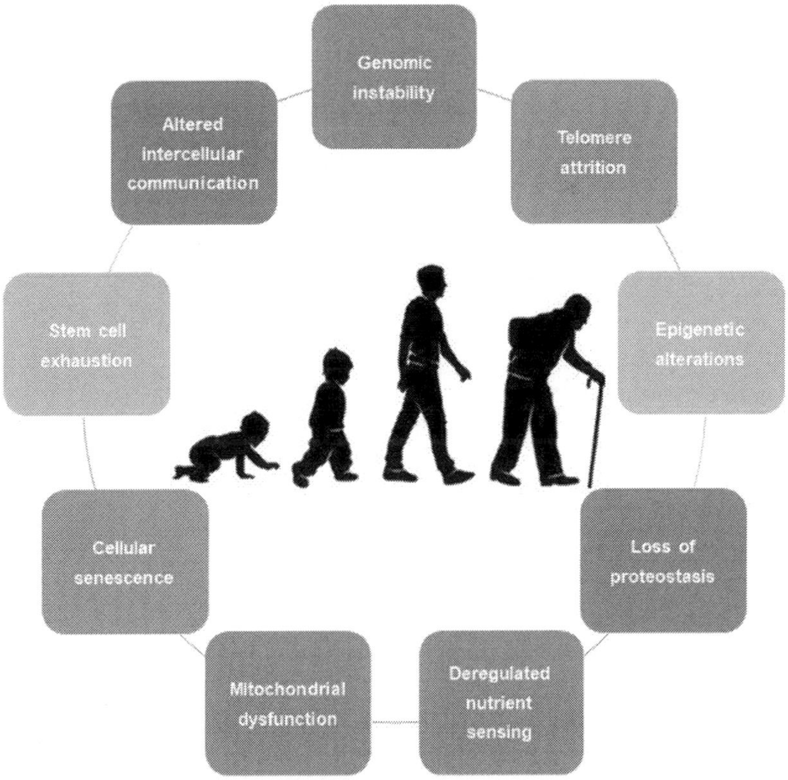

Rebelo-Marques, De Sousa Lages, Andrade, Ribeiro, Mota-Pinto, Carrilho and Espregueira-Mendes, CC BY 4.0, via Wikimedia Commons

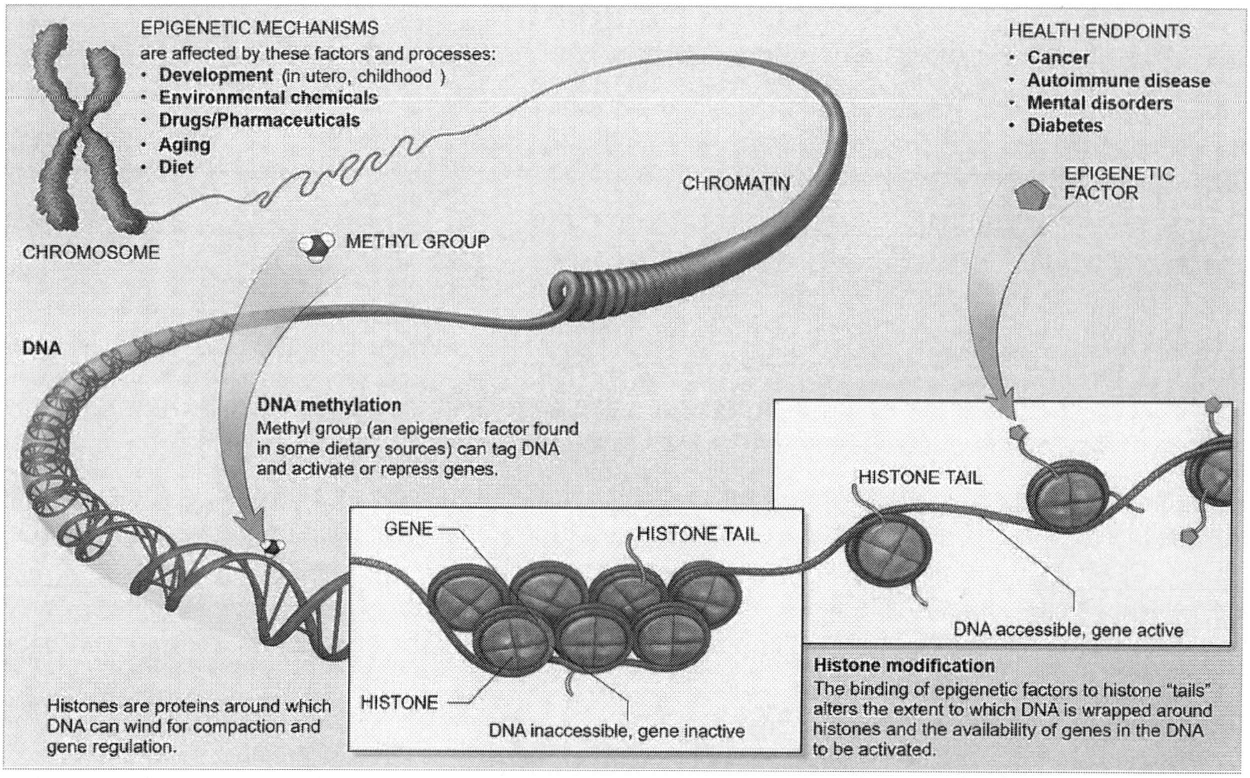

Fig. 4.8 – Factors affecting gene expression/activation by methylation and histone modification

Image courtesy of National Institutes of Health, Public Domain, via Wikimedia Commons

The tissue types included: subcutaneous adipose, tibial artery, left ventricle of the heart, lung, skeletal muscle, tibial nerve, skin, thyroid and whole blood. The ages of the participants ranged from 20 to 70 years, both male and female. A down-regulation of electron transport chains in the heart and adipose tissue, and up-regulation of inflammatory responses and cell death in the arteries was also present as a function of aging. [77](J. Yang, et al., 2015)

The most significant finding across several tissue types (adipose, artery, heart, lung, and blood) was down-regulated **mitochondria** in aging genes.

This research team noticed 'co-aging coefficients' being particularly significant with heart, lung, and blood. If one of these tissues appeared young in someone, there was a high probability that the other related tissues would also appear young. Nonetheless, they also found that aging in the arteries and nerves were usually related, and much more common in the older participants. In 2013, Daniel Glass and a large group of researchers studied tissue-specific changes in fewer tissues but with a larger sample size of over 800 post-mortem individuals who were female twins between 30 and 85 years of age.

This team analyzed tissue from abdominal skin, subcutaneous adipose tissue, brain, and lymphoblastoid cell lines. Although there were predictable age-related changes in skin tissue related to fatty acid metabolism, there weren't across-the-board changes in genes of the older population. The programming concerning aging does not appear to be inherent, but very much epigenetic in its tissue specificity. [78] (Glass, et al., 2013) They also found increased inflammation with age.

In 2018, Stephen Frank & Jonathan Houseley report a list of clear physiological outcomes considered to be the hallmarks of aging:

- Down-regulation of genes encoding mitochondrial proteins
- Down-regulation of the protein synthesis machinery
- Dysregulation of immune system genes
- Reduced growth factor signaling
- Constitutive responses to stress and DNA damage
- Dysregulation of gene expression and mRNA processing

Two factors that seem to dovetail on one another as vital to the aging issue, are the cumulative damage to DNA which reduces gene expression and generates mutations, coupled with the reduction in efficiency of the repair process, perhaps due to limited energy. [79](Frank & Houseley, 2018) There is some agreement that cells age differently in different tissues, but the blood tends to show signs of aging across the board. Since it has been shown in one study to be co-aging among blood, heart, and lung tissue, it could be that the originator is in the blood. Given that heart disease is the number one killer for men and women in most ethnic groups, this deduction seems to be true. The World Health Organization estimates that almost 18 million people per year perish from heart disease.

Regarding biological clocks, Frank and Houseley state that, "*Unfortunately, there is not a clear relationship between differentially expressed genes in these transcriptional clocks, and differentially methylated sites in the epigenetic clocks. Nor, in fact, is there any strong bias in the function of genes that contain differentially methylated sites. Therefore, the epigenetic clock is in itself unlikely to be the direct driver of aging, but rather it should be considered that epigenetic and gene expression changes provide parallel read-outs of the aging process.*"

Changes in **mitochondria** function are seen across species during aging. These researchers go on to say that, "*The change most consistently reported in aging transcriptome studies is a down-regulation of mitochondrial protein mRNAs, particularly nuclear-encoded components of the electron transport chain (ETC) and mitochondrial ribosome proteins.*" (Fig.4.9)

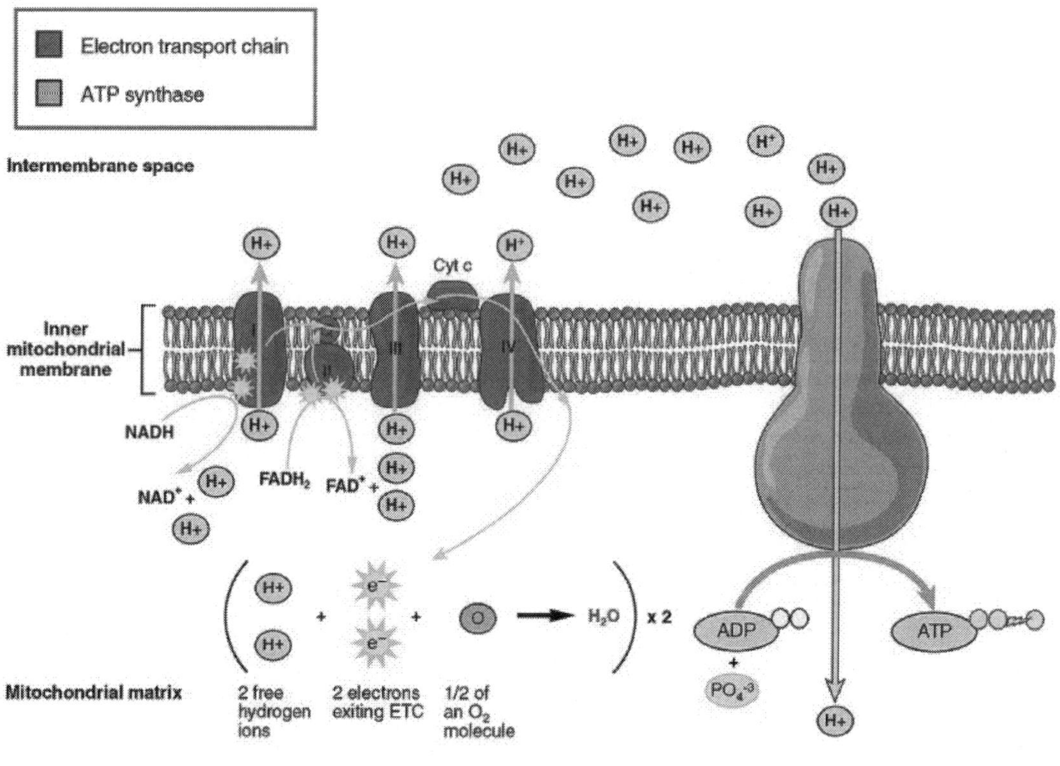

Fig. 4.9 – The electron transport chain

There is a series of four protein complexes that lead to the creation of ATP in the ECT (electron transport chain).The entire process is called oxidative phosphorylation which is directly related to cellular respiration and necessary for the life and function of every cell.

Image courtesy of OpenStax College CC By 3.0 via Wikimedia Commons

Energy is released in a cell by breaking down organic molecules. Most of the energy is dissipated as heat or used to pump hydrogen ions (H+) into the intermembrane space and create a proton gradient. Electrons are transported between the protein complexes shown in red (Fig. 4.9) by way of the energy produced during sugar metabolism and its byproducts, NADH or $FADH_2$. (Robert A. Lue, 2017) CoQ10 participates in one of the stages of this process. (Maria Ahmed et al., StatPearls, 2021)

Protein complexes gather the energy produced by the electron chain and use it to pump protons into the intermembrane space where electrons are transferred to a CoQ10 molecule. Those electrons are either cycled back into the protein complexes or shuttled forward to protein complex 4, where a molecule of oxygen is combined with two molecules of water. Our breath helps this transfer process to continue, as cellular respiration and the production of ATP or ADP would not be able to happen without oxygen.

As mentioned earlier in the text, micro-neurocurrent and frequency-specific application of infrared light have been shown to increase activity in mitochondria by several-fold. Cold stimulation (ice bath, cryotherapy, etc.) and caloric restriction as in intermittent fasting have all been proven to be beneficial for mitochondrial functioning and the production of ATP. The ETC pathway is the most important one for producing ATP. CoQ10 is one of the electron carriers involved in this process and is often recommended as a supplement for mitochondria support.

Other options include Creatine, Alpha lipoic acid, arginine, carnitine, riboflavin, thiamin, vitamins C and E, and folinic acid. ("Dietary Supplements for Primary Mitochondrial Disorders," NIH, 2020) Other sources recommend PQQ (pyrroloquinoline quinone), which has been said to stimulate mitochondrial biogenesis. Some have even called it the fountain of youth, perhaps because it has been found to also stimulate nerve growth factor and protect brain cells against damage, among other benefits. [80](Dr. Edward Group, 2019) R-Lipoic Acid, L-Carnitine, and L-Carnitine Tartrate have also been shown to improve mitochondrial function.

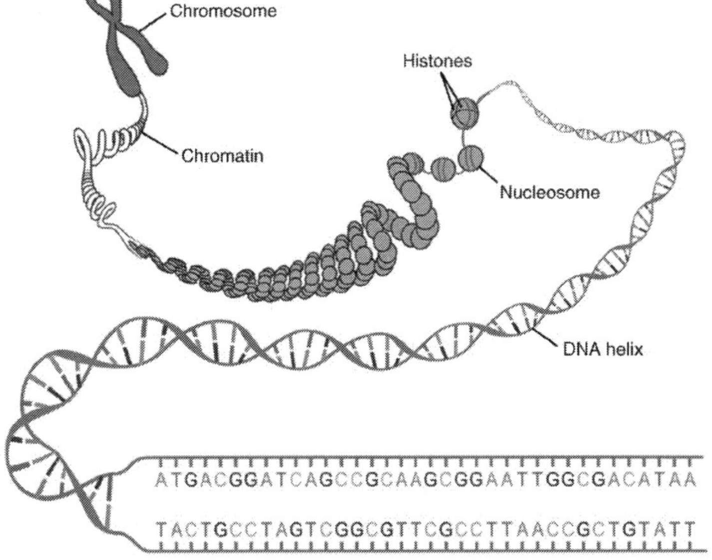

Fig. 4.10 – DNA base pairs coiling into wrapped histones or nucleosomes condensed into chromosomes

Many lifestyle factors impact how one ages, and whether the actual chromatin (protein, RNA and DNA in the nucleus of a cell) structure of the cell will be altered. The primary protein components of chromatin are called 'histones', which help organize DNA into bead-like structures called nucleosomes. (Fig. 4.10) There are 147 base pairs of DNA that are wrapped around a set of 8 histones. (Cell News, 2017) Further folding of the nucleosome can create a chromatin fiber, which can be coiled and condensed to form chromosomes. The multi-purpose chromatin enables DNA replication, transcription, DNA repair, genetic recombination, and cell division to happen.

TELOMERES AND SENESCENT CELLS

A couple of decades ago there was a focus on telomeres, the structures at the ends of chromosomes, as a predictor or indicator of aging. Their function is to protect the chromosome from damage. However, when they shorten and can no longer replicate, the cell cannot divide in the same way and becomes senescent – a vulnerable, inactive stage right before the cell dies. (National Human Genome Institute) Recent studies are investigating this area again to discover ways this 'canary in the mine' can help forestall if not reverse disease processes associated with aging. (National Institute on Aging, July 2021)

Senescent cells increase with age, and as they compromise our immune function, the body becomes less able to cope with stress, it heals more slowly, and they may contribute to cognitive decline. (Fig. 4.11) These types of cells have been connected to cancer, diabetes, osteoporosis, cardiovascular disease, stroke, Alzheimer's, dementia, and osteoarthritis. [81] (NIH, 2021) It was discovered by Hayflick and Moorehead in the 1960s that a cell can only replicate so many times before it becomes senescent, because the telomeres shorten and can no longer function.

It has become a hot topic for research to see if adding senolytics that help the body remove senescent cells can reverse certain age-related conditions. Initial studies with mice have been promising. Fisetin is a naturally occurring senolytic agent and anti-oxidant in fruits and vegetables that stimulates apoptosis in senescent cells. For therapeutic purposes, there would most likely need to be a particular dosage and frequency of these particular foods in order to make a noticeable difference, but it's an experiment well worth the task of discovering about the details for effectiveness.

Jerry Shay PhD, from the UT Southwestern Medical Center defines telomeres this way:

"A telomere is a repeating DNA sequence (for example TTAGGG) at the end of the body's chromosomes. (Fig. 4.12) The telomere can reach a length of 15,000 base pairs. Telomeres function by preventing chromosomes from losing base pair sequences at their ends. They also stop chromosomes from fusing to each other. However, each time a cell divides, some of the telomere is lost (usually 25-200 base pairs per division).... Telomere activity is controlled by two mechanisms: erosion and addition. Erosion occurs each time a cell divides. Addition is determined by the activity of telomerase."

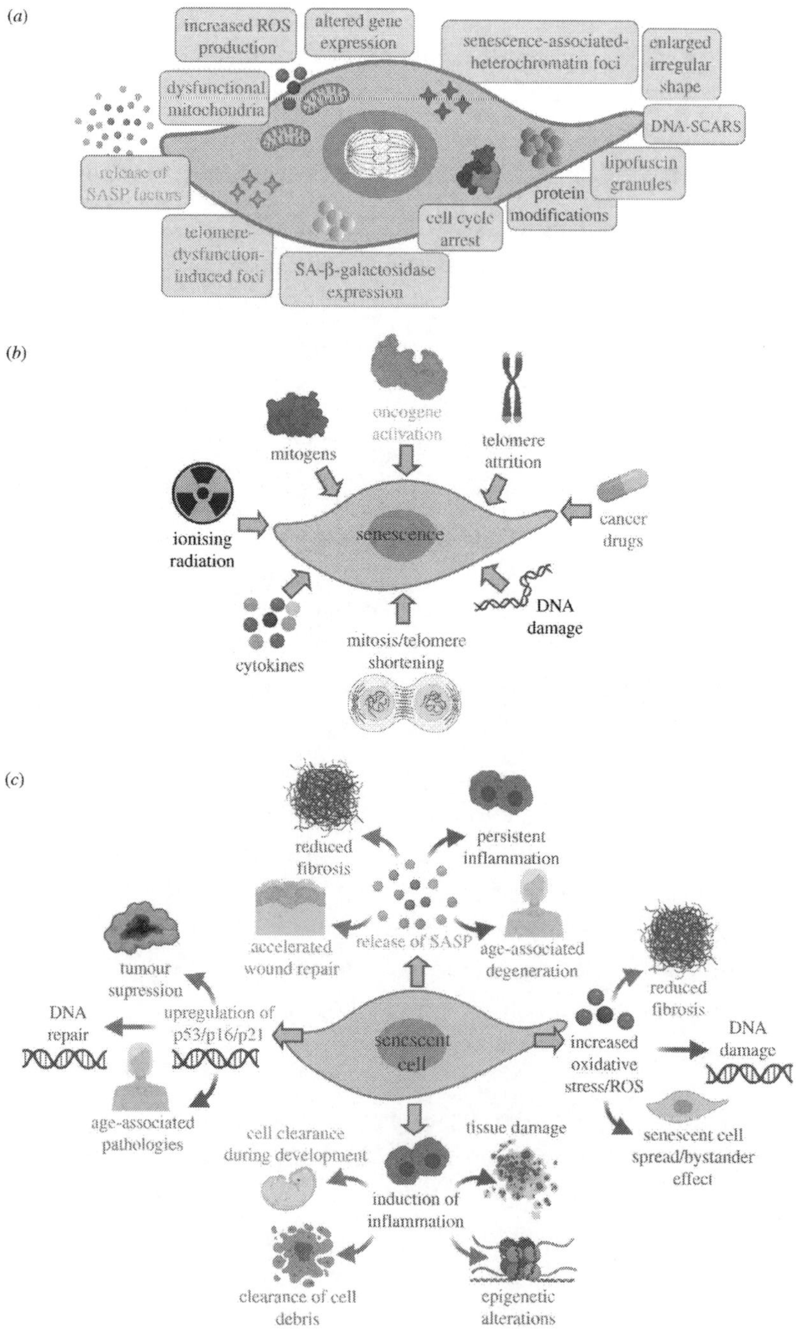

Fig. 4.11 – The body's response to senescent cells

Some senescent cells resist apoptosis, but in doing so they harm neighboring cells. As we age, the body isn't as efficient in removing dysfunctional cells, which weakens the immune system and potentially serious illness. (National Institute on Aging, July 2021)

Image courtesy of Sonia S. Elder and Elaine Emmerson published by The Royal Society, CC 4.0 via Wikimedia Commons

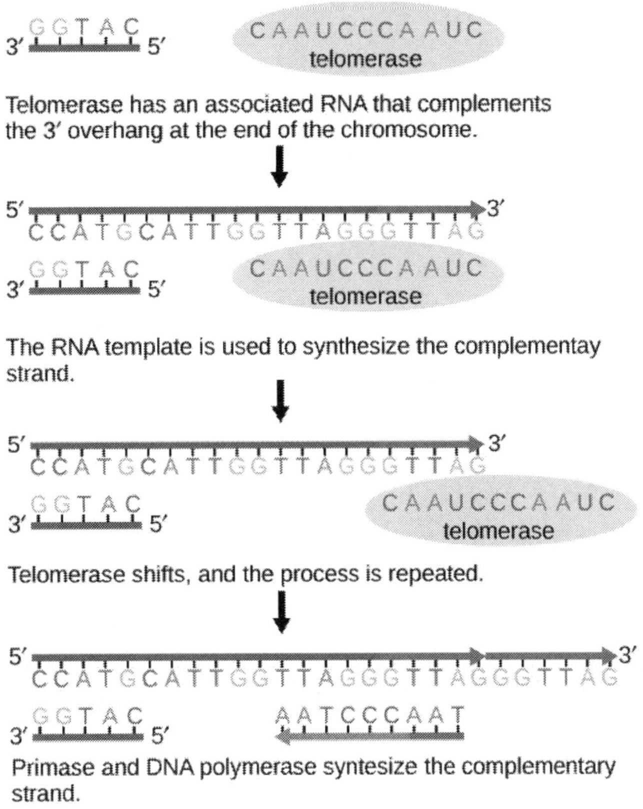

Fib. 4.12 – Series of base pairs that are copied and regulated by the enzyme telomerase.
Courtesy of National Institute of Health, Public Domain via WikiMedia Commons

Genetic information, Shay explains, "is really just a series of bases called Adenine (A), Guanine (G), Cytosine (C), and Thymine (T). These base pairs make up our cellular alphabet and create the sequences, or instructions needed to form our bodies. In order to grow and age, our bodies must duplicate their cells (mitosis)." When telomeres are too short, problems can result, but they can also become too long whereby they become fragile and also subject to problems.

Another intriguing prospect is to regrow telomeres. Marina Rossi and Myriam Gorospe report that, "Noncoding (nc)RNAs are emerging as major regulators of telomere length homeostasis." [82](Rossi and Gorospe, 2020) There is an RNA molecule known as TERRA (telomeric repeat-containing RNA), which appears to help regulate telomerase - which regulates telomere length - and chromatin remodeling during cellular development and differentiation. (Luke and Lingner, 2009) Similar to 'junk DNA', non-coding RNA was assumed to not have a role until recently when functions other than coding were becoming identified.

Mattick and Makunin report that, "Although it has been generally assumed that most genetic information is transacted by proteins, recent evidence suggests that the majority of the genomes of mammals and other complex organisms are in fact transcribed into ncRNAs many of which are alternatively spliced and/

or processed into smaller products. (Fig. 4.13)These ncRNAs include microRNAs and snoRNAs (many if not most of which remain to be identified), as well as likely other classes of yet-to-be-discovered small regulatory RNAs, and tens of thousands of longer transcripts, most of whose functions are yet unknown." [83](Mattick and Makunin, 2006)

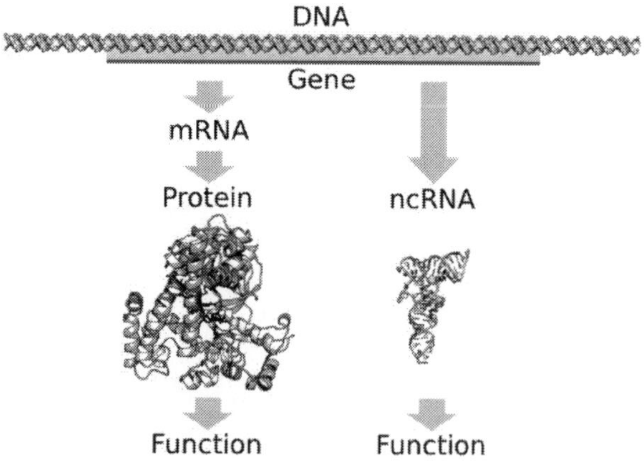

Fig. 4.13 – Example of micro RNA and non-coding RNA
Thomas Shafee CC BY 4.0 via Wikimedia Commons

Another team of researchers from Stanford University School of Medicine are looking at a different way of treating age-related diseases and genetic conditions using a modified RNA coding sequence called TERT, an active compound of telomerase. So far, they've been able to successfully lengthen telomeres by 10%, or 1,000 nucleotides. [84](Honor Whitman, 2015) Seeing that treating muscle cells with TERT produced 3 times more cell divisions than untreated cells left researchers, Ramunas and Yakubov, optimistic for the possible benefits in improving conditions like muscular dystrophy.

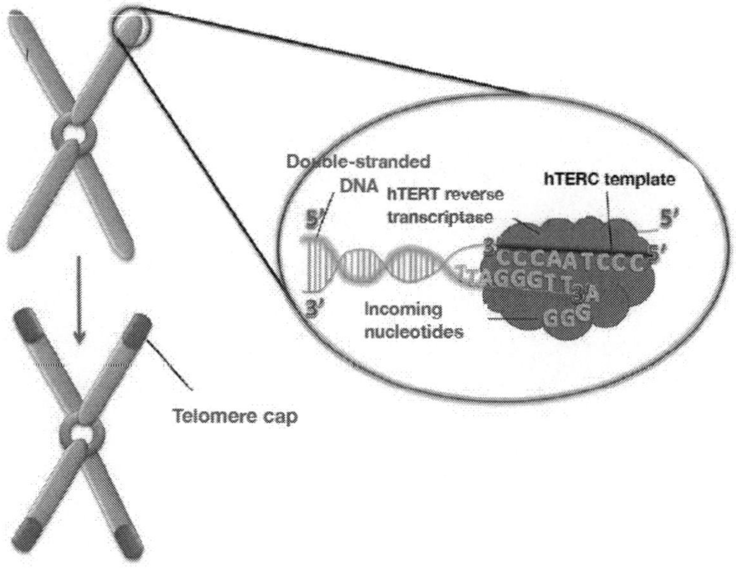

Fig. 4.14 – Example of telomere activity at the ends of chromosomes, whereby when they become too short and the senescent cell does not self-destruct, this regulation becomes unstable. Telomerase and hTERT can then become tumor promoters and act to promote the life of the cancerous cell. (Leão et al, 2018)
Image courtesy of DevelopmentalBiology CC BY-SA 3.0 via Wikimedia Commons

Frej Fyhrquist and Peter Nilsson report that although active telomerase inhibits telomere shortening in certain cells, they also inhibit it in cancer cells, facilitating proliferation. (Fig. 4.14) [85] (Fyhrquist & Nilsson, 2015) They also reported that it's possible that women have a longer life expectancy because estrogen activates telomerase and inhibits telomere shortening. These researchers are making the connection that there is likely a link between telomere function and vascular aging – a primary tissue that showed cellular decline across the board in tissue aging studies.

EXERCISE

Exercise, particularly interval training, has been shown to increase telomere length. Efficiency of eliminating waste and reduction of oxidative stress has been cited as reasons that exercise extends telomeres. (Masood A. Shammas, 2011; Samuel S. Aguiar et al., 2021) A separate study found that those who are in their 50s who have run at least 50 miles per week for 35 years have the telomeres of a 20 year-old. (Mortis, 2022)

Long distance runners showed the greatest extension of telomeres, but those who run or do moderate exercise consistently a few times per week have telomeres that look the same as marathon runners. *[86](Zoe Corbyn, 2017)*

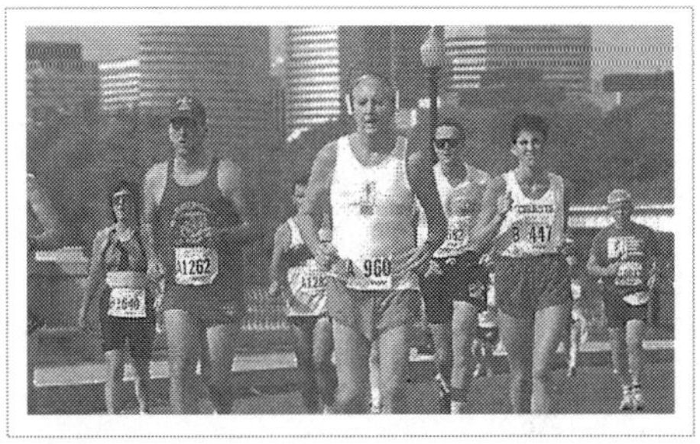

Author, Jeremy Mortis, also finds that saturated fat and processed meats can add 10-14 years to a lifespan. Although Omega 3s are consistently promoted as being healthy for the brain and other functions, he does not recommend getting them from fish. Stress is a reliable source of shorter telomeres at any age; however, early trauma has been shown to shorten telomeres more than trauma experienced as an adult. Studies show that shortened telomeres are associated with Muscular dystrophy, Type 2 diabetes, osteoporosis, cardiomyopathy, heart disease, and is a causative factor for pulmonary fibrosis.

That said, just a few minutes of meditation each day can lengthen telomeres.

Elizabeth Blackburn, a Nobel Prize winner, admits that chronic stress can be a factor, depending upon how a person relates to it, but that being sedentary is proving to be reliably worse. She reports that anything that is in general harmful for health is harmful for telomeres. A study in 2014 by the Karolinska Institute in Sweden (published in Epigenetics) showed that exercising regularly – in this case 4 times a week for 45 minutes – developed genes in the participants that were associated with insulin response, inflammation, and energy metabolism. [87](Renee Morad, 2017) Movement is proving to be the best medicine for one and all, but there are also many offerings from Mother Nature on this topic of protecting DNA and empowering epigenetics.

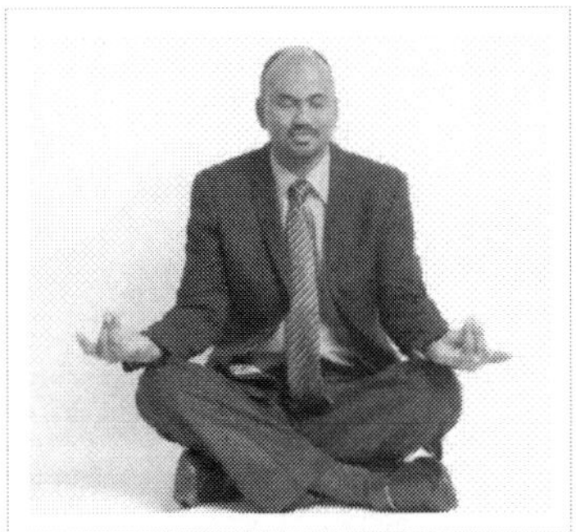

Chapter 5

Courtesy of Pixabay

Epigenetics and diet

As mentioned earlier, food is information and carries with it substances that interact with the cell nucleus. The types of food, such as junk food and certain fats that have an impact on fetal health during pregnancy, are the same ones that can alter genetic expression as an adult. From this point of view, food offers potential beyond the perspective of nutrition. Janos Zempleni, a molecular nutritionist at the University of Nebraska, is one researcher who is very excited about the possibilities of how far the diet dimension can reach in determining health outcomes. Once he discovered that certain plants we eat could potentially switch genes on and off, he redirected his path of study.

Zempleni and his team, hoping to find a way to deliver cancer drugs reliably into certain cells, began to focus on how the system takes up and delivers milk exosomes; with exosomes being used as a protective shield around the microRNAs. [88](Kristina Campbell, 2020) Without the protective shield, the miRNAs disintegrate in the gut. Lin Zhang, initially published the study in Cell Research that inspired colleagues to investigate further. She noticed that cells released from the gut's epithelial lining can secrete the microvesicles needed to protect and transport the miRNAs from food. In her study, the food was rice, and the miRNA delivered the substances at its own discretion.

Zhang states, "*Given that exogenous miRNAs in food, or miRNAs that are 'added' into the food, can enter the circulation and various organs of animals and play a role in regulating the physiological or pathophysiological conditions, food-derived exogenous miRNAs may be qualified as a novel nutrient component, like vitamins and minerals*." [89](Liz Shang, et al., 2012)

She describes microvesicles (MV) as being shed from almost all cell types under both normal and pathological conditions. *"They bear surface receptors/ligands of the original cells, and have the potential to selectively interact with specific target cells and mediate intercellular communication by transporting bioactive lipids, miRNAs, or proteins between cells,"* explains Zhang.

Methylation and DNA

> The fact that foods can alter specific mechanisms in our DNA and its communications regarding regulatory and maintenance functions is very significant.

DNA methylation has been looked at for a while for its relationship to cancer and a possible doorway for a cure. In 2017, Klecker and Nair defined methyl groups as, "highly stable, consisting of a central carbon atom bonded to three hydrogen atoms." Bailey Kirkpatrick defines methylation as, "*a well-known epigenetic mechanism characterized by the attachment of a methyl group to DNA by an enzyme called DNA methyltransferase (DNMT), which stifles gene expression*." [90](Baily Kirkpatrick, 2018)

Dr. David Jockers describes methylation as, "one of the most essential metabolic functions of the body. Methylation is a controlled transfer of a methyl group (one carbon and three hydrogen atoms) (Fig. 5.2) onto proteins, amino acids, enzymes, and DNA in every cell and tissue of the body in order to regulate healing, cell energy, genetic expression of DNA, liver detoxification, immunity, and neurology."

> Without balanced methylation, Jockers notes that the body's adaptation to life's stressors isn't adequately regulated. This imbalance can lead to dysfunction and diseases like diabetes, multiple sclerosis, chronic fatigue, cardiovascular disease, cancer, and more. *[91](Dr. David Jockers, 2022)*

Jockers lists the significant and vital biological processes involving methylation as:

- Turning genes on and off
- Processing chemicals and toxins
- Building neurotransmitters
- Building immune cells
- Synthesizing DNA and RNA
- Producing energy (i.e. CoQ10, Carnitine, and ATP)
- Producing protective coating on nerves/myelination

Methylation regulates gene expression by recruiting proteins involved in gene repression, or by inhibiting the binding of transcription factors to DNA. (Moore, 2012) During development, methylation and demethylation support differentiated cells becoming stable and unique in their DNA methylation pattern, which then regulates tissue-specific gene transcription. Lisa Moore explains that, as far as its function in the nervous system goes, if this process is altered with environmental risk factors during pregnancy, "such as drug exposure or neural injury, mental impairment is a common side effect." [92](Lisa Moore, et al., 2013)

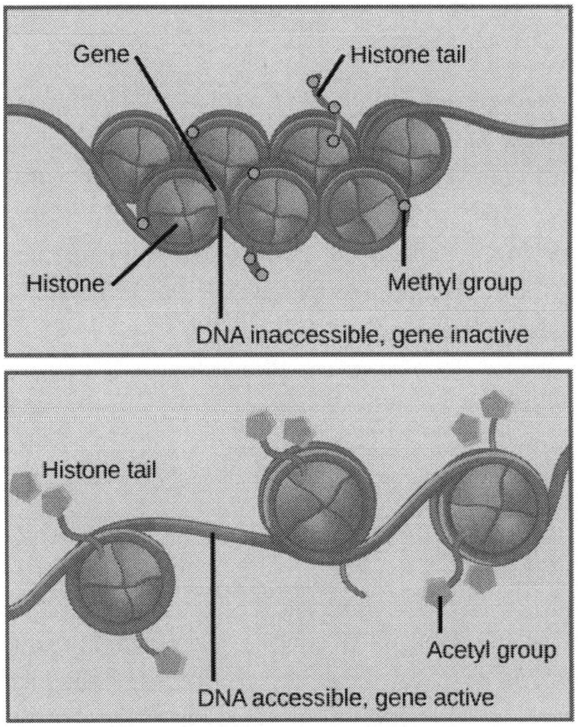

Methylation of DNA and histones causes nucleosomes to pack tightly together. Transcription factors cannot bind the DNA, and genes are not expressed.

Histone acetylation results in loose packing of nucleosomes. Transcription factors can bind the DNA and genes are expressed.

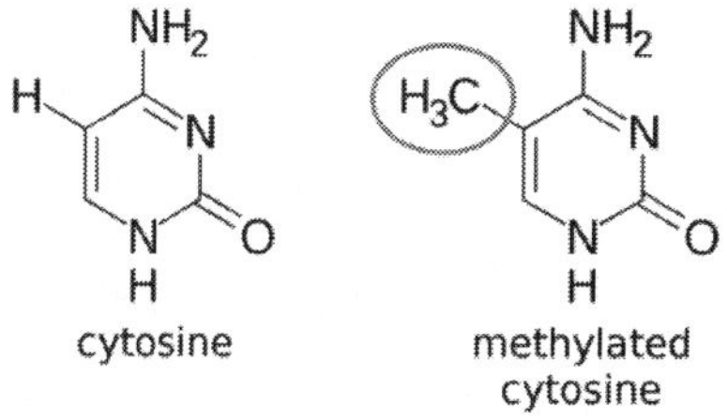

Fig. 5.2 – Methylation: the transfer of one carbon and 3 hydrogen atoms onto a protein

Fig. 5.1 – Illustration of genes being suppressed or expressed based upon the wrapping of the histones

Courtesy of CNX OpenStax CC BY 4.0 via Wikimedia Commons

Moore and others have reported that the DNA being wrapped around histone proteins very tightly can limit the expression of a gene. (Fig. 5.1) What remains to be clarified, are the conditions under which DNA methylation silences gene expression, and when it helps promote expression; when it is inherently tissue-specific, and when it is not. She goes on to say that, *"Although methyl groups have low reactivity, they still impart a sizable influence on their surroundings, thereby affecting cellular functions."*

Superoxide Dismutase and cell protection

There are ways to protect the cells from damage; to support the body's own mechanisms for maintenance, balance, and repair. Nutritionist Alex Swanson has found that longer life is often related to reduction of oxidative stress in the mitochondrial DNA. His approach to protecting the mitochondria has a few steps. One is to support the function of Superoxide Dismutase 1 and 3, which "*is an **enzyme** that protects cells from increased oxidative stress and free radical damage to cell structures like membranes, mitochondria, DNA, and proteins. SOD1 is located in the cytoplasm, binds copper and zinc, and is one of two isozymes responsible for destroying free superoxide radicals in the body. If you have a mutation in SOD1 or SOD3, make sure you're getting enough zinc and copper.*"

Dietitian Toby Amidor explains that copper "*helps make energy, connective tissue, and blood vessels. It also helps maintain the nervous system and activates genes.*" He added that it would be rare to find a copper deficiency in this country since it is freely available in many common foods like cashews, oysters, chick peas, dark chocolate, and potatoes unless one had a mutation in the Superoxide Dismutase family, or those with celiac or Menkes disease. [93](Toby Amidor, 2020)

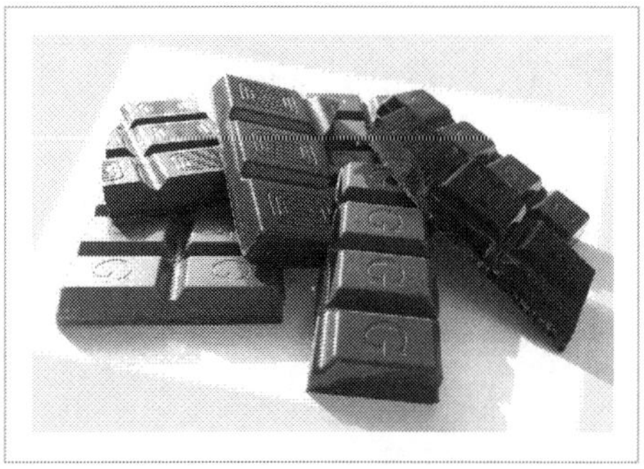

Swanson goes on to say that the mushroom **Cordyceps** may improve the activity of SOD in red blood cells, brain, and liver, and that foods with manganese, folate, and those packed with flavonoids could also protect the inside of the cell from oxidative damage. This researcher is focused on certain genotypes who may have inherited weaknesses or mutations that led them to needing supplementation to avoid the diseases that follow deficiencies. Nonetheless, including foods that support the health of the cell is a good idea. Swanson states,

"When your cell membranes and mitochondria are strong, it is difficult for viruses, bacteria, toxins, mold and chemicals to create disease."

Fats and the cell membrane

Swanson recommends dietary cholesterol to support the cell membrane's balance, permeability and fluidity; polyphenolic fruits and vegetables, choline to inhibit the binding of calcium to the arterial walls, vitamin E to decrease vascular lesions even when cholesterol levels are high, and the avoidance of fried foods, sugar, and vegetable oils. [94](Alex Swanson, MS, 2015)

Dr. Aaron Ernst reports that, *"Cholesterol adds rigidity but maintains flexibility. Glycolipids are also found in your membranes – acting like hair-like projections to allow for sensation and communication as well as stability of the membrane. (Fig 5.3) Sterols are also found in the membrane - waxy-like molecules that again help with the stability and communication within the cell membrane.*

The Standard American diet is essentially devoid of healthy phospholipids, cholesterol, glycolipids and sterols." Ernst emphasizes that the cell membrane is made up of fats, so whatever fats we eat becomes the cell membrane.

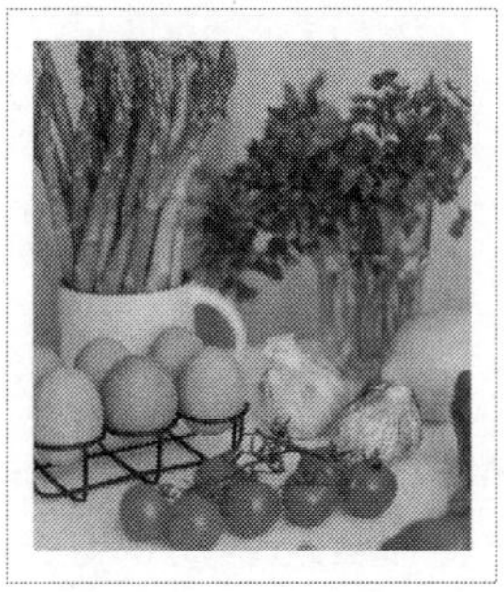

Toxins are attracted to fatty tissues and are fat soluble, so being exposed to, or ingesting toxins while eating harmful (trans) fats will wind up damaging the cell membrane. Not only will the downstream cascade of signaling be compromised, but the cell's ability to release the toxins will be also. He lists organic, pasture-raised eggs and the liver of grass-fed, pasture-raised animals as the best source of phospholipids, or high quality supplementation of Phosphatidylcholine, Phosphatidylinositol, or Phosphatidylethanolamine. [95] (Dr. Aaron Ernst, 2019)

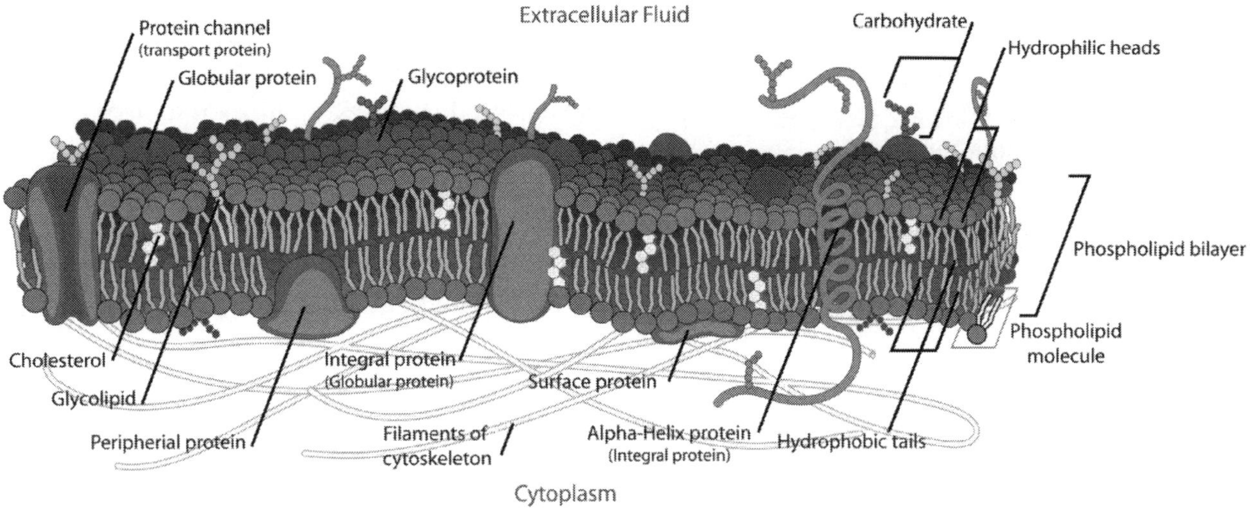

Fig. 5.3 - The principle components of the plasma membrane are lipids (phospholipids ad cholesterol), proteins, and carbohydrate groups that are attached to some of the lipids and proteins (integral and peripheral). A phospholipid is a lipid made up of glycerol, two fatty acid tails, and a phosphate-linked head group. Cholesterol is found alongside phospholipids in the core of the membrane. Proteins account for about 50% by mass, lipids 40%, and carbohydrates (on the outer surface attaching to proteins to form glycoproteins or lipids to form glycolipids), represent about 10%. (Khan Academy, "Structure of the plasma membrane"

Image courtesy of LadyofHats Public domain via Wikimedia Commons

THE IMPORTANCE OF ENZYMES

Paula Rothstein of Ann Arbor Holistic Health states that, "You are what you can digest." Her emphasis is on the need to either consume a largely raw diet for longevity, or to add digestive enzymes to every meal. She reports that undigested or partially digested cooked or processed foods can remain in the intestines for months, wreaking havoc on the body.

Rothstein went on to say, "***Enzymes** are energy catalysts that are essential to the successful occurrence of over 150,000 biochemical reactions in our bodies, particularly involving food digestion and the delivery of nutrients to the body. Enzymes help convert food into chemical substances that pass into cell membranes to perform all of our everyday life-sustaining functions... It is estimated that 80% of diseases start in the intestinal tract.*" (Paula Rothstein, "Enzymes: A Dead Diet's Necessary Companion,")

Ornsbee is an Associate Professor in the Dept. of Nutrition, Food, and Exercise Sciences and Interim Director of the Institute of Sports Sciences and Medicine at Florida State Univ. He differentiates types of fat in terms of their impact upon the cell membrane. He states, "*Saturated fats and trans fats are much more rigid than unsaturated fats, and they cause membranes to be much more rigid than is optimal, potentially limiting the functionality of the cells.*" [96](Michael Ornsbee, PhD, 2020)

An erroneous popular belief, according to these researchers, is that digestive enzymes remain in the stomach. When traced with radioactive dye, they were actually located in the liver, spleen, kidneys, heart, and other vital organs. They serve many functions around the system, including breaking down and carrying away toxins and microbes, delivering nutrients and hormones, supporting immune function, purifying the blood, and balancing cholesterol and triglyceride levels to name a few. (Rothstein, 2022) Rothstein believes that the body's enzymes are only meant to digest a portion of the food we eat, and the enzymes inherent in food in its raw state are designed to digest the rest. Cooking food destroys most of these inherent enzymes in food, thereby straining and draining the body's resources when the digestive demand is 100%.

> Michael Ornsbee, PhD, posits that, *"The foods you eat have a major influence on your cellular function because they ultimately become your cells."*

FATTY ACIDS AND OMEGA 7

The body requires fatty acids for good health. Gęgotek et al. found that **Sea Buckthorn** (*Hippophae rhamnoides L.*) oil was able to enhance the level of phospholipid and free fatty acids in skin cells, as well as enhance anti-oxidant activity. (Agnieszka Gęgotek, et al., 2018) The Omega 7 oil found in Sea Buckthorn was also shown to increase telomerase activity and speed wound and tissue healing for those suffering from burn injuries and treated with skin grafts, which is a significant finding. (Yosuke Niimi et al., 2021) Omega 7 is a monounsaturated fatty acid (MUFA), meaning that it has just one unsaturated carbon bond in the molecule. Other monounsaturated fats include olive oil, peanut, safflower and sesame oils. Palmitoleic acid is a long chain fatty acid belonging to the Omega 7 group and is reported to provide benefits for the arteries, cholesterol levels, and blood sugar.

Omega 7 is not an essential fatty acid since it is produced in the body, but adding it rather than saturated fats into the diet would be beneficial. Macadamia nut oil and avocado oil are other sources of this nutrient, along with salmon, herring, and mackerel. It also provides anti-inflammatory benefits as well as cellular rejuvenation for the skin. Maria Dudau reports that Sea Buckthorn seed oil has protective qualities against the potential damage from the sun's UV rays (Dudau et al., 2021) Beata Olas expressed that the seeds, berries, leaves and bark of the Sea Buckthorn oil all have medicinal properties. Much of the benefits come from the unsaturated fatty acids, phytosterols, vitamins A and E. (Beata Olas, 2017)

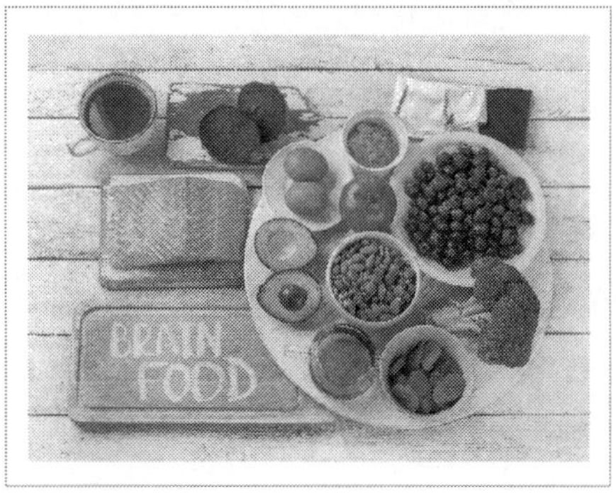

Other unsaturated fatty acids have extensive benefits as well. For example, oleic acid helps to reduce blood pressure, docosahexaenoic acid (DHA), and eicosapentaenoic acid (EPA) help to prevent cardiovascular diseases and cancer, [97](Alisa Zapp Machalek, 2013) while omega 3 fatty acids show measurable changes in cell membrane content within days in tissues like the retina, brain, and myocardium. [98](Marc E. Surette, PhD, 2008)

Surette clarifies in his article, "The science behind dietary omega-3 fatty acids," that any other source than fish or fish oils, such as the α-linoleic acid from plants, is not well absorbed by the body and they do not produce the biological activity that omega 3's from fish do.

Surette goes on to say that certain cellular changes are activated by omega 3 fatty acids. Some changes include signaling between all the cells in the body, (including those involved with gene expression) while supporting the function of membrane-associated proteins that are in direct contact with the lipid bilayer. Apparently the Western diet in general has far less than the recommended daily intake of this essential nutrient that the body cannot produce on its own. Tuna, salmon, and cod are good sources, but since two servings per day would be needed to achieve the desired levels the body needs, taking supplements is usually advised.

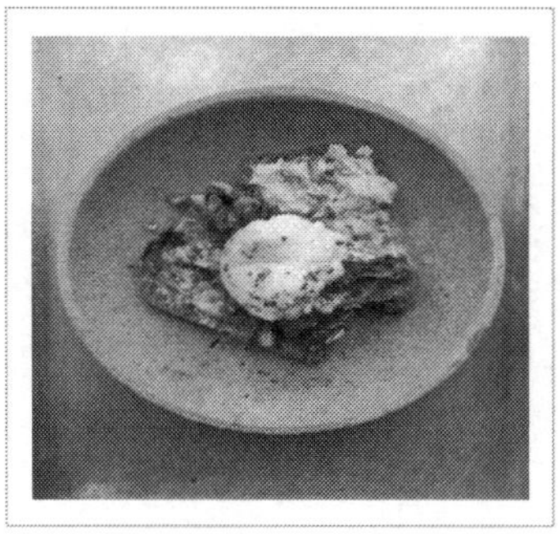

As far as cellular communication and regulation are concerned, mono and polyunsaturated fats and fatty acids are better for the cell membrane than saturated fats. Dr. Wei Min, in her research in 2017 (in cooperation with the NIH Biomedical Imaging and Biomedical Engineering) that compared the two, her team noticed that saturated fat created stiff areas in the cell's endoplasmic reticulum (ER). According to Min, the ER is a *"large, complex structure that makes and transports substances the cell needs. The behavior of saturated fatty acids once they've entered cells contributes to major and often deadly diseases."*

That being said, a diet consisting mainly of polyunsaturated fats will make cell membranes too loose, which is also not good. Dr. Mark Heisig recommends include one-third each of saturated, polyunsaturated, and monounsaturated to achieve the perfect balance. (Heisig, 2019) The brain is about 60% fats, some of which is saturated. Similar to the conflicting evidence around the polyunsaturated canola oil, there is also conflicting evidence on the benefits of coconut oil and other saturated fats as they have a tendency to raise LDL cholesterol.

The main concerns related to canola oil are that it is often a genetically modified plant, and that the heating, bleaching, and deodorizing process destroys the Omega 3's and transforms a portion of the oil into a trans fat. According to Dr. Crosby, unless it is a virgin, cold-pressed oil, they are all processed in this way and will have a percentage of trans fats. *[99](Dr. Guy Crosby, 2022)*

Soybean oil, which is prevalent in salad dressings, has the highest amount of trans fats after processing. Another concern about canola oil is that it contains a high amount of Omega 6, which can be inflammatory when not in balance with Omega 3. It has also been shown in some studies to impair memory. The concern about saturated fat is only valid when looking at numbers on a chart as opposed to actual health outcomes. A study of 458 men with a diet higher in saturated fat that produced higher LDL levels had a lower incidence of heart disease, coronary artery disease and death than those on a diet higher in unsaturated fats. [100](Jillian Kubala, MS, 2019) Corroborating research suggests that people with diets higher in saturated fats live longer. Autopsies show that those with the highest cholesterol are not necessarily the ones with the most heart disease. Studies also show that those who included saturated fat in their diets reduced their rates of dementia by 36%. (Dr. Gregory Jantz, 2016) This issue has not been revisited for decades, in terms of the established recommended numbers for cholesterol levels.

Traditional Native Alaskans were found to have a diet 'remarkably high in fat', but the sources were mainly from fish. This group of over 500 Yup'ik Eskimos had a much lower incidence of heart disease and chronic diseases in general. (Andrea Bersamin, PhD, et al., 2019) Those from the same region who transitioned to a more Western diet began experiencing similar incidences of chronic disease and obesity. In fact, of all the instances where artherosclerosis and heart disease were potential outcomes of life behaviors or diet, looking at it from a cellular communication perspective, high cholesterol was not mentioned as a factor in any of the studies mentioned here.

Looking at fats as a crucial component of epigenetics, it would be helpful to understand how they are involved in the flow of communication and what might interfere with it. From this perspective, experts point out that fats and fatty acids are an integral part of the microbiome, a huge regulator of inflammation, and are intimately connected to the brain. Because the standard American diet is rife with inflammatory triggers, this is a vital part of restoring health.

Dietitian, Judith Thalheimer, RD, reports that all oils have a few different types of fatty acids, which are classified by the length of their carbon chains. For example, the gut ferments fiber to produce short chain fatty acids (SCFA), which have less than 6 carbons. SCFA act as anti-inflammatories, play a key role in neuro-immune modulation, and are suspected to be involved in the gut-brain axis crosstalk. The three types of SCFA are butyrate, propionate, and acetate. Butter has a small amount of butyrate, and apple cider vinegar is a good source of acetate. Propionate forms when carbohydrates are broken down by bacteria. It has the potential to reduce cholesterol and fat storage, as well as acting as an anti-cancer and anti-inflammatory agent.

Coconut is a source of medium chain fatty acids, which is why MCT oil from coconut oil has become so popular. Medium chain triglycerides also have a long list of health benefits, including anti-fungal and anti-inflammatory properties, improved cognition, weight loss, and more. Long chain fatty acids have 14 or more carbons and are in most oils. Their benefits vary according to the balance of the Omega 3-6-9 ratios in them, but in general, most oils that have long chain fatty acids have many benefits.

Arachidonic acid, or Omega 6, is only helpful in smaller amounts. (Elizabeth Brown, 2018) It's worth repeating, that most vegetable oils are imbalanced in the direction of Omega 6, and after processing, may possess trans fats. Cold-pressed, organic, virgin oils are going to be the safest choice for the cell membrane, and optimum cellular communication. Olive, avocado, sesame, safflower, and walnut oils are the most stable at high temperatures. (L. Panoff, 2021)

Saturated fats have no double bonds. Sources of monounsaturated fats — which have one double bond — include olive, peanut and avocado oils, almonds, hazelnuts, and pecans, pumpkin and sesame seeds.

Polyunsaturated fats — which have more than one double bond — can be found in sunflower, flax, and walnut oils, as well as in fish. (Harvard School of Public Health, 2022) The Omega 3s found in fish are more readily used by the body, but because it would be difficult to eat enough on a regular basis to fulfill the body's needs, it's good to supplement. Studies continue to produce new findings and the key, as usual, seems to be finding what works best for your system that helps keep it in balance.

THE ROLE AND BENEFITS OF BROWN FAT

The body has three types of fat – all very different from what we consume — each with a different function. The most prevalent is white fat, which is under the skin, around the organs, and in bone cavities. It stores energy, secretes hormones, and serves as insulation. Beige or pink fat is in and around white fat. It burns calories and at times generates heat. Brown fat is the type that babies have that generates a lot of heat and energy. (Dr. Anna Hernandez, Osmosis, November 2020)

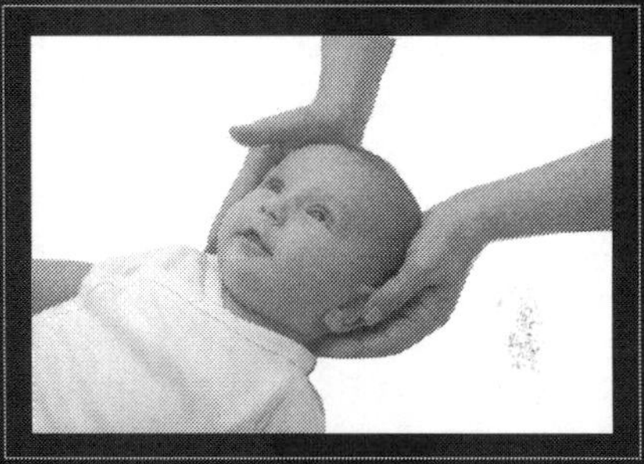

The fat's color is dependent upon the levels of blood and iron-containing mitochondria. (Bailey, 2019) The biggest danger to adipose tissue functioning correctly is obesity, in which case it becomes inflammatory and dysfunctional. (Alan Chait and Laura J. den Hartigh, 2020) Injuries or blunt trauma can also damage adipose tissue, resulting in a cyst or necrotic tissue that forms a hard lump of dead cells, but isn't harmful. A small percentage of breast lesions are necrotic tissue that may be a little frightening. (Rachel Nall, 2017)

A study done in 2009, involving 50,000 patients concluded that the people with the most brown fat had the least prevalence of chronic disease - particularly hypertension, type 2 diabetes, and coronary artery disease.

Exposure to cold increases brown fat. (Haridy, 2021) According to Regina Bailey, in her 2019 article on, *"The Purpose and Composition of Adipose Tissue," "Adipose tissue acts as an endocrine system organ by generating hormones that influence metabolic activity in other organ systems. Some of the hormones produced by adipose cells influence sex hormone metabolism, blood pressure regulation, insulin sensitivity, fat storage and use, blood clotting, and cell signaling."* [101](Bailey, 2019) She goes on to describe adiponectin, one of the hormones produced by fat tissue, *"which acts on the brain to increase metabolism, promote the breakdown of fat, and increase energy use in the muscles without affecting appetite."*

The main perspective presented in this text that has a bias, is the one that encourages you to discover how to enhance cellular communication, and to understand what disrupts it, because every experience will be deeply processed at the macro and micro level. Every experience will contribute to your overall health and quality of life.

Leaning into the behaviors that support optimum flow of information throughout the system, and limiting the ones that restrict, alter, or damage the structures responsible for that flow is the understanding and awareness I hope to cultivate with the information provided here.

FOOD AS MEDICINE FOR CANCER

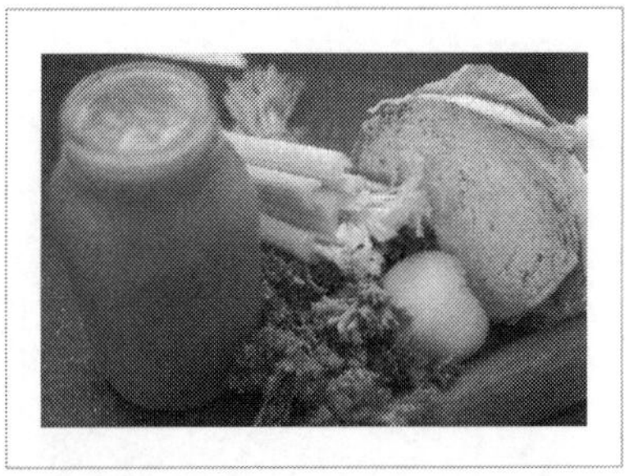

It is difficult to look for alterations and disruptions to cellular communication without turning up scores of articles reporting cancer as an outcome. Since it's become such a widespread issue, there are also scores of researchers trying to find answers. Some researchers have found helpful information for us. Nishat Fatima and her team concur that, *"Flavonoids are naturally occurring phenol compounds which are abundantly found among phytochemicals and have potentials to modulate epigenetic processes. Knowledge of the precise flavonoid-mediated epigenetic alterations is needed for the development of epigenetics drugs and combinatorial therapeutic approaches against cancers."* [103](Nishat Fatima et al., 2021)

Bailey Kirkpatrick mentioned in her article on the subject, that *"plant flavones have been connected to (helpful) changes in DNA methylation across the whole genome and on particular genes."* Kirkpatrick includes blueberry juice and vitamin C to potentially inhibit methylation issues for the MTHFR and DNMT1 gene in humans. [102](Bailey Kirkpatrick, 2018)

FLAVONOIDS ARE THE SUPERHEROES FOR THE CELLS

Nishat Fatima explains that there are several subgroupings of flavonoids which may have slightly different effects on the cell. A few of them that you may have already heard of include **flavanols, flavones, isoflavones**, and **anthocyanidins.** They are found in a variety of foods like fruits, vegetables, nuts, some grains, dark chocolate, and many types of tea, (flavan-3-ols) as well as coffee. **Citrus** contains flavanones, which are anti-inflammatories. This is also a property of flavones, which are found in foods like parsley, celery, chamomile and peppermint. Isoflavones are mainly in soy products, whereas anthocyanins that are responsible for the rich color in red and purple foods, and can be found in strawberries, blackberries, or red and purple grapes, for example. (Watson, Healthline, October, 2019)

Flavonoids have health benefits that are analgesic, antioxidant, antibacterial, antiviral, hepatoprotective, apoptotic, cytostatic, anti-allergic, and hormone balancing. (Kumar and Pandey, 2013) They can also promote the enzymatic activity of detoxifying cells, and stimulate the activity of tumor suppressing genes. The **catechin** type of flavonoid found in green tea (EGCG) mentioned earlier, is well established for its anti-proliferative, anti-angiogenic, pro-apoptotic and anti-invasive properties. (Singh et al., 2011)

EGCG (Epigallocatechin Gallate) has been studied specifically in its roles of inducing prostate cancer cell death (Lee et al., 2012), promoting tumor suppression and apoptosis in breast cancer cells (Lubecka et al., 2018), and suppressing metastasis in hepatocellular carcinoma (Kang et al., 2021) The specificity with which EGCG influences methylation and histone acetylation hasn't been spelled out here, but rest

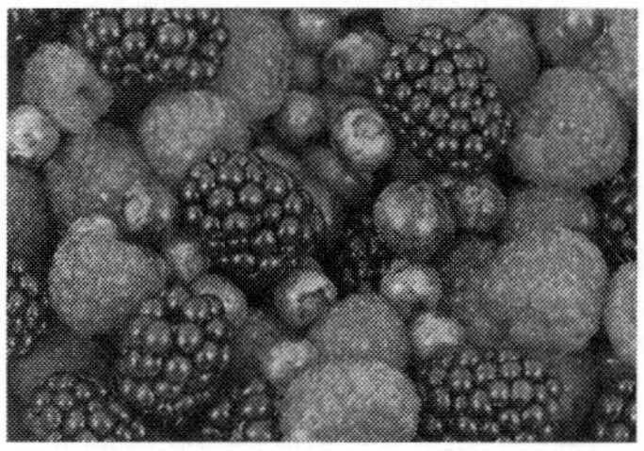

assured that when there's a claim that foods can help sustain and regain health, the levels that they can operate on are deeply targeted and therapeutically specific biochemically.

Nishat Fatima claims most biologists agree that mutations in the replication of DNA are inevitable as the body ages, whether it be a spontaneous error or caused by environmental and lifestyle exposures. Nevertheless, she believes that 10% or less of the cases of cancer that evolve are hereditary. She cites the stats for 2020 as being over 19 million cancer cases, of which 10 million died, which is a drop by 30% from 2018. Fatima admits that in either case — nature or nurture — particularly if in the early stages of mutation, cancer is reversible.

Kaempferol is a flavonoid and phytoestrogen that we don't hear too much about under the flavanol subcategory. It interferes with several signaling pathways required for the survival of breast cancer cells, along with ovarian, gastric, lung, pancreatic, and blood cancers. It also stimulates apoptosis in glioma cells. (M. Shields, 2017) It can also promote apoptosis for pancreatic cancer cells, but also has anti-metastatic properties by downregulating VEGF, thereby limiting blood supply to those cells. Some say that the higher your intake of these types of polyphenols is in your diet, the lower your chances are of contracting cancer. [104](Brian Bender, PhD, 2018)

Brian Bender lists the top 10 vegetables highest in kaempferol as being

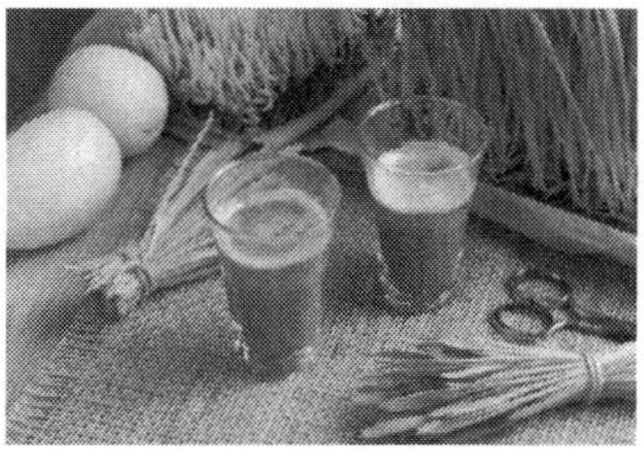

1. Watercress
2. Mustard greens
3. Arugula
4. New Zealand spinach
5. Kale
6. Endives
7. Radish seeds
8. Dock
9. Garden cress
10. Turnip greens

The top 10 fruits with the most kaempferol include

1. Blueberries
2. Gooseberries
3. Watermelon
4. Kiwi
5. Strawberries
6. Apricots
7. Elderberries
8. Blackberries
9. Peaches
10. Cherries

Although plentiful in a variety of foods, kaempferol has very low bioavailability, as does quercetin**.** (DuPont, et al., 2004, Dabeek and Marra, 2019) Promising research is underway to coat the outer layer of injected kaempferol with nanoparticles that prevent its degradation in the liver so it can be used effectively as a cancer treatment. (Chen, 2013) **Quercetin** is also a flavonol and has gained popularity recently as a preventative measure for COVID-19. It has proven to act as a tumor suppressor by down-regulating certain methylation concentrations and modulating the expression of chromatin (material that chromosomes are made of containing RNA and DNA) modifiers in cervical cancer. It also promotes apoptosis and non-proliferation in pancreatic cancer cells. Quercetin is a prebiotic, feeding the friendly

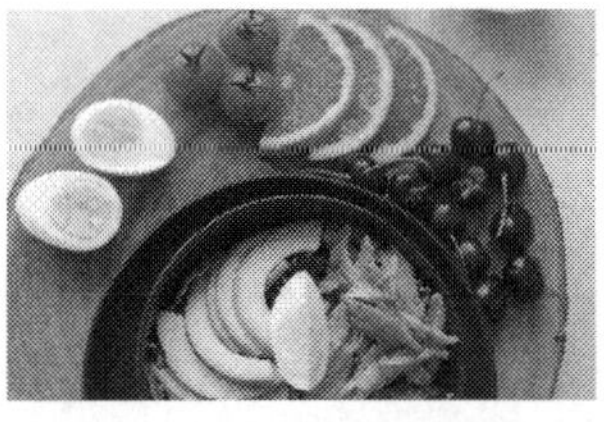

bacteria in the gut, which lends itself to immune support. It also acts as transport for zinc getting into the cells, which inhibits viral replication.

Quercetin can be found in high concentrations in capers and red onions, and also in shallots, red apples, grapes, berries, cherries, scallions, kale, organic tomatoes, broccoli, Brussel sprouts, cabbage, citrus, asparagus, almonds, pistachios, black and green tea, green and yellow bell peppers, and buckwheat. (Lindsay Boyers, 2021) Myricetin is a seldom spoken of flavonoid that, along with being an anti-inflammatory, antioxidant, and antimicrobial, is also neuroprotective. There are additional properties that have been studied regarding its potential to perform in antidiabetic, immunomodulatory, cardiovascular, anti-hypertensive, and anti-cancer roles. (Yasaman Taheri et al., 2020) Like the other flavonols, myricetin can be found in tea leaves, berries, onions, and several vegetables. **Fisetin**, mentioned earlier in the text, is also a flavonol.

Luteolin is a flavonoid that has been studied for its potential benefits in neuropsychiatric and neurodegenerative conditions. Although flavonoids are plentiful in fruits and vegetables, they are frequently not absorbed beyond 10% and quite a bit more than that is needed for optimum benefits to be realized. Luteolin has anti-inflammatory and anti-oxidant properties that serve the function of the microglia surrounding the nerve cells, but also inhibits auto-immune cell activation and stimulates apoptosis of damaged cells. (Theoharides, 2015)

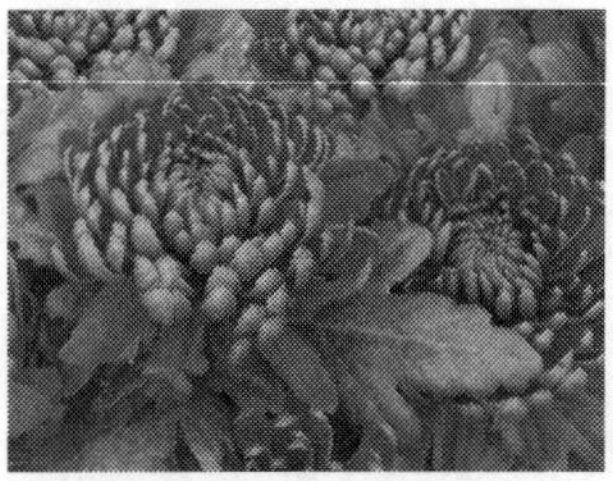
Chrysanthemum

It can also protect against cancer by inhibiting invasion, metastasis, and angiogenesis (formation of new blood vessels) by inhibiting kinases, reducing transcription factors, suppressing cell survival pathways, regulating cell cycles, and inducing apoptosis. (Yong Lin et al., 2008) Celery, parsley, broccoli, onion leaves, carrots, peppers, cabbages, apple skins, and **chrysanthemum** flowers are rich in **luteolin**. It has been used traditionally in Chinese medicine for several diseases, and is particularly useful in the neuroprotective capacity because it can pass through the blood-brain barrier. **Curcumin**, one of the powerful 243 compounds in turmeric, has been used for centuries in Ayurvedic medicine. It was studied extensively more recently in the West regarding its effectiveness in combating inflammation, oxidation, and cancer, among other things. Hassan describes some of the many interactions of curcumin like this: "Curcumin may also act as an epigenetic regulator in neurological disorders, inflammation, and diabetes. Moreover, curcumin can induce the modification of histones (acetylation/deacetylation), which are among the most important genetic changes responsible for altered expression of genes leading to modulating the risks of cancers." (Hassan, 2019)

Hyper and hypo-acetylation have both been found in cancer cells. Curcumin is active in the inhibition of DNMTs (DNA methyltransferaces), regulating and modifying histone acetyltransferases, regulating miRNAs, and in binding transcription factors to DNA. Curcumin has been found to regulate several important signaling pathways that modulate cell survival, govern anti-oxidant properties, inhibit cancer cell proliferation, and induce apoptosis via caspase activation. [105](Faiz-ul Hassan et al., 2019) A few of the cancers this polyphenol has been shown to influence in a beneficial way through a variety of strategies include prostate, leukemia, pancreatic, bladder, and lung cancers.

Even though ingesting turmeric (more absorbable with bioperine/pepper) can help prevent cancer, curcumin also helps cancer patients during chemotherapy by disarming the avenues of resistance and by turning on the pathways that activate inherent tumor repressor genes like P53. Curcumin can also help with insulin sensitivity, arthritis, wound healing, circulation, and immune function. It is also nutritious, containing iron, manganese, B6, fiber, copper, and potassium. (Times of India, August, 2019)

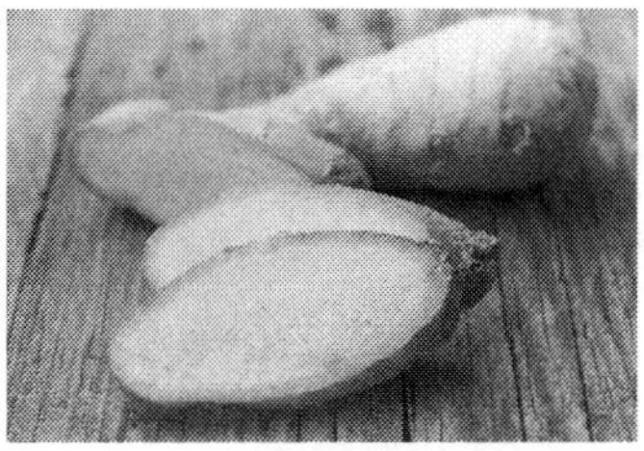

Ginger

Tumeric is in the ginger family, both belonging to the Zingiberaceae family and coming from the rhizome, or root of the plant. Some have found ginger to have well over 400 compounds, and it has been cultivated for millennia for its medicinal benefits. Along with tulsi, turmeric, and cinnamon, ginger is able to impact the chromatin (contents) in a cell's nucleus and regulate epigenetic mechanisms, particularly histone 3 acetylation. (What is Epigenetics, May 2, 2017)

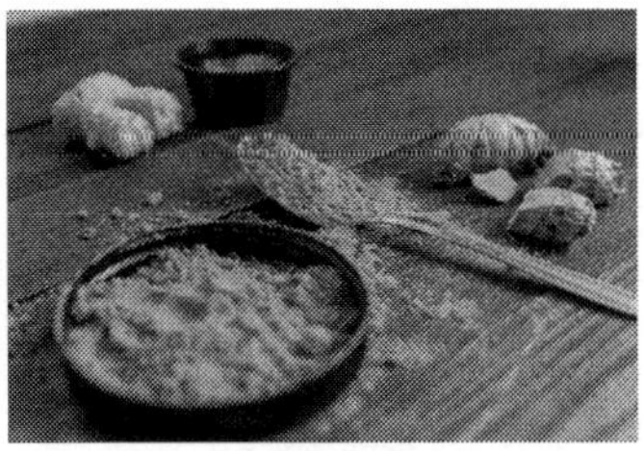

Turmeric

Apparently **ginger** can affect the way thousands of genes are expressed as well as facilitate their ability to be expressed by relaxing the tightly knit structure of the histone so that the transcription process of copying a strand of DNA onto RNA is made easier. It's been known for its gastrointestinal and anti-inflammatory benefits, and is recently being studied more thoroughly for its ability to shrink tumors.

The bioactive ingredient in cinnamon has also been found to suppress a tumor's growth, ability to migrate and invade tissue, as well as in some cases stimulate autophagic cell death. *(Tae Woo Kim, 2021)*

PHENOLIC ACIDS AND GENE MODULATION

Phenolic acids, such as cinnamic, coumaric, ferulic, caffeic, chlogenic, and rosmarinic acids have very powerful therapeutic benefits. They are usually included in the compounds of quinic, shikimic and tartaric acid in foods that have been frozen, sterilized, or fermented. [106](Angeles Carlos-Reyes et al., 2019) Carlos-Reyes and his team intended to discuss "*the mechanism by which these natural compounds modulate gene expression at the epigenetic level and describe their molecular targets in diverse types of cancer. Changes in DNA sequence are caused by mutations, amplifications, or deletions...but also by modifications of chromatin with no alterations in DNA sequence.*" He goes on to express that many compounds found in fruits and vegetables due to the phytochemicals that can regulate the expression of oncogenes and tumor suppressor genes.

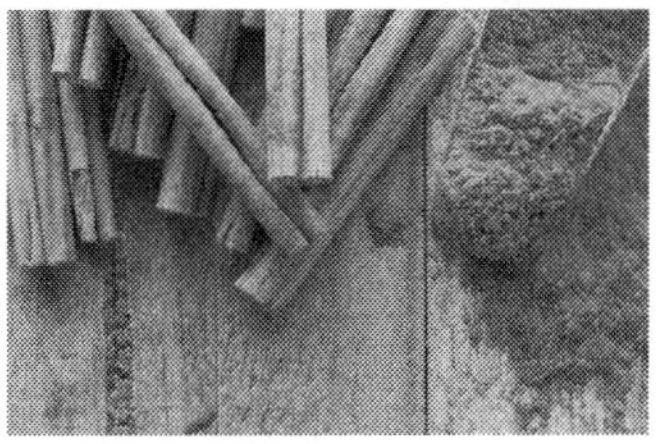

Cinnamon

Phenolic acids can be found in just about every food group, like whole grains, seeds and oils from seeds, herbs, herbal beverages, red wine, fruits and vegetables. (Anoma Chandrasekara, 2019) They often also have anti-oxidant, anti-viral, anti-inflammatory, and antimicrobial properties. They are the major components of most berries, mainly in benzoic and cinnamic acid derivatives. (P. Padmanaban, 2016) For example:

Cinnamic acid derivatives include (Hüseyin Boz, 2015; MedicineNet, 2021;):

- P-coumaric acid: barley, wheat, oat, corn, panax ginseng, carrots, and tomatoes
- Caffeic acid: coffee, wine, apples, artichoke, berries, and pears
- Ferulic acid: marjoram, blueberries, oats, fresh dates, hard wheat, dark chocolate
- Chlorogenic acid: coffee, prunes, tomatoes, eggplant, tea, apples, blueberries

Benzoic acid (excess can irritate the belly) derivatives include (Zeece, 2020, Oaks, 2012):

- P-hydroxybenzoic acid: cranberries, blackberries, prunes, cinnamon, cloves
- Salicylic acid: apricots, cantaloupe, guava, raisins, avocado, red grapes, alfalfa, broccoli, sweet potato, almonds, cucumber, pine nuts, pistachios, olives, green pepper, cumin, paprika, turmeric, dill, oregano rosemary, thyme (grace ibay, 2013)
- Gallic acid: blueberries, walnuts, flax seeds, apples, watercress, strawberries, tea, herbs, pomegranates, witch hazel, onions
- Ellagic acid: strawberries, raspberries, blackberries, pomegranate, walnuts, pecans

ANTI-CANCER FOODS AND COMPOUNDS

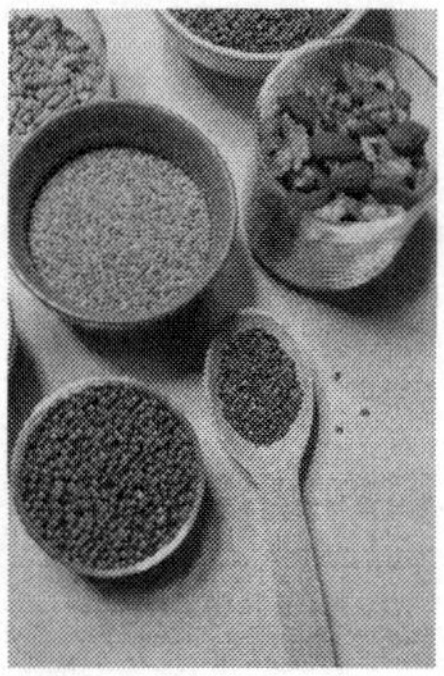

There are other food categories being studied for the anti-cancer properties, such as lignans (i.e. flax seeds) and sulforaphanes (i.e. cruciferous veggies, radish, mustard). The medicine cabinet in our kitchens can help protect or heal cells from damage to the cell membrane or to the DNA, whether by oxidation or inflammation, by restoring tumor suppressor genes, blocking infiltration pathways, helping with detoxification, stimulating apoptosis, stimulating killer T cells, or by regulating the methylation process and gene expression. The Cancer Research Institute estimated in 2015 that 1 in 2 men and 1 in 3 women will receive a diagnosis in their lifetime.

Approximately 1 million per year are diagnosed as of 2020, and about half of them survived. It could be that a paradigm shift into viewing the body as a multi-dimensional transducer of several types of information could help retain health or reverse disease processes. Starting from conception and birth processes, setting up a scenario where the outer and inner environment of the child support cellular communication, builds a healthier foundation for their entire life.

The late Dr. Nicholas Gonzalez, who helped many people recover from cancer, had a refreshingly unique approach and perspective to correcting imbalances. In a 2015 interview he described the need for an individualized diet that fits the metabolic tendencies of that particular person. He explained that there are so many controversial diets out there; one with a focus on carbs, another on plants, another fats, another Mediterranean, and so on, that it would be confusing for the average person.

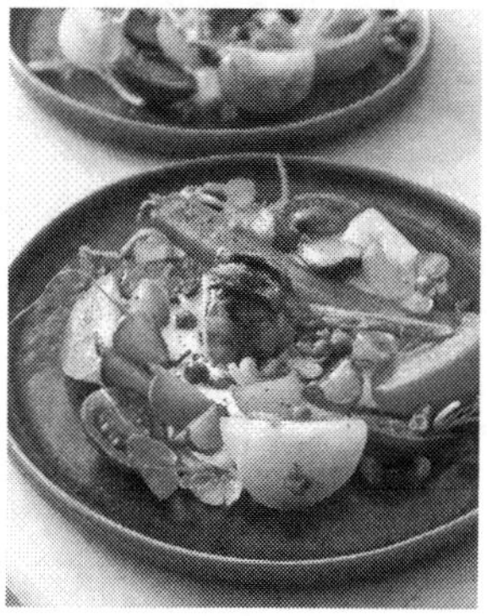

His approach is to get the autonomic nervous system in balance. Gonzalez stated that, *"We believe that disease occurs when the autonomic nervous system is out of balance. After all, that controls all physiological and biochemical processes in the body. It is the ultimate regulator of metabolism in the body. And when that's out of balance, you end up with serious problems."* This approach is aligned with the view of some of the early osteopaths mentioned earlier in this text, and Dr. Gonzalez credits Francis Pottenger, Sr. and Ernst Gelhorn as early proponents of this position.

Gonzalez goes on to say, *"And what we're trying to do with diet and supplements is to bring an out of balance autonomic system into balance. For example, if a person comes in with a strong sympathetic nervous system, they need to be on a plant-based diet. They need to be on certain supplements like beta carotene and the B vitamins thiamine, riboflavin, niacin, pyridoxine, and folic acid. They don't do well with B12, choline inositol, PABA, and pantothenic acid. They do well with high doses of C and high doses of D. They do terribly with calcium, but great with magnesium.*

"Other patients come into us who have a parasympathetic system. And these are the patients with a weak sympathetic system. And these are the patients that will thrive on a meat diet. They need lots of fatty red meat.

They do really well with it. That helps bring the strong parasympathetic system down a bit and builds up the weak sympathetic system. Fatty red meat has certain nutrients in it that have a very strong effect on the autonomic nervous system... They don't do well on high doses of C or high doses of D. They do well on E; they do well on calcium."

Dr. Gonzalez performed various nutritional analyses on his patients to determine which type of nervous system was predominant in them, but he then said that he could generally tell by how they presented due to many years of experience. *"For example, patients that get the typical solid tumors like tumors of the breast, lung, stomach, pancreas, colon, liver, uterus, prostate always have a strong sympathetic system and weak parasympathetic system. People that get the traditional blood borne or immune cancers — leukemia, myeloma, or sarcomas which are genetically related to the immune cancers like connective tissue cancers —they need to be on meat. These are the people that will thrive on a ketogenic diet."*

In Japan, doctors are allowed to use any treatment they find that works for their patients, giving them enormous flexibility to explore new options. Some doctors are aware of the limitations of having very little or no instruction in medical school on nutrition, (because natural cures cannot be patented) so not much has been passed on to the patients about the countless benefits of specific foods, herbs, and teas that can help them return to health. Another doctor mentioned that Carnegie and Rockefeller, along with the AMA, have made efforts to shut down the larger homeopathic colleges, as they were not promoting pharmaceutical interventions.

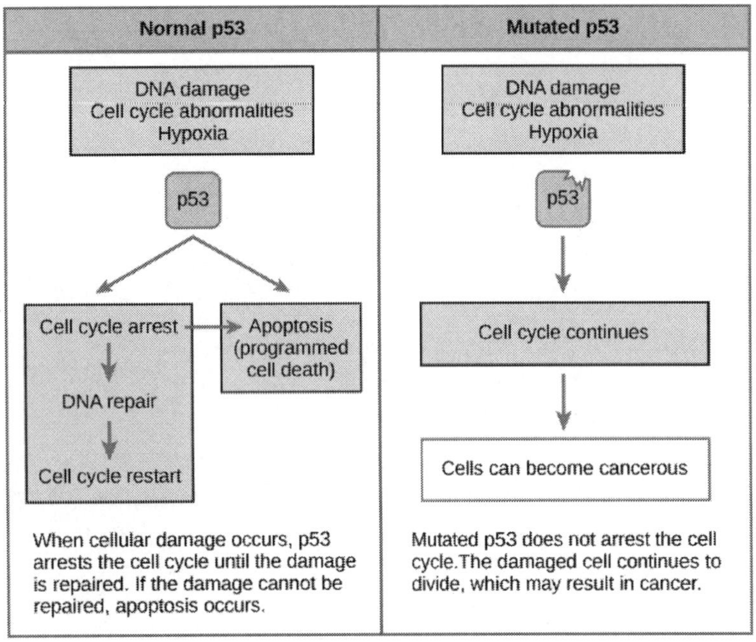

Fig. 5.4 – Function the P53 gene

Courtesy of CNX OpenStax 4.0 via Wikimedia Commons

One Japanese doctor who has successfully treated brain, lung, pancreatic, breast, liver and bladder cancers described his treatment as being **liposomal P53**. He states, *"Most of the patients suffering from cancer have a P53 mutation. That P53 mutation causes chemotherapy resistance and radiotherapy resistance. So P53 therapy can eliminate this resistance. Furthermore, P53 can work to stop the cancer cell cycle and induces apoptosis."* It also works because P53 is positively charged and cancer cells are negatively charged, so they are attracted to each other. One of the anti-cancer properties of curcumin is the ability to activate the tumor suppressing gene, P53.

Noa Rivlin, et al., found that mutation or inactivation of the P53 gene was present in 10% to 100% of cancers. (Fig.5.4)They describe the role of this gene as being able to induce cell cycle arrest, DNA repair, regulate senescence and apoptosis, cell cycle arrest. P53 also acts as a tumor suppressor and master regulator of various signaling pathways involved in the process. When this gene mutates, it can become part of the problem and actually promote tumor growth as it becomes a cancerous cell itself. [107](Noa Rivlin, et al., "Mutations *in the p53 Tumor Suppressor Gene,"* Genes & Cancer, April 2011)

One of the ways that this gene can mutate in early stages of cancer, according to researcher Panagiota Markaki, is due to carcinogen exposure in the form of the mold micotoxins, Aspergillus flavus and Aspergillus parasiticus, or AFB_1.

There have been instances of AFB_1 in olives and cold pressed olive oil, so daily consumption could prove to facilitate an accumulation of this mycotoxin, which tends to adversely impact the liver. *[108](Markaki, 2010)*

K.A. Wilson et al. have called it a *"worldwide health concern due to the contamination of foods such as peanuts and corn, as well as cosmetics. AFB_1 causes adverse health effects, such as liver cancer, and is a contributing factor to the etiology of hepatitis."* (Wilson, et al., 2016) It's best to check the label for a stamp of approval from a national or international organization. It could also be helpful to periodically consume supplements that are able to kill mold and fungus or parasites in your system.

The buildup of mold, fungus, and their mycotoxins has been an issue for several foods, particularly corn, nuts, and grains while they are being stored. Several essential oils have compounds that can have an impact on AFB_1, such as **geraniol**. It is contained in over 250 essential oils, including some well- known ones like lavender, rose, geranium, lemongrass, and palmarosa. **Palmarosa** is nearly 70% geraniol, whereas rose has around 10%. Diffusing geraniol into the storage container for grains delayed the onset of the mycotoxin for up to a week, but did not kill it or prevent it. Coriander and dill essential oils degraded AFB_1 by 66% - 93% depending upon whether or not it was irradiated. (Xi Tang et al., 2018)

Parsley and Dill

Parsley, dill, coriander, and celery essential oils were tested against AFB_1 and found to be nearly completely effective against the aflatoxin depending upon the dosage of the application. The stronger the dose, the more effective the treatment, particularly for coriander and parsley, which were able to achieve 100% inhibition, while the other two showed a 65-75% reduction. **Ajowain** essential oil was also able to block 100% of AFB_1 growth, clove, lemon, bitter orange, and bergamot were at 96-98% effective. (Restuccia, 2019) Oil of cinnamon has chemical constituents that make it a powerful antimicrobial and also very effective against fungus. (Jasmyne Brown, 2021) While the oils are more potent, ingesting them in food form could also potentially inhibit mold and fungus mycotoxins in the body. The oils have been used for fumigation during food storage, and could be used in diffusers in the home or office.

Reishi mushroom varieties

We shouldn't leave the discussion on foods for fighting or preventing cancer cells from developing without covering a few mushrooms with this characteristic. **Chaga** mushrooms are able to stimulate apoptosis in tumor cells, inhibit proliferation, and provide anti-mutagenic properties as well. Turkey tail mushrooms contain polysaccharides which are able to target and attack tumor viruses and inhibit several cancer triggering mechanisms in the body. (Adored Beast Team, 2021) They also beef up the immune system by increasing the production of immune cells. **Reishi** mushrooms also have polysaccharides and are able to activate natural killer cells, slow the growth of tumor cells, and trigger programmed cell death. (Bollinger, 2021)

CARCINOGENS AND PREVENTATIVE MEASURES

There are some foods that contain toxins before they reach your table, and some that have carcinogens added to them. There are about 2500 chemicals added to foods to modify flavor, color, stability, texture, or cost, and possibly 12,000 other chemicals that come into direct contact with food, like packaging, processing, etc. (NCB!, 1983) Here's a short list of the first type with associated cancers (Christian C. Abnet, 2007):

- Aflatoxins, metabolites of *Aspergillus* fungus (seeds, nuts, grains, corn); liver
- Alcohol, ethanol metabolites (alcoholic beverages); several types of cancer
- TCDD, Dioxin; liver, lung, thyroid, non-Hodgkin's lymphoma

- Acetaldehyde; alcohol, auto exhaust, smoke; several cancers
- Benzo(a)pyrene; smoked meats, coffee, oils, grilling; several cancers
- Nitrosamine: smoked/preserved foods, alcohol, dairy; several cancers
- Maté, hot herbal drink over 1 liter/day; head, neck, mouth, esophagus cancer
- Fusarium moniliforme, fungus in corn, maize; esophageal cancers
- Ochratoxin A, molds in grains, beer, livestock feed; liver, kidney cancers
- PhIP, an amine from cooking meat at high temp; intestine cancers
- Acrylamides, found in drinking water; no specific cancer sites determined

Skin care ingredients that are carcinogenic include (HealthyOne Family Medicine):

- Coal tar, in hair dye, shampoos, and skin ; skin, lung, kidney, bladder cancers
- Parabens, lotion, shampoo, shaving cream, make-up, spray tan; breast, skin
- Parabens can also disrupt hormones and impact reproduction abilities
- Triclosan, in anti-bacteria soaps, toothpaste, shampoos; skin cancer
- Formaldehyde, skincare, nail polish, lotions, shower gel, hair straighteners
- Contaminated talc, with asbestos, in cosmetics

Additional ingredients that could be hazardous or cancerous (Scott Faber, 2020):

- Quaternium-15, releases formaldehyde
- Dibutyl phthalate, developmental toxicant and endocrine disruptor Heavy metals, lotion, shampoo, foundation, makeup; carcinogen
- Metals include cadmium, chromium, D&C Red, aluminum, polyvinyl acetate
- PFAs, polyfluoroalkyl substances linked to cancers
- M and o-phenylenediamine in hair dyes can cause DNA damage, cancer
- Mercury

A few more not on the above lists that are considered hazardous and harmful (Cancer Active, 2016):

- BHA and BHT
- Perfume (Fragrance)
- PEG compounds
- Petroleum
- Siloxanes
- Sodium Laureth/Lauryl sulfate; can stop hair growth, irritate skin, hurt the eye
- BPA in plastics, is an endocrine disruptor
- Toluene, in nail enamel, hair gel, hairspray, perfumes; neurotoxin, xenohormone

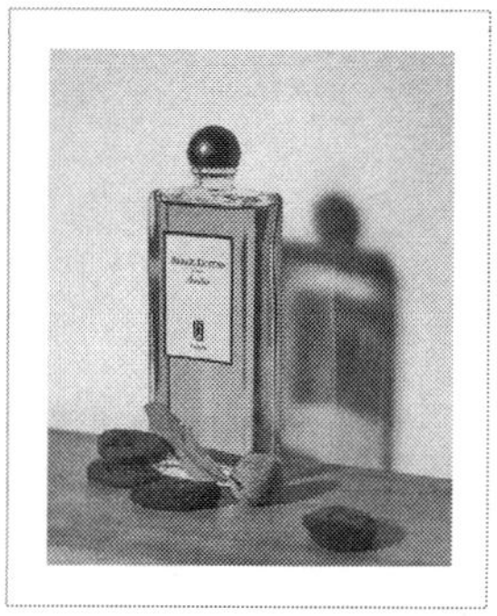

- Fluoride, in tap water, toothpaste and mouthwash; unsafe to swallow
- Propylene Glycol, form of mineral oil – used in antifreeze, sun screen
- Talc, in baby powder and blush; risk of ovarian and endometrial cancer
- Xylene, or dimethylbenzene, nail varnish; liver damage, respiratory issues
- DEA, TEA, MEA, in products containing nitrates; carcinogenic
- Vitamin A as retinyl palmitate, skin cream/lotion, sunscreen; skin cancer
- Oxybenzone is under review – in sun screens
- PPD or paraphenylenediamine, in hair dyes; bladder cancers
- Phenacetin, facial hair bleach, hair color, and depilatory products; breast tumors
- Crystalline silica, lipstick, gloss, eye shadow, liner, lotion, shampoo; lung cancer

The American Lung Association warns about breathable toxins that include aerosol spray products of any kind, air fresheners, chlorine bleach, detergents, dishwashing liquids, rug and upholstery cleaners, furniture and floor polish, and oven cleaners. Cleaning products are also laced with dozens of irritants that can worsen asthma and allergies, or create them. Pet flea and tick treatments have similar ingredients to pesticides so can be harmful to pets as well as to humans.

> A study of 3,500 people around the world revealed that using spray cleaners just once a week led to an average of 40% increased risk of developing asthma *(Zock, 2007).*

The list goes on and on. This is one of the areas, like diet, that is greatly connected to epigenetics. A huge part of that equation is what we take into our bodies, exposure to environmental toxins, and how we respond to stress. Not all roads lead to cancer, but also to numerous other imbalances that affect auto-immune conditions, metabolic conditions, cognitive or emotional disorders, chronic pain processes, and can also greatly influence the quality of life. Luckily, the body is always listening and ready to respond anew to whatever information is coming its way, and can also modified by how we interpret and respond to the information or experience.

For just about every dysfunction listed, there are also numerous options to prevent or correct the imbalances using the signaling capabilities of scores of foods, supplements, herbs, and spices, some of which are dose-dependent. Some work best combined with allopathic approaches, by either protecting healthy cells or enhancing apoptosis and non-proliferation of mutant cells. Eastern doctors have been described as focusing on 'the wave' rather than on the particle, like in Western medicine. They are more likely to integrate food, herbs, nutrition, the flow of energy harmonics and blood, as well as the psycho/emotional state of the person into the Western therapeutic process, rather than just focusing on the cancer cells.

Dr. Yu-Cheng Kuo speaks about the internal exercise of t'ai chi which doesn't get the heart rate up, but increases circulation of blood and energy through gentle, flowing movements while decreasing activity in

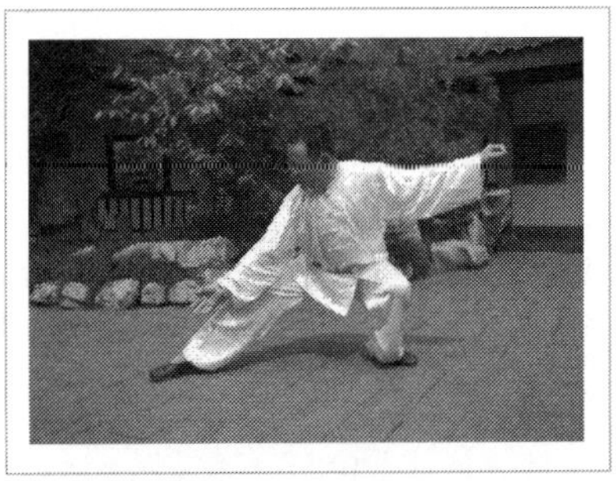

the brain and reducing stress. He also spoke about cancer being a dynamic process that may benefit more from altering the treatment regimen based upon the current status of the cells and pulses. With 384 herbs at their disposal, there are many combinations to use that can address the ways in which the mutated cells may strategize in order to survive.

Doctor Pan Nien Chung, who also uses Chinese Medicine, mentioned that there are special methods for addressing cancer stem cells whereby the urine can be tested afterwards to verify that the cells are being excreted. This is a rare technique that takes quite a while to learn, but using the energy made available from this solar alignment technique while stimulating 4 main acupuncture points, the stem cells are excreted en mass through the urine. (Ty Bollinger, Truth About Cancer, 2014) Of 244 patients using this method for various types of cancer, only two died. That rounds down to less than 1% compared to around 50% mortality rate in the U.S. so far.

Dr. Huang Chien-Jung reiterates the importance of **spinal alignment** so that optimum meridian flow is possible. From other points of view, the nervous system is in direct contact with the immune system that directly relates with the lymphatic system, which returns us to the blood and urine so that toxic elements can be excreted. Other doctors from Asia emphasized **detoxing** as a major component for curing any major or chronic disease, along with the use of a few key herbs and mushrooms. **Megadoses of vitamin C,** both intravenous and/or liposomal have been an adjunct to treatment in some cases. The doctors recommend using the foods that grow in your general area, but here's a partial list of those that have been found to be effective, mainly in combination with other treatments and dose-dependent:

- Ginseng
- Reishi and
- Cordyceps mushrooms were among those mentioned, in addition to Antrodia Camphorata.
- Papaya seeds/leaves
- Cassava root (B17)
- Artemisinin (from wormwood)
- Periwinkle flower
- Mistletoe
- Soursop leaves (tea)
- Solanacae (in Devil's Apple, eggplant, green peppers)

Revitalizing the system after the detox or chemo was a key aspect of their patients' treatments. There are scores of treatments for cancer that don't involve chemotherapy, or that can enhance the effectiveness of chemo if one has chosen that treatment and is noticing less than ideal results. Some doctors mentioned finding parasites as a key issue that was slowing down their immune response, and others note silver/

mercury fillings as a component that can make healing sluggish. Candida or mold toxicity may be overloading the system's resources, and any other condition that could compromise the efficacy of the gut, including lingering low-grade infections in the mouth.

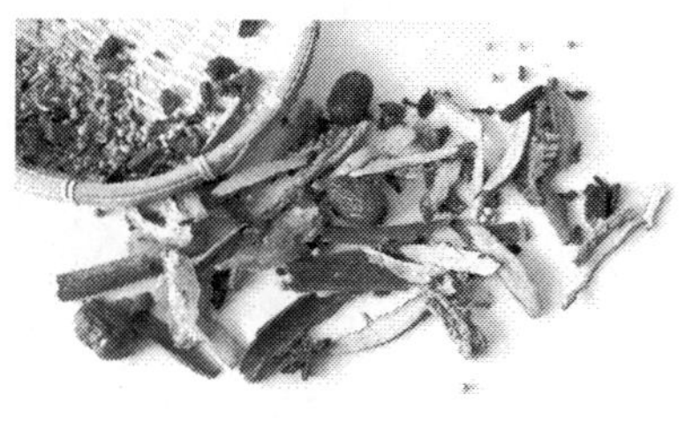

Chinese herbs

It's best to integrate any of these approaches that resonate with your body on a regular basis rather than wait until a major illness has erupted in the body. There is an enormous amount of research on the breakdown of communication in and between the cells, and it nearly always leads to the growing phenomena of cancers or degenerative, metabolic, and autoimmune diseases. The ways in which the system processes information is profoundly intricate and complex. It's like a language that has discreet rules of grammar with an extensive vocabulary that is coded for specific ears to hear. Much of the language is still a mystery with rules that are flexible and rigid at the same time. It seems that we can take any type of internal discomfort as part of that language. Remember that where the discomfort is may not be the cause.

The body is always listening to us. The system prioritizes our point of view even if it's subconscious. It was interesting to see that in order to cure the eczema on my ankles I had to use a comprehensive approach addressing several aspects of the contributors to the rash as though I was curing a disease. No single approach was successful, and no lasting approach was possible until I eliminated the source irritant. This was a seemingly simple expression on the surface that was actually reflecting a myriad of changes that were happening at the molecular level inside my system.

The first layer that may have compromised all the others was the gritty, ropey, strained, scar tissue in both ankles and feet. There are thousands of nerve endings in the feet that weren't able to function at an optimum level all those years. I doubt that anyone, including me, would have suspected this as part of the issue. This will be the challenge for all of us: to look at the possibility of old, forgotten issues as still being in tissue memory and potentially slowly altering the efficacy of the whole.

Many times when I ask a client about their accidents, falls, injuries, or surgeries, they initially say they have none. Then when I say, "Never?" they'll say, "Yes, lots, but that was a long time ago." It's very often a surprise and a paradigm shift to turn towards the idea that there can be lingering, impactful influences from events happening 10, 20, or 30 years ago. The symptoms today may be different than the original ones, and could even be showing up in a different area of the body. When you think of the body as a continuum of fabric, an interlinked matrix that flows information through itself every millisecond and nanometer, the idea isn't so far-fetched.

That speaks to the fact that many areas of imbalance happened before the result of eczema erupted. Quite a bit of effort had to go into correcting all the layers of communication that had been altered; it wasn't immediate going in or going out. It followed a circuitous path into the altered cellular processes, and the return to balance was like retracing all the steps along the path that couldn't self-correct. Much research is dedicated to intervening at one of those steps in an attempt to prevent an unfavorable outcome, but it seems that a combined approach might be indicated.

The epigenetics of diet suggests a similar theme. The over-arching recommendation is to protect the cells from damage that will interfere with their ability to communicate efficiently and accurately. Communication happens in a variety of ways, so addressing foods that can protect the nerves, the vascular system, the bones, the skin, the organs and glands would all be helpful.

I have noticed over months and years since the major eczema outbreak and subsequent smaller ones after ingesting chicken, that the 'protection blend' I made has always been the most effective. It also works well for any little skin tag, odd bump, or mysterious pin-head size hard spot. Essential oils and medicinal butters operate on multiple levels based upon their chemical profile, but are more known for a particular property based upon the amount of a specific constituent. The majority of the ingredients in this most effective blend functioned to block the proliferation of mutant cells, or are known to be cytotoxic to them.

Although many other more serious conditions can arise through faulty cellular information transfer caused by diet, there are also growing numbers of atopic dermatitis or systemic contact dermatitis, which is the canary in the mine in many cases. The dermatologist called my eczema 'contact dermatitis' and felt it would respond easily to a mild, topical cortisone cream. It did not. It took four years to resolve. Dr. Rajani Katta and Megan Schlitche, BSc report that, "Foods may trigger rapid, immunoglobulin E-mediated hypersensitivity reactions or may lead to late eczematous reactions. While immediate reactions occur within minutes to hours of food exposure, late eczematous reactions may occur anywhere from hours to two days later." In my case, it took years before the reactivity expressed itself in that way.

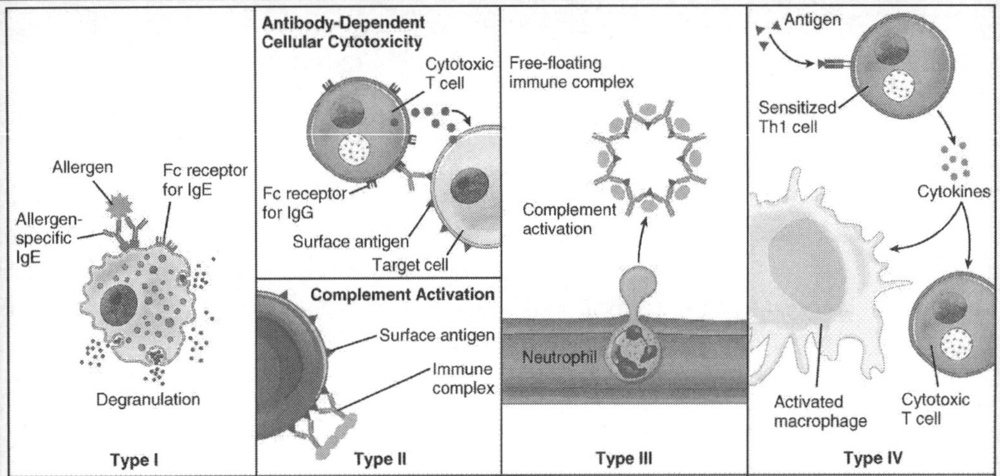

Type I	Type II	Type III	Type IV
IgE-Mediated Hypersensitivity	**IgG-Mediated Cytotoxic Hypersensitivity**	**Immune Complex-Mediated Hypersensitivity**	**Cell-Mediated Hypersensitivity**
IgE is bound to mast cells via its Fc portion. When an allergen binds to these antibodies, crosslinking of IgE induces degranulation.	Cells are destroyed by bound antibody, either by activation of complement or by a cytotoxic T cell with an Fc receptor for the antibody (ADCC)	Antigen–antibody complexes are deposited in tissues, causing activation of complement, which attracts neutrophils to the site	Th1 cells secrete cytokines, which activate macrophages and cytotoxic T cells and can cause macrophage accumulation at the site
Causes localized and systemic anaphylaxis, seasonal allergies including hay fever, food allergies such as those to shellfish and peanuts, hives, and eczema	Red blood cells destroyed by complement and antibody during a transfusion of mismatched blood type or during erythroblastosis fetalis	Most common forms of immune complex disease are seen in glomerulonephritis, rheumatoid arthritis, and systemic lupus erythematosus	Most common forms are contact dermatitis, tuberculin reaction, autoimmune diseases such as diabetes mellitus type I, multiple sclerosis, and rheumatoid arthritis

Fig. 5.5 – Immune sensitivity - possible outcomes of food allergies that remain unchecked

Moderate to severe reactions are more common in children and infants, but there are also incidents of food reactivity in adults. Reactions can occur in the skin, the lungs, esophagus, eyes, nose, digestive system, or nervous system, making it more challenging for anyone to identify to source. Hence, the need for awareness of what symptoms to look for and which foods are commonly suspect. That said, my father was allergic to strawberries, my aunt to chalk dust and newspaper ink, and my mother to cigarette and cigar smoke. Since it can vary widely, it may be more useful to be aware of the areas in the body where sensitivities most often manifest.

The most common food allergens are often listed on packaging as being eliminated: soy, corn, wheat, milk, eggs, and peanuts. Sensitivities to Balsam of Peru is also common. It can be found in fragrances or in foods that contain similar compounds - like vanilla, cinnamon, cloves, some liquors, condiments, citrus, chocolate and tomatoes. Any of these could trigger a reaction that expresses in a systemic, recurring dermatitis. Propylene glycol is another common allergen that is found in many toiletries, sauces and salad dressings. Symptoms improve dramatically by removing the irritant from the diet. (Katta and Schlichte, 2014)

There is some controversy over what constitutes an actual food allergy vs. a food reactivity, and studies are still underway to clarity the difference. In general there are currently two categories of response: IgE (immunoglobulin) and non-IgE mediated (a chemical reaction that doesn't involve the immune system.) Food sensitivity testing is not always the best measure since false positives do happen, food intolerances don't trigger the immune system, and responses aren't always immediate. The histamines released by the reaction to the allergen, according to author, Fatima Fahs in June of 2022, can create symptoms as widespread as itching, diarrhea, dryness, discoloration of the skin, swelling, hives, blisters, abdominal cramps, vomiting, wheezing, a drop in blood pressure or tightening of the throat. Many foods contain histamines, but most say that it's a particular protein in trigger foods that create the reaction.

There is a cascade of reactions at multiple levels of the messaging process, including transcription, mRNA processing, translation, phosphorylation, and degradation.(Laure Escoubet-Lozach, et al., 2002) (Fig.5.5) It's best to take care of the symptoms right away and decipher the source of the irritant before more serious health conditions develop. Chronic inflammation can be a setup for countless other issues in the body and in the case of eczema, it appears that one of the key communication systems — the skin — has become compromised.

Cellular modification is unavoidable because toxins are everywhere in modern society, but there are remedies. Certain foods we discussed can prevent or repair the damage, and eliminate senescent or damaged cells. Limiting the foods and products known to be toxic to the cells and their ability to function (eliminate the phrase in red) also seems like the best preventative measure. There are a few more key areas of communication at the level of the transcription process, (please add this comma) whereby the alteration of those particular genetic signaling proteins is most significant for health outcomes. The few transcription factors mentioned here are fundamental to several 'decision-making' processes in our bodies which I feel can also be modulated by conscious participation. The ones I'll focus on as we go along will be those most related to skin and bones, as they are significant in their influence, but also palpable.

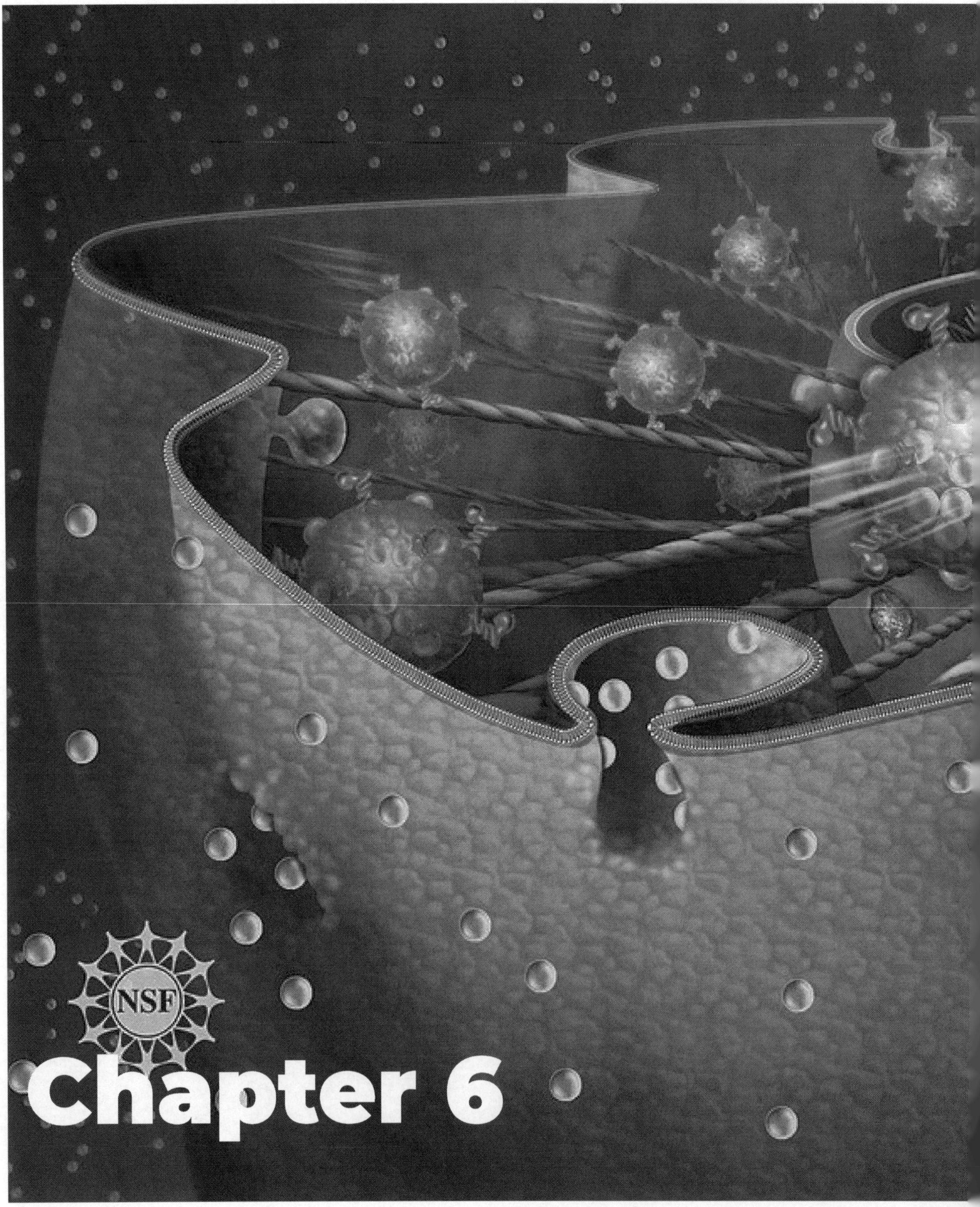

Chapter 6

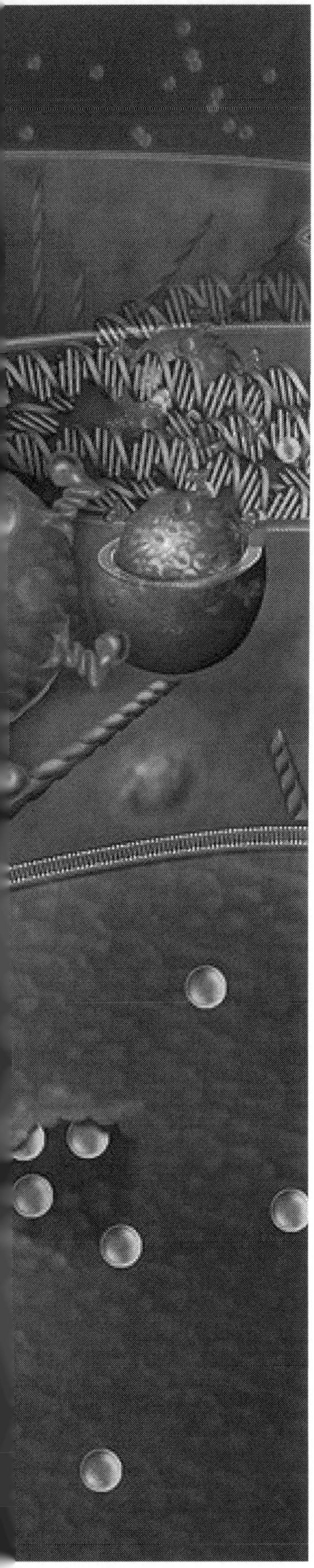

Transcription Factors and Your Health

We covered some of the initial embryological signaling involved in the proliferation and function of various cells as our bodies are being formed. These same transcription factors in the fetus continue to be significant contributing factors in the health of adult bodies. Their ability to communicate accurately with one another is crucial throughout our lifetime. The function of these proteins is to copy a sequence from DNA to RNA which can control the extent to which a gene may be expressed.

Most transcription factors use transcription pathways that will either activate or inhibit their function by determining which signal is sent, or how it is regulated by co-factors. [109](Sally Robertson, B.Sc., 2019) Robertson describes a key enzymatic aspect of the process as, "*Using DNA as a template, an enzyme called RNA polymerase catalyzes the chemical reactions that enable the production of RNA. Transcription factors determine where, when, and how effectively this enzyme functions.*"

In fact, most transcription factor pathways involve kinases, which are enzymes that activate, speed up, or silence/deactivate the action of a transcription protein. The transcription process often happens using the transfer of a phosphate group to other molecules, which is called phosphorylation; the most common form of signal transduction. (Enjalbert, 2003)

Mitsis, et al., offered an overview of the complex process: "*Gene expression is an intricate process and involves the coordination of multiple dynamic events, which are subject to multi-level regulation. Those regulatory levels include the transcriptional level, the post-transcriptional level, the translational level, and the post-translational level.*" He goes on to confirm that gene expression is only partly inherited, and is largely responsive to outside stimuli. [110](Thanasis Mitsis, et al., 2020)

Transcription factors are under continual scrutiny within scientific communities in order to better understand exactly which aspect of the communication process is most significant in an activating, generating, deactivating, or in a regulatory capacity. They are so central to the function of our cells, that being able to uncover more specifics in what influences their 'decision-making' process, could be invaluable in the prevention and treatment of a number of diseases. Hopefully, we can also gain a better understanding of the reasons for why dysfunctions happen.

Transcription factors and endocrine disruption

The National Institute for Environmental Health Sciences created a list of known chemicals that interfere with the body's hormones and are linked with "developmental, reproductive, brain, immune, and other problems." They mention that even a small amount of exposure can have far-reaching biological effects and are unsafe.

> *"This leads scientists to think that endocrine-disrupting chemical exposures, even at low amounts, can alter the body's sensitive systems and lead to health problems."*

The list they provided includes:

- Bisphenol A (BPA) - used in many plastics and in epoxy
- Dioxins - found in herbicide production and paper bleaching
- Perchlorate - a by-product of aerospace and pharmaceuticals landing in water
- PFAS - Polyflouryl substances used in manufacturing and textiles
- Phthalates - found in packaging, cosmetics, toys, and medical devices
- Phytoestrogens - from plants like soybeans
- PCB - used to make electrical equipment, hydraulic fluids, lubricants, plastics
- PBDE - used to make flame retardants for household products
- Triclosan - often found in anti-bacterial products like hand sanitizers

Multiple studies over the last 20 years have linked DNA methylation changes, altered mRNA expression, altered Notch signaling, and more, in humans and animals exposed to DES (Diethylstilbestrol). DES — a synthetic form of estrogen — "was given widely to women for 30 years to prevent complications during pregnancy, and to prevent miscarriage and premature labor." (National Cancer Institute, October, 2021)

> However, it was discovered in the 1950s that it was ineffective for its intended use, but continued to be prescribed for another 20 years. As a result, daughters of women prescribed DES during pregnancy continued to have elevated risk for adenocarcinoma, breast cancer, and pancreatic, cervical, and vaginal cancers.

This is just one example of life-threatening facts being withheld from the public by the medical community, and makes it even more important that we become our own health advocates.

Dr. Nasha Winters, inspired by her own journey with cancer, listed a few other endocrine disruptors that can either 'mimic, block, interfere with production of, or modify the body's sensitivity to hormones' as delineated by the Environmental Working Group (EWG). For example, atrazine is a common toxic herbicide that winds up in drinking water that, like perchlorate, can be filtered out. Lead, which can also lead to birth defects, can cause kidney and brain damage, high blood pressure, miscarriage, and hearing loss. The most common sources of lead poisoning are from old homes with lead paint, lead water pipes, and some environmental sources that wind up in the soil.

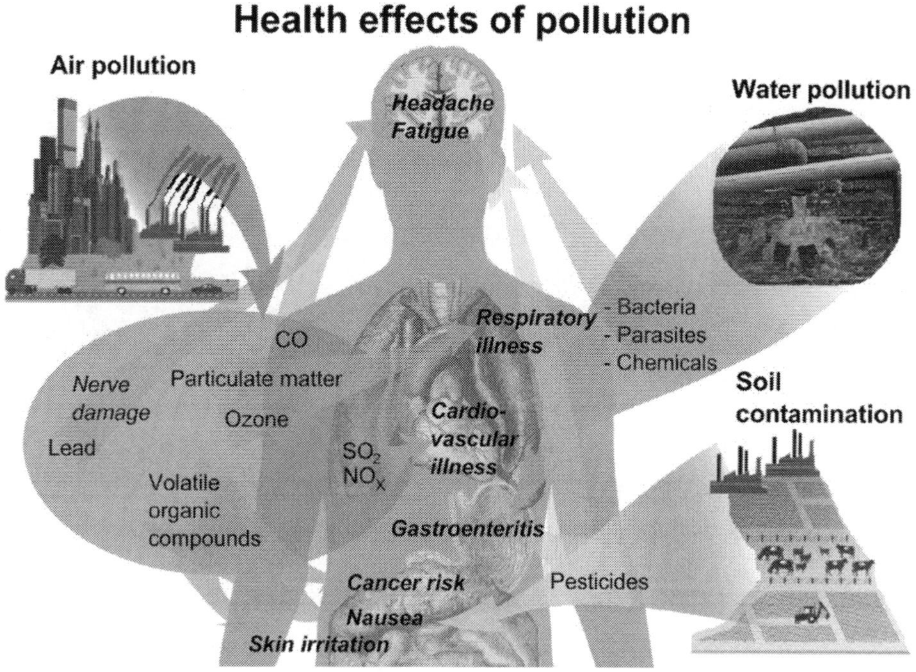

Fig. 5-1 – Potential health outcomes of environmental contaminants

Winters also lists arsenic, which can be sourced in water, soil, and in or on certain contaminated food. Arsenic is an endocrine disruptor that is known to elevate risks for certain types of cancer and cause glucocorticoid (sugar metabolism) and immune suppression issues. (Fig. 5.1) Mercury, often found in fish, coal burning factories, and vaccines, can wind up in the fetal brain and impact its development. Both can be avoided after becoming aware of the dangers.

While ongoing studies continue to evaluate the impacts of these chemicals on breast tissue, the uterus, fat cells, male reproductive tracts, and the liver, the burden also lies upon the consumer, particularly when optimizing safety during preconception, prenatal, and lactation periods.

Changes in purchase practices and dietary intake can make a huge difference in the health of the entire family for generations to come.

Sonic Hedgehog (Shh)

There are presently over a thousand transcription factors, and the specificity and complexity of how they all work in tandem may take a few more decades to pin down. There is some agreement on a few areas of engagement that can have far-reaching impacts on serious health conditions. The Shh protein (Fig.5.3) becomes a chemical signal that's involved in cell growth, cell specialization, and the patterning of the body. (Medline Plus, National Library of Medicine) (Fig. 5.2)

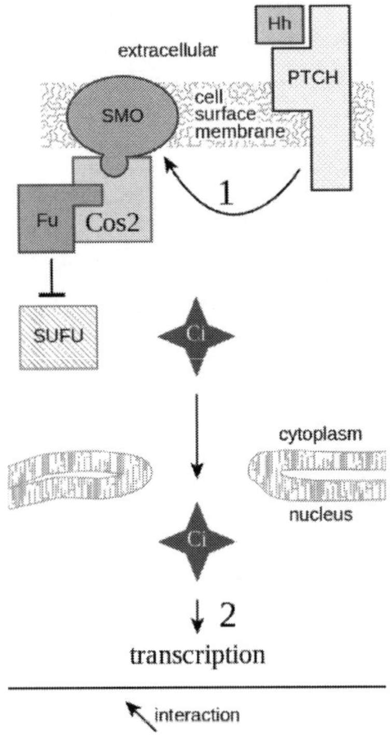

Fig. 5.3 – Example of Shh pathway whereby Shh binds to PTCH transmembrane receptor which can either signal SMO to activate target genes Fu and Cos2 that may be further modulated downstream by SUFU, or it may use Ci (Cubitus interruptus) as possibly a more direct nuclear suppressor or activator. (Ohlmeyer and Kalderon, 1998)

Courtesy of Erdélyl-Belle Boglàrka PhD.

It seems that this gene is also largely responsible for the early bilateral forebrain organization, including the telencephalon and diencephalon, as it has been seen along the ventral midline expressing bilaterally. The dorsoventral fates are derived from the neural crest and appear to be mediated by members of the BMP (bone morphogenetic protein) family. [111](Lumsden and Graham, 1995)

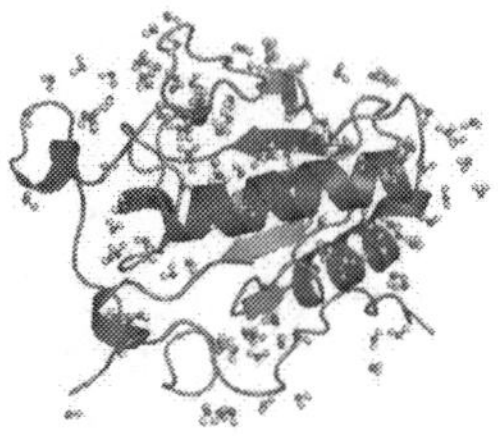

Fig. 5.2 - Rendering of Sonic Hedgehog

Shh has also been found to be expressed in the polarizing region of mesenchymal cells involved in spatial relationships - like the distance between the thumbs and forefingers, and the width of the limb buds. [112](Tickle and Towers, 2017) The fact that this protein arises out of the ventromedial aspect of the notochord and initiates the formation of the spinal cord, forebrain, and eyes is generally accepted. (Lumsden and Graham, 1995). In the adult, deregulation or mutation of this pathway plays an important role in cancer.

Finding ways to block Shh pathways is a major focus in cancer treatment in recent years. [113] (Yu-Chen Huang, et al., 2013) Over-expression of this pathway is implicated in many cancers, and tumor cells have been found to secrete Shh and promote its own growth. Carballo finds the Shh signaling pathway to be a *"valid therapeutic goal for pancreatic, prostate, breast cancers, and is of particular interest for the potential treatment of brain tumors."* [114](Gabriella Basile Carballo, et al., 2018)

Given that Shh has a function directly related to the homeostasis and maintenance of normal stem cells, being able to curb its activity when it has gone rogue and has begun to perform the same function for cancer stem cells is a significant discovery. This research finding has positive implications for cancer outcomes like medulloblastomas, hepatocellular carcinomas, glioblastomas, pancreatic, breast, multiple myeloma, prostate, colon, skin, bladder and gastric cancers. (Anna G. Vorobyeva and Aleister J. Saunders, 2016; Omenetti, et al., 2011) As Shh is expressed in the brain and in the liver, taking protective care of these systems could help prevent Hh mutations.

> Right now, it's clear that **environmental toxins** (Fig. 5.1) can disrupt Shh pathways, create sex hormone signaling disruption, possibly block androgen receptor activity, and create feminized male genitals. *(Johansson & Svengin, 2020)*

There have been studies that experiment with using any compound to deactivate or disrupt the pathways, but research is scarce on what actually disrupts signaling besides toxins. Nonetheless, reversing the damage is of utmost importance. So far, the **natural compounds** Huang and his team [113](Yu-Chen Huang, et al., 2013) have been able to verify are able to repress proliferation or stimulate apoptosis in some of the aforementioned tumor types are:

- Cyclopamine from the corn lily plant,
- Curcumin from turmeric,
- Epigallocatechin-3-Gallate from green tea alone or with quercetin
- Isoflavone Genistin from soy,
- Resveratrol from grapes, berries, and other polyphenol-laden foods,
- Zerumbone from a tuberous root
- Norcantharidin from blister beetles
- Arsenic trioxide known in Chinese Medicine

SOX Family

Daniela Grimm and her team of researchers described the SOX family of proteins as also being implicated in several types of tumor formation - namely, breast, prostate, renal cell carcinoma, thyroid, gastrointestinal and lung, brain, and skin tumors, as well as in their metastasis. They are involved in the regulation of numerous biological processes so their deregulation can be problematic. The SOX family of transcription factors, through the HMG (high mobility group) domain and their role in DNA binding, provide regulatory functions in cellular development, cell-fate decision, and differentiation of the embryo. [115](Grimm, et al., 2020). They have also been found to regulate other signaling pathways, such as Shh, Notch, Wnt, and Hippo. (Kelsie Thu et al., 2014)

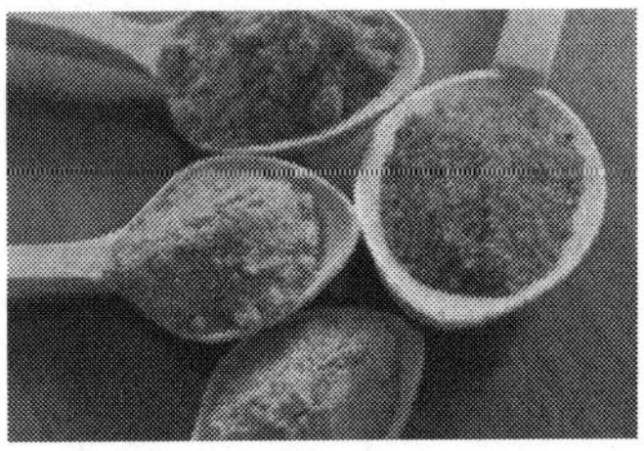
Curcumin

The 20+ SOX transcription factors also play a crucial role in development related to the retina, the cardiovascular and central nervous systems, cartilage differentiation, and sex determination. Going forward therapeutically, part of the conundrum in developing intervention protocols, is that depending upon a variety of factors – such as the cellular environment and methylation process – certain SOX proteins can act either as a tumor suppressor or generator. In a healthy cellular environment, these genes can play a role in tissue homeostasis/regeneration, and apoptosis of unhealthy cells. What determines which way each gene will express are being scrutinized one by one, but studies at this time are mainly in relation to which factor's over-expression tends toward specific cancers.

In 2021, Milena Stevanovic and a group of researchers were able to report the double-sided factors regarding specific Sox transcription factors, brain homeostasis and neurogenesis discovered over recent years. They cited numerous influencers on glial cell proliferation, which are neuronal stem cells that provide mechanical, metabolic, and trophic support to neurons in the adult brain. Deregulation of the Sox family functions is related to neurodegenerative conditions. Some factors that become imbalanced include neurotrophic factors, transcriptional programs, inflammatory cytokines, cell cycle regulation, neurotransmitters, and hormones. Deregulation can often be attributed to stress, aging, alcohol abuse, and neuron loss after injury. [116](Milena Stevanovic et al., 2021)

Charles Murray emphasizes the role in cellular communication by saying, "*Many of the diseases that place the greatest burden in society are, at their root, diseases of cellular deficiency. Heart failure, diabetes, stroke, hematological disorders, neurodegenerative disorders, most cases of blindness and deafness, spinal cord injury, osteoarthritis, and kidney failure all result from the absence of one or more critical populations of cells that the body is unable to replace.*" [117](Murray and Keller, 2008)

One interesting study focused on what could eradicate cancer stem cells (CSC), since they are often responsible for therapeutic interventions being unsuccessful. In 2013 Huang et al. looked at a few combined allopathic and natural options, such as **curcumin**, which has been shown to enhance CSC apoptosis and dampen their ability to resist drug treatments. In addition, ceramide, a secondary lipid messenger often included in skin care products, has also been shown to activate apoptotic pathways when another drug (Tamoxifen) is used alongside it to inhibit ceramide's enzyme-induced metabolism out of the cell. [118](Chen, Ke, et al., 2013)

Several studies over the years have verified that curcumin, a phytochemical in turmeric, is effective against CSC.

In 2019, Arpan De and his group of researchers reported that curcumin "*has recognized activity against cancer stem cells and affects several signaling pathways. Many molecules targeted by curcumin also regulate the circadian timing system that has effects on carcinogenesis, tumor growth, and metastasis. It is well tolerated by individuals ingesting it for possible cancer prevention or in combination with conventional cancer therapies, and it shows low toxicity toward noncancerous cells at low dosages.*"

The author cautions that curcumin has low bioavailability, and may interfere with conventional treatments. Collaboration is encouraged using complimentary medical approaches that "work in concert with daily physiological cycles controlled by the circadian timing system, because cancer cells are subjected to daily hormonal and neural activity that should be considered when timing optimal curcumin treatments." [119](Arpan De, et al. 2019)

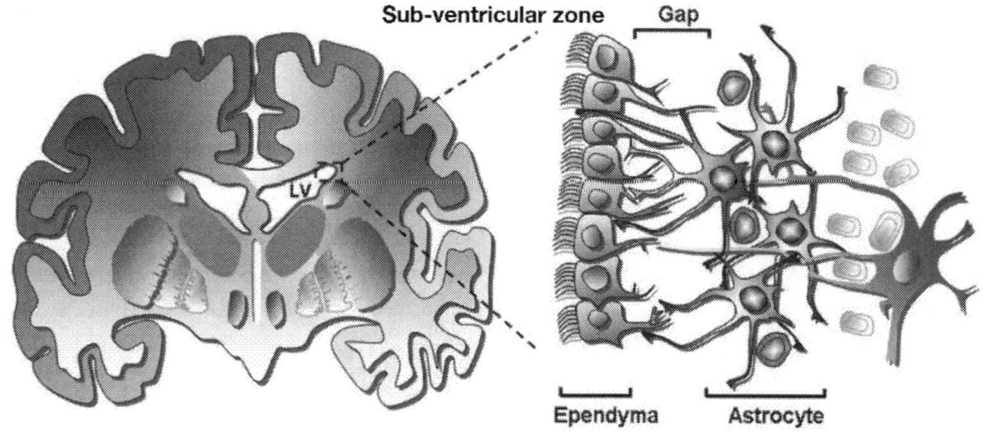

Fig. 5.4 – Illustration of the subventricular zone where SHH signaling is expressed

Image is an Oscar Arias-Carrion derivative work: Copper Kettle CC BY 2.0 via Wikimedia Commons

A very significant report by Gabriella Carballo and her team, is that neurogenic stem cells are found near the lateral ventricles of the brain in the **subventricular zone**, (fig. 5.4) as well as in the hippocampus. Chronic stress is known to stimulate cell death in the hippocampus, so it could, by association, also impair Hh signaling. Shh signaling activation determines the balance between active and quiescent stem cells, which is the regulatory function of these 'neural niches' where the stem cells are generated and differentiated. Gaining a better understanding of the signaling processes in mutated cells that are resistant to treatment is the current focus of researchers. If they are able to understand and manage that part of the process, the hope is that cancer stem cell signaling will then not be used to protect or to multiply those cells.

So far, we have covered the findings that several foods, herbs, and spices can stimulate cancer cell death, apoptosis of senescent and mutated cells, as well as to discharge cancer stem cells. Toxic exposures, or certain foods — like trans fats, processed meats, and additives — can alter the functioning or make-up of the cell membrane and other transport or signaling mechanisms. Those alterations can generate oxidation and/or damage of the cells. Certain types of movement and manual therapy can open the flow of fluids, oxygen, nutrients, and energy through the system, as well as help to optimize the flow of information by way of the nervous system, fascia, skin, joints, and other methods of transmission.

Yubing Sun, a researcher from the University of Michigan in Ann Arbor, reports that physical forces can and do indeed have a direct impact at the level of molecular communication. He states,

"Physical factors in the local cellular microenvironment, including cell shape and geometry, matrix mechanics, external mechanical forces, and nanotopographical features of the extracellular matrix, can all have strong influences in regulating stem cell fate.

Stem cells sense and respond to these insoluble biophysical signals through integrin-mediated adhesions and the force balance between intracellular cytoskeletal contractility and the resistant forces originated from the extracellular matrix." [120]*(*Yubing Sun, et al., 2012)

The researchers go on to say that cell shape is a potent regulator of cell growth and physiology. In fact, it serves as a signal to set stem cell activity in motion upon a deformation of the normal shape, as is true for bone and adipose cells. Muscle and vascular cells also use mechanical force as a cue to be on alert for regulatory action. The mechanical regulatory pathways, MAPK/ERK, are shared by several transcription factors so it wouldn't be a great leap to consider that movement and manual therapy can have an influence on these pathways.

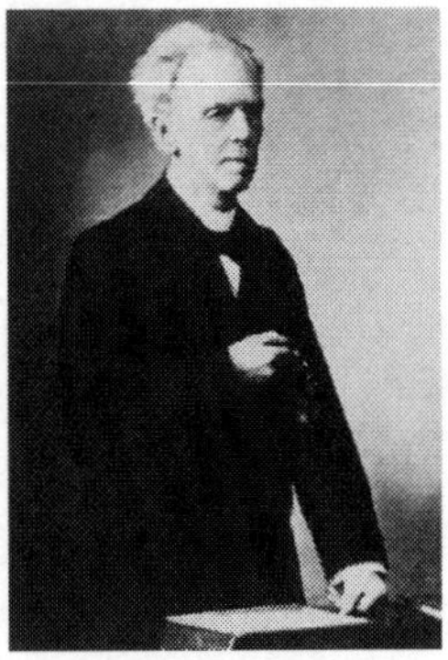

Fig 5.5 - Ernst Neumann in 1895

Mariona Nadal-Ribelles finds that, "*Modulation of gene expression in response to the extracellular environment is one of the main mechanisms that determine cell fate. MAPKs (mitogen-activated protein kinases) have thus emerged as fundamental transcriptome regulators that function through a multi-layered control of gene expression, a process often deregulated by disease, which therefore provides an attractive target for therapeutic strategies*." [121](Mariona Nadal-Ribelles, et al., 2018) Cancer is a very unique process that should be taken on a case-by-case basis as to whether or when to apply manual therapy.

The subject of mechanical signaling, or mechanotransduction, will be covered in much greater detail in the next chapter, but suffice to say that it's the foundation of movement as medicine. One of the main outcomes of movement and manual therapy is increased balance and integration in the body. Balance is crucial at every level of communication, as the over- or under-expression or regulation of any chemical, hormone, ligand, nutrient, or metabolic process can lead to illness. There is one more transcription factor that is also very involved in a number of fundamental processes throughout the system that is worth mentioning again, and that is bone morphogenetic protein (BMP).

Perhaps one day there will be research done on how movement improves cellular signaling at the level of specific transcription factors, but in any case, it's likely there are many micro corrections happening every time we exercise. Many key processes in the body involve, or are regulated by a function related to the bones. After understanding and appreciating what those functions are a little more, we can move into how to apply this knowledge in everyday life.

Ongoing Discoveries about the Properties of Bones

As early as 1868, Ernst Neumann of Prussia (Fig.5.5) recognized the hematopoietic properties of bone marrow, and not long after noticed lymph stem cells. He is credited with arriving at the distinction between red marrow cells and yellow, fatty marrow cells and the fact that they had different functions. (Barry Cooper, MD, 2011) For many decades, bone was believed to provide structural support as it regulated its own turnover process to remodel itself. In the 1950s to 60s, researchers were realizing that the acid/alkaline balance in the body was being somewhat regulated by the secretion of calcium from bones, even raising the question whether a more acidic diet contributed to osteoporosis. (Lynda Frasetto, 2018)

The answer to that question turned out to be that acidosis does stimulate osteoclast activity and bone resorption. (Arnett, 2008; Yuan, 2016; Bushinsky and Frick, 2000) In the 1970's, it was discovered that toxins (including lead, mercury, and other heavy metals) exposed to in childhood could remain in the bones for as long as thirty years and be released into the bloodstream later in life, such as during pregnancy. (Libby McDonald, 2007, William Morrison, MD, 2017) However, a diet rich with vitamins and minerals acts to buffer the absorption of lead into the intestines, and in some cases, also protects the bones. (Kresser, 2019)

A group of researchers found that the adipose tissue that sequesters OCPs (organochlorine pesticides) and releases them over time due to their long half-life, may release them more quickly in unintentional or aggressive weight loss programs. OPC's are neurotoxic and they do reach the brain. In fact, serum levels of OPCs in the blood of Alzheimer's patients matched the levels in their brains. [122](Duk-Hee Lee, et al., 2018) Toxins released from the bones can also reach the brain, and may be a reason that dementia often follows osteoporosis.

Although a study in Germany with nearly 60,000 participants who were followed over 20 years showed a positive correlation with osteoporosis and dementia, the mechanism of action for this association wasn't fully explored. [123](Karl Kostev, et al., 2018) Every other study includes women at a higher risk than men, possibly due to the association with estrogen loss, inflammation, and osteoclast activity. However, Kostev's study showed men at a higher risk for dementia related to bone loss. Another possibility is that the decline in muscle mass that accelerates bone loss is accompanied by reduced exercise, which leads to less circulating BDNF and slower neurogenesis.

Even though every researcher offers a disclaimer in the beginning of whatever they're about to report, admitting that there are mechanisms of action that are complex and not yet completely understood, the last 50 years have yielded an impressive amount of new information about the multiple interdependent and crucial functions of bone. Recently, bone's role as an endocrine organ has come center stage, along with it being heralded as possibly the most significant source of mechano-sensory input in the body. Delving into the molecular aspects of how it interacts with other systems will paint a better picture of what is being used to wield the extensive influence it exerts.

Bone Morphogenetic Proteins

BMPS AND BONE FRACTURES

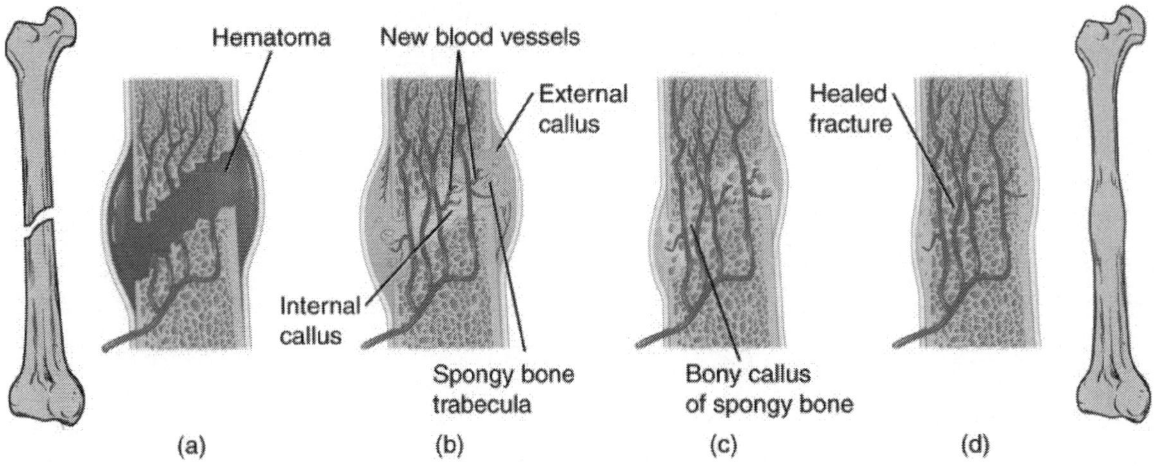

Fig 5.6 – Stages of healing in a long bone

Image courtesy of OpenStax College CC BY 3.0 via Wikimedia Commons

There was a long gap from the revelation by Dr. Jacob Van Meekeren in 1668 to the discovery by Dr. N. Senn in 1889 that a decalcified substance from bone marrow could heal aseptic bone. It was even much later when Urist repeated the finding in 1965 and labeled the substance bone morphogenetic protein. Over the next few decades the various BMPs were found to be biochemically related to the transforming growth factor β (**TGF-β**) family. After being identified and coded according to function, the role of BMPs was seen to extend far beyond proliferation, differentiation and potential for bone repair. BMPs have many regulatory functions in other cells as well.

BMPs are involved in a *"wide range of biological activities in various cell types, including epithelial cells, mesenchymal cells, endothelial cells, monocytes, and neuronal cells." (Miyazono and Shimanuki, 2008)*

BMP-2 is seen in large amounts in lung, spleen, and colon, and less but significant amounts in the heart, brain, liver, skeletal muscle, pancreas, kidney, prostate, ovaries, and small intestine. (Fitzgerald, et al., 2002) Because it has been observed to be involved in fracture repair (Fig. 5.6) and in the production of bone and cartilage, BMP2 has been experimented with for its possible assistance in bone grafts. It has so far had sketchy but promising results for bone grafts, and was somewhat successful for cervical spinal fusions. Noteworthy are the reports of reduced rates of osteoarthritis after surgery when BMP-2 was used. (Winn, 2017)

That said, post-operative adverse events suggest caution in isolating a particular protein expecting it to produce the same results by itself in the role it otherwise plays in concert with many other co-factors. Aaron W. James, MD reported that side effects like life-threatening swelling, tumors, ectopic bone formation, bone resorption, inflammation, and inappropriate adipogenesis have accompanied the use of BMP-2 in place of bone grafts. [124](James, et al., 2016) Surgery itself is a trauma, so post-surgical guidance about how to minimize those after-effects would be very beneficial even without the use of BMP-2.

WORKING WITH SHOCK AND TRAUMA

Another option would be to enhance or stimulate the system's propensity to read the tissue field, and to mobilize its own sequence of repair mechanisms. Injuries, surgeries, and prolonged illness have been known to create a type of sensory-motor amnesia; a trauma/freeze response that could be preventing the body's proper assessment and response to the healing process. We've seen this so many times in somatic education and manual therapy. It can be corrected when taken into consideration as an initial step in the stages of recovery. Checking for unresolved forces is a key factor.

It could also be useful to have a collaboration of perspectives in the difficult-to-mend or chronic pain scenarios so they could be more successful. In one situation, an orthopedic chiropractor and I worked together to reestablish smooth functioning in a patient following a hip replacement. The reeducation process included gait training after alignment and other biomechanical forms of balance and integration were offered into her system. From a somatic education perspective, a system needs to be able to sense itself accurately in order to make appropriate changes.

If inherent systems are not engaging in the repair process yet, or a condition has become chronic, most likely the body's energy and attention is engaged in another process that the system views as a priority, or it is 'shut down' so to speak, and can't mobilize its resources. There are often forces still at work that need to be resolved in order for energy and attention to proceed towards the primary symptom.

In one instance, with a client who was in chronic pain years after a fall off a cliff, the pressure from the muscles of the pelvic floor and sacral attachments were unyielding. (Fig. 5.7) She'd landed on her feet, sustained compression fractures in several vertebrae, and needed a rod in her mid-back. While the system is still in a state of 'limbo' with dysregulated, restricted fluid patterns, the primary lesion may continue to be underneath the surface 'noise' generated by the agitated nervous system producing symptoms in many areas.

Although the majority of her pain was near the screws attaching the rod to her body, the source was further down. Much of the force from the fall was still situated in her pelvic floor, limiting the degree of motion her spine was still capable of. (Fig. 5.7) In particular, the **iliococcygeus muscle** and **sacrotuberous ligaments** were binding the action of her low back and pelvis after the hip flexors and hip rotators were released. When the pressure from those long-held, deeper muscles was reduced, and the ligaments were balanced, she said she felt great and was able to function much more easily without pain. Although it was tempting to assume the area of all the hardware was responsible, her body revealed that further down in the tissue field was locked, fluids were restricted, minimalizing the levels of interaction that needed to happen between cells for fuller, freer functioning to happen.

The center of gravity often captures longitudinal forces due to the horizontal anatomy in the area at a few different vantage points. The broad ligament would be another place to look for ensnared forces as it runs laterally, attaching the female reproductive structures to the ilium. There is a possibility that balancing trapped forces in the tissue fields is a primary step in a healing process. These tissue and fluid fields are the domains where trophic substances and regulatory information need to be transmitted. Lingering pain and restriction could be reflections of the unresolved trauma, which also has a biomechanical and neurophysiological manifestation.

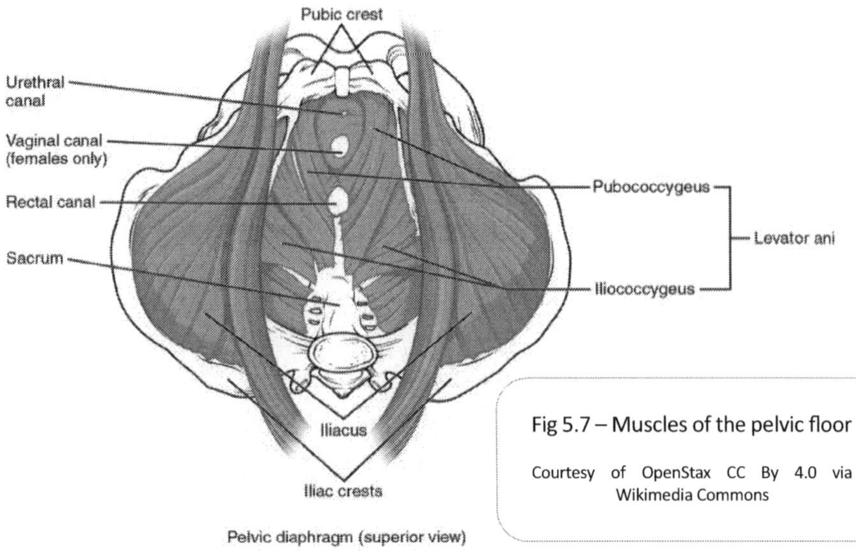

Fig 5.7 – Muscles of the pelvic floor

Courtesy of OpenStax CC By 4.0 via Wikimedia Commons

> I greatly admire the success story of the 'dancing molecules' researchers, whereby a severe spinal cord injury was restored by using an injection included in nanofibers that mimicked the action of 100,000 molecules. [127]

The molecules were moving; they were dynamic like the body is in its natural state. The materials injected included a facsimile of the ECM, and had receptor sites built into it. This may be that the most promising direction for future research to deepen its understanding about the therapeutic use of cellular communication. It provides a whole template the system needs in order to recognize itself in its natural, fully functional state, using a language that it can decode and respond to in kind.

It could be useful to consider the entire environment as part of the process rather than looking for the absence or addition of a single molecule. Looking at the process as a whole from start to finish, as being a conversation that the system is having with itself in the form of a dynamic, biochemical profile of that patient's system, may be revelatory. Perhaps the correct chemistry is present but not interacting due to any type of stagnation that could suppress the system while in the residuals of shock. It could be that a resetting the barometer would be a useful place to begin, instead of assuming that the system is able to take care of that step on its own.

Shock is clinically defined as a restriction of blood flow whereby the cells don't receive essential oxygen and nutrients, and are unable to remove metabolic waste products. Many other symptoms appear in serious cases. (Walters, 1967, Basu, 2021, Bononno, 2011) Severe cases can be life-threatening, but mild to moderate cases leading to pain and dysfunction are generally overlooked. Presentations of unresolved shock may vary based upon the initiating incident. A burn will be different from a fall, which will be different from surgical interventions, or traumatic brain injury, or the layers of emotional trauma, a head-on collision, and so on. Lingering scars may not take a form that's visible.

Perhaps what is needed can become clearer based upon the understanding of where the breakdown in communication happened. Up to now, almost everyone I see as a client who has been in chronic pain presents with stagnation in the fluids (CSF, lymph, and blood) with restricted motion in the major organs and imbalances (malalignment) in the spine and cranium that limit primary respiration. Once these imbalances and restrictions are corrected, the body's proprioceptive sensing is often back online and can more fully utilize its own resources to heal.

Erythropoietin (EPO) is a tissue and neuroprotective cytokine and glycoprotein kidney hormone that is usually known for its role in stimulating red blood cell production, but is now under investigation as a potential assistant in spinal cord injuries. It is derived mainly from the renal cortex, but is also produced in small amounts in the liver, brain, bone marrow and spleen. From the perspective of Alfredo Gorio and his team of researchers, saving neurons (oligodendrites) from death in a serious injury is a major focus. They found that retaining myelination and blood flow has been able to restore motor function much more quickly in the case of an aneurysm or major spinal contusion in animal models by using recombinant EPO injections and their receptors. [125](Carelli et al., 2017, Gorio et al., 2002) It has also been found helpful in bone and cartilage repair, (Wan et al., 2014) and shown to reduce inflammation and cell death, thereby perhaps being useful in neurodegenerative diseases. (Federica Rey, et al., 2019) From the biochemical aspects of the healing process, using interventions that facilitate regeneration using precursors that can jumpstart the natural cascade of signaling is also optimal and very promising.

BMPS AND NEUROGENESIS

Gabriel Jensen et al. find that BMP signaling is critically important for the development of both the central and peripheral nervous systems, along with neurogenesis. It is possible that this is the 'how' as to the connection of bone loss and dementia, since it has been shown that exercise stimulates **BMP4** signaling in the hippocampus and dentate gyrus. (Kessler, 2017) One study reported the dysregulation of **BMP6** in the hippocampus of Alzheimer's patients, with an over-expression of BMP6 mRNA. However, further testing by this group of researchers revealed that the presence of Amyloid β plaques created a 25% increase in BMP6 and other proteins. (Leslie Crews, et al., Journal of Neuroscience, 2010)

> Jensen goes on to say that over a half dozen BMPs and their receptors are found in the lateral ventricles, choroid plexus, the sub-ventricular zone, hypothalamus, medulla, hippocampus, olfactory bulbs, cortex, and striatum of adult mammal brains, accentuating their role in neurogenesis, astrogliogenesis, and gliogenesis.

BMP7 has been shown to stimulate neurogenesis and be a protector in stroke and severe injury. It is suspected that BMP6 may also have a similar role. BMP6 and BMP7 have both been seen in the meninges. (Barneda-Zahonero et al., 2009) **BMP12** and **BMP13** have been found in the spinal cord, but not the brain.

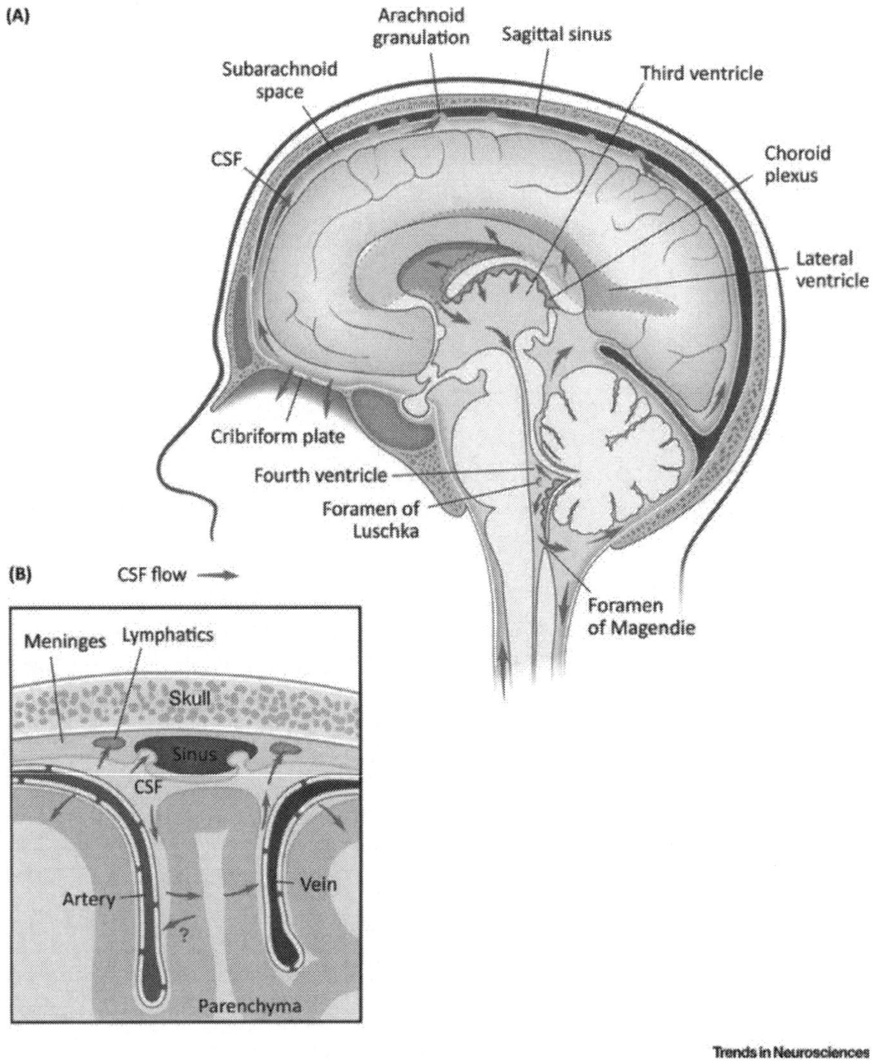

Fig. 5.8 - Diagram of the circulation of cerebral spinal fluid in the brain

Image Courtesy of OpenStax CC BY 4.0 via Wikimedia Commons

Jensen mentions that, "BMPs also have the potential to influence brain regions far from where they are expressed, due to the brain's ventricular transport system...As BMP7 has been found to circulate within the cerebrospinal fluid, BMP7 may be produced in the choroid plexus and bind to cells at the brain-CSF interface." (Fig. 5.8) Using rodent examples to investigate the role of BMPs in spinal cord injuries, Al-Sammarraie and Ray's in vitro study revealed that **BMP2, 4, and 7** '*increased in neurons, microglia, oligodendrocytes, and neural stem cells after the spinal cord injury, promoting differentiation of* ***astrocytes*** *(Fig.5.9) and inhibiting differentiation of oligodendrocytes.*' Her team attempted to clarify the roles of these particular BMPs' signaling in 'neuronal and/or glial cell proliferation, differentiation, survival, apoptosis, autophagy, and inflammation in spinal cord injuries.' [126](Nadi Al-Sammarraie and Swapan K. Ray, 2021)

Northwestern University is experimenting with a promising, novel therapy for spinal cord injuries that has yielded great results in vitro and in mice so far. It has combined a functional, cellular communication approach with an injectable nanotechnology that has been successful in reversing paralysis. Samuel Stupp, who is founder of the Simpson Querrey Institute for BioNanotechnology and its research arm, Center for Regenerative Nanomedicine, explains the method this way:

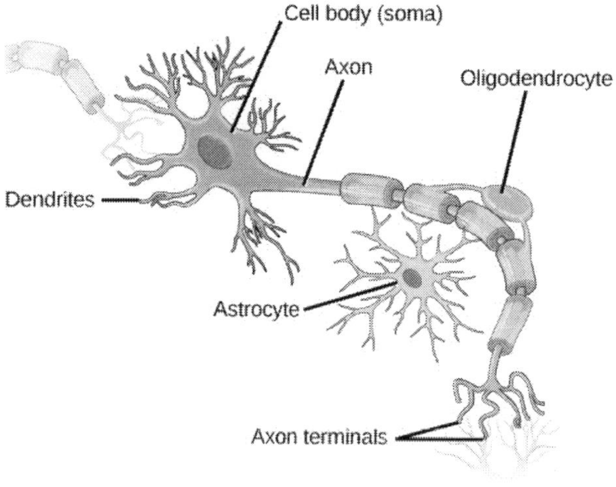

Fig. 5.9 – Illustration of astrocytes and oligodendrites

CNX OpenStax CC BY 4.0 via Wikimedia Commons

"Injected as a liquid, the therapy immediately gels into a network of nanofibers that mimic the extracellular makeup of the spinal cord. By matching the matrix's structure, mimicking the motion of biological molecules and incorporating signals for receptors, the synthetic materials are able to communicate with the cells. Receptors in neurons and other cells constantly move around. The key innovation in our research which has never been done before is to control the motion of more than 100,000 molecules within our nanofibers." [127](Samuel Stupp, 2021)

The widespread expression and regulatory functions of BMPs and their ability to have balancing effects throughout the body is in support of the healing potential of cranial osteopathic approaches at a cellular level. Stupp's findings are also in support of the perspective that reeducating the system using/inputting patterns of movement that represent the normal coordinated activity can trigger a reset, similar to the 'restore' function on a computer. Jensen and his team report that, *"In addition to the CSF and vasculature expression of **BMP2, BMP3, BMP4, BMP5, 6, 7, BMP8b**, and **BMP8,** they have been identified along the ependyma of the ventricles and throughout most hypothalamic regions."*

Included in manual therapy for the brain's nuclei, as well as in Biodynamic Cranial work, is a focus in the areas of the thalamus, and hippocampus, the 3rd and 4th ventricles, along with balanced CSF flow in and around the brain and through the spinal cord. Those unfamiliar with the potential of these gentle methods may not easily understand how balancing the 'fluid body' and levels of activation in the brain can have such far-reaching effects. Unpeeling the cellular level of communication can demystify and validate why these methods are beneficial. The health benefits may be more than we imagined and more easily explained by BMP functions.Jensen and his group of researchers also focused on the probability that metabolism and weight loss are also regulated by this group of transcription factors. They state that, *"We and others have highlighted the roles of **BMP7,** and **BMP8**, as well as BMP receptor 1A in reducing weight by modulating hypothalamic signaling, appetite, and sympathetic outflow to adipose depots.*

The current worldwide obesity pandemic highlights the importance of understanding BMPs in the context of both neural plasticity and energy balance regulation, as BMPs directly impact body weight, food intake, and energy expenditure, at least in part through the plasticity of the hypothalamus." [128](Jensen, Leon-Palmer, and Townsend, 2021)

Due to the presence of numerous BMPs in the **arcuate nucleus**, (Fig.5.10) which circulates signals of hunger and satiety based upon stored energy and nutrients, and the ependymal cells of the third ventricle where tanycytes are located, Jensen is building upon the theory that some aspects of obesity and the difficulty in losing weight is regulated by BMPs in the brain. Jensen states that, "*Our work as well as the work of others has demonstrated that BMPs and their receptors are important for the regulation of energy balance both by acting in the CNS to regulate appetite, and by stimulating sympathetic activity in brown adipose tissue (BAT), as well as promoting the development and production of heat producing, calorie-burning brown adipocytes.*

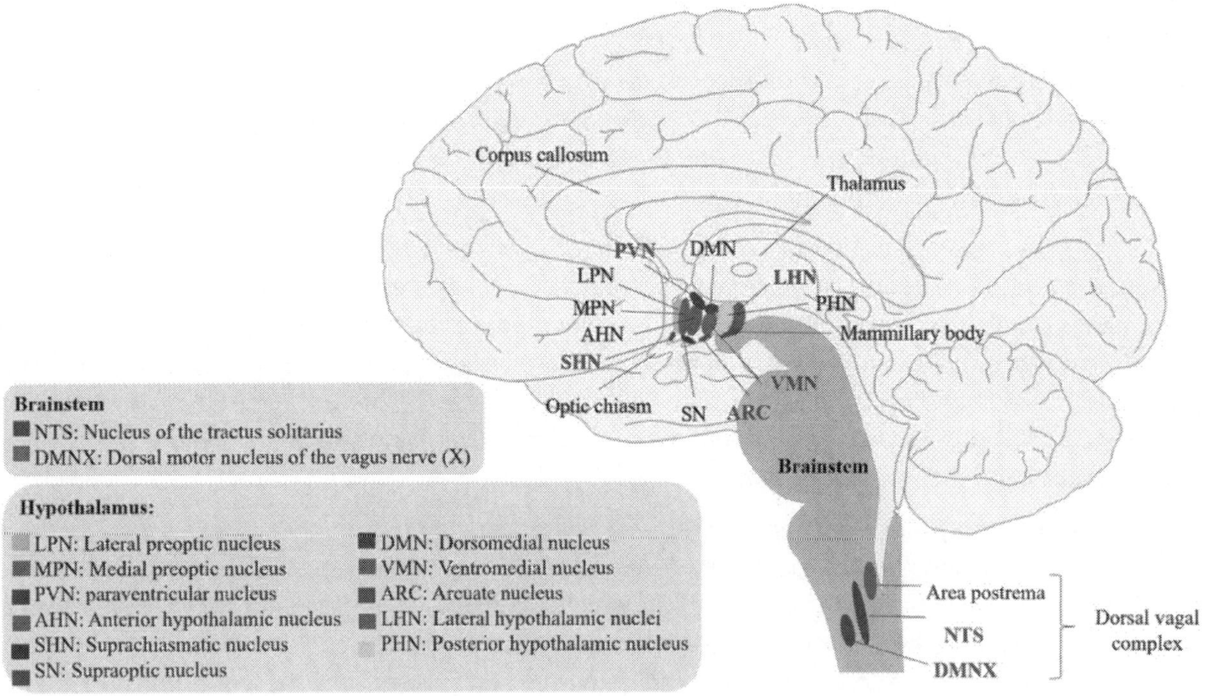

Fig. 5.10 – Arcuate nucleus and hypothalamic regions, brain stem Various BMPs bind to receptors and are stored, regulated, and phosphorylated in Smad proteins before being transported to transcription co-factors and before being activated for gene expression in the cell nucleus.

The ability of BDNF (Brain-derived neurotrophic factor) signaling in the hypothalamus to regulate appetite, as well as energy expenditure via sympathetic innervation of adipose tissue may be dependent upon changes in hypothalamic neurogenesis."

Much of how bone morphogenetic proteins continue to function in adulthood is still being investigated. Their role in the proliferation, differentiation, and regulation of osteoblasts and chondrocytes has been clarified, and many of BMPs' functions in the brain and nervous system are coming into view. There is still much to learn about the complex interactions with the endocrine system, the kidneys, pancreas, liver, urogenital system, and cardiovascular system. It has already been pointed out that the circulation of certain BMPs in the cerebrospinal fluid gives them access to distant target sites, and apparently the same is true for the circulatory system.

Nicholas Morrell, et al reported that, *"Several BMPs, including **BMP6, BMP9, and BMP10** also circulate in blood, and have the potential to exert effects on distant tissues and organs.*

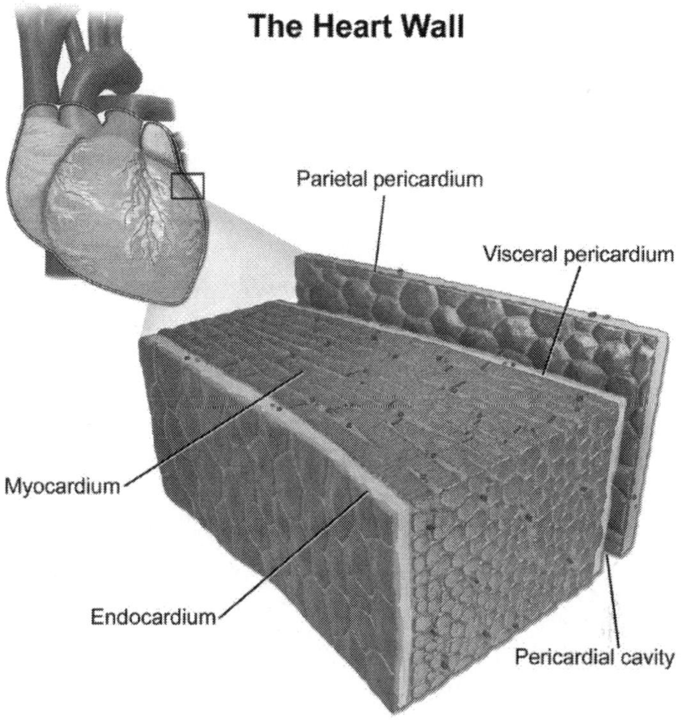

Fig. 5.11- Illustration of the pericardium and endocardium

Image courtesy of Blaus.com staff (2014) "Medical gallery of Blausen Medical 2014" WikiJournal of Medicine 1(2); CC BY 3.0, via WikiMedia Commons

BMPs thereby function as an important endocrine regulator of cardiovascular, metabolic, and hematopoietic function. As a group, these molecules have essential roles in vasculogenesis, cardiomyogenesis, ventricular compaction, valve formation, and maintenance of the integrity of the pulmonary and lymphatic circulation."

What is also fascinating, is that BMPs are often named as being located and involved in epithelial, endothelial, and, in this case epicardium cells. (Fig.5.11) Morrell states, *"The epicardium has been shown to serve as an important reservoir of cardiac fibroblasts and vascular smooth muscle progenitors in the developing heart, and plays an important role in cardiac repair after injury."* [129](Morrell et al., 2016) These authors also found that BMP signaling mutations are implicated in pulmonary arterial hypertension, vascular calcification, tumor angiogenesis, and anemia, in addition to participating in the repair of the heart post infarct. Releasing and balancing forces in the pericardium with a myofascial method could protect the action of the BMPs in this region and support protective mechanisms at the cellular level.

BMPs are located in numerous epithelial cells, acting to protect them from oxidative stress, and to otherwise perform a regenerative function, including around the eye and heart. (Bei Du, et al., 2020; Dronkers et al., 2020) There is some evidence that BMPs are also involved in the regulation of skin inflammation (Sconnochia, et al., 2021), skin cell regeneration, pigmentation, and hair follicle regulation. (Singh, 2012; Botchkarev, 2003) They are also found to act on a variety of lymphoid and myeloid cells to promote anti-inflammatory responses. BMP7 is secreted by dendritic cells, so dysregulation in the nervous system could likely trigger dysfunction in signaling downstream.

As recently as 2021, Hua Mao and a team of researchers report that BMPs are also active at the layer of the endothelium in adult mammals. They state, *"More than 100 million U.S. adults are now living with diabetes or prediabetes, a condition that, if not treated, often leads to Type 2 diabetes within 5 years. BMP-binding endothelial regulator* ***(BMPER)*** *adapts endothelial cells to inflammatory stress in diverse organ microenvironments. Both global and endothelial cell-specific inducible knockout of BMPER cause hyperinsulinemia, glucose intolerance, and insulin resistance without increasing inflammation in metabolic tissues in mice*." [130](Hua Mao, et al., 2021)

It appears then, that BMPs are involved in regulating glucose metabolism, but also plays a role in regulating the immune system. Michal Kuczma reports that, "*Recently, BMPs were found to regulate cells of the innate and adaptive immune system. BMPs are involved in thymic development of T cells at the early, double negative, as well as later double positive stages of thymopoiesis*." (Kuczma and Kraj, 2015) Lauren Browning and her team describe BMPs as 'immunoregulatory cytokines.'

They state, *"Thus, we establish that BMPs, a large cytokine family, are an essential link between stroma tissues and the adaptive immune system involved in sustaining tissue homeostasis by promoting immunological tolerance." (Browning, et al., 2020)*

Bone morphogenetic proteins are involved in numerous regulatory functions in several organ systems along with those directly connected to bones and connective tissue. There are many types of research currently underway related to the therapeutic use of BMPs (i.e. BMP2 and BMP7) but very few have obtained FDA approval. Explorations have happened on non-union long bone fractures, pelvic fractures and in place of bone grafts in certain facial reconstructions. But due to the expense, sophistication of the complex signaling interactions involved between systems, and potential side effects, more study is needed before their use becomes more commonplace. Products that are beginning to show up on the market for internal use, and the long term consequences of trying them may not be available. Studies have not yet been done to guarantee their safety for internal or external use, but the therapeutic potential is very promising. ``

Similar to the uppermost layers of structure and function, the innermost microenvironment is also intricately interconnected and interdependent. It can be useful to consider that a mishap at the nanomolecular level can be reflected in numerous categories of discomfort and disease in various stages. This is one reason to respond to the initial signs of discomfort in any system. These signaling systems are regulatory, so if one becomes over or under expressed, it impacts a protein or pathway that alters the homeostasis of downstream targets.

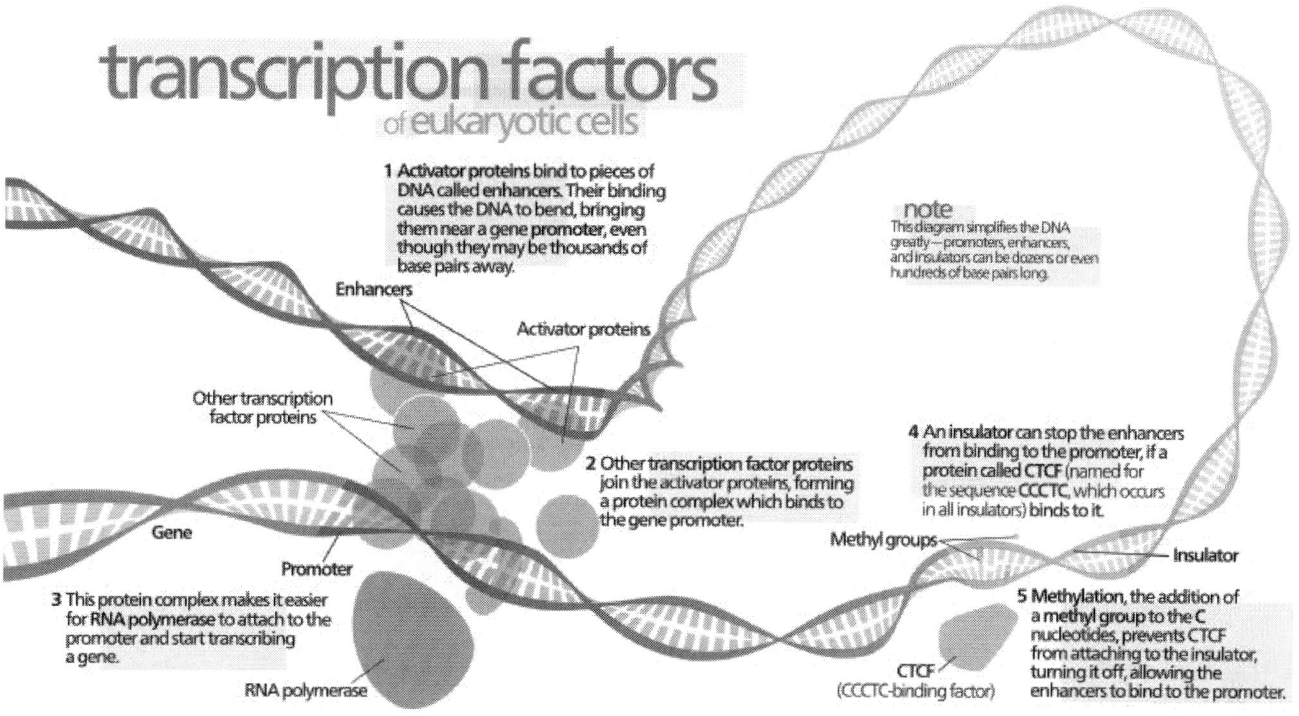

transcription factors
of eukaryotic cells
1 Activator proteins bind to pieces of DNA called enhancers. Their binding causes the DNA to bend, bringing them near a gene promoter, even though they may be thousands of base pairs away.
note
This diagram simplifies the DNA greatly—promoters, enhancers, and insulators can be dozens or even hundreds of base pairs long.
Enhancers
Activator proteins
Other transcription factor proteins
2 Other transcription factor proteins join the activator proteins, forming a protein complex which binds to the gene promoter.
4 An insulator can stop the enhancers from binding to the promoter, if a protein called CTCF (named for the sequence CCCTC, which occurs in all insulators) binds to it.
Methyl groups
Insulator
Gene
Promoter
3 This protein complex makes it easier for RNA polymerase to attach to the promoter and start transcribing a gene.
RNA polymerase
CTCF
(CCCTC-binding factor)
5 Methylation, the addition of a methyl group to the C nucleotides, prevents CTCF from attaching to the insulator, turning it off, allowing the enhancers to bind to the promoter.

Mikäel Haggström, used with permission, Public Domain via Wikimedia Commons

For example, Milena Stevanovic et al. stated in 2021 that, "SOX proteins influence survival, regeneration, cell death, and control homeostasis in adult tissues. Distinct SOX members determine down-stream processes of neuronal and glial differentiation. Deregulation of specific SOX protein activities is associated with neurodegenerative diseases." Alessia Omenetti et al., find that Hh signaling pathway modulates wound healing responses in a number of adult tissues and is particularly involved in the regeneration of the liver and GI tract.

Omenetti's team also found a variety of tissues synthesize the Hedgehog protein in response to tissue construction or remodeling, including the ovaries, testes, and peripheral nerves. The Wnt signaling pathway is also used in tissue remodeling for systems other than skin. Steinhart and Angers reported in 2018 that, "Human genetics data perhaps best highlight the crucial role of Wnt-β-catenin signaling in bone tissue homeostasis." So BMPs are not working alone in this function.

The signaling pathways are as important as the ligands that use them, as the target receptors that are intended in the regulatory process. The transcription factors on their way to the cell nucleus are only as effective as the coherence of every step along the way, including the matrix and the cell membrane. Although the biological processes involving transcription factors are very complex and conserved throughout our lifetime, the takeaway is that their activity is profoundly influenced by the lifestyle factors mentioned in the text. That's the good news that places us at the helm of that fluid, sometimes elusive thing we call 'health'.

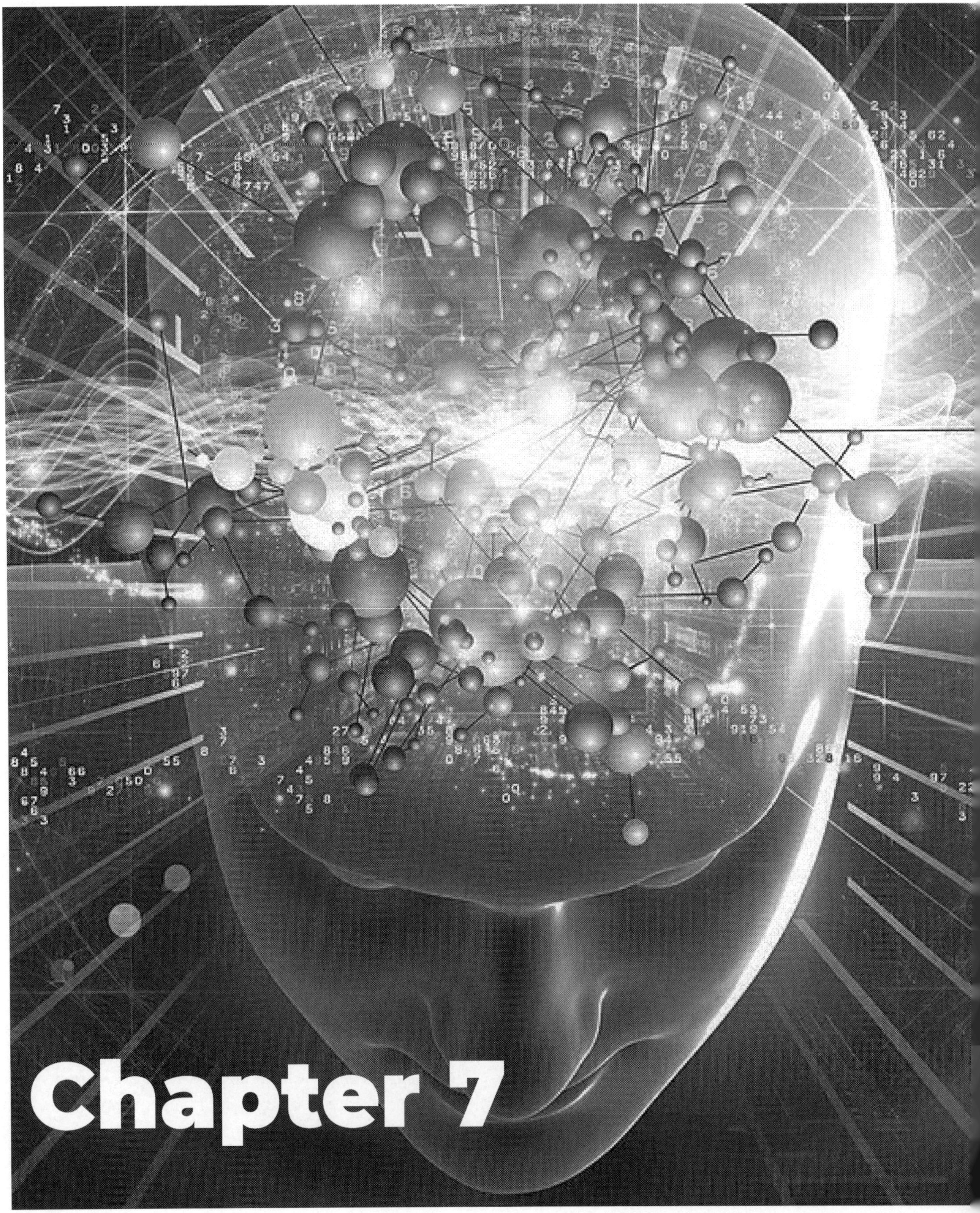

Chapter 7

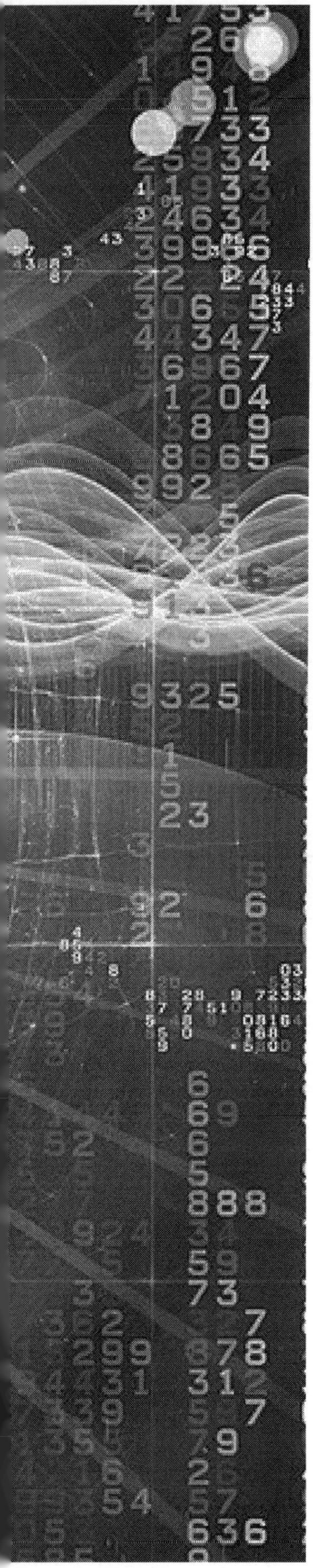

Crosstalk between Bones and Other Systems

Organs and our Bones

KIDNEYS, LIVER, AND PARATHYROID

There is an intimate relationship between the **kidneys** and the bones, aside from their initial embryogenetic interactions. This is most likely why in Chinese medicine it is said that the kidneys govern bones. BMP7, which is able to stimulate the production of new bone, and has been used to heal fractures, treat osteoarthritis and disc degeneration, is produced in the kidneys. Low levels are produced in the bones, but the main source for this vital protein comes from the kidneys. In addition, 90% of **EPO (erythropoietin)**, a glycoprotein, kidney hormone, and cytokine that has a role in neurogenesis and in the regulation of red blood cell production in bone marrow, is produced by the kidneys; in the renal cortex and outer medulla. (Fig.7.2) [131](Wei, Yin, and Xie, 1016)

The **liver** also maintains crosstalk with bones through signals generated by **osteopontin**, osteocalcin, and **osteoprotegerin**. Musso and his team postulated that dysfunction within the interactions between bone, the liver, and adipose tissue could result in non-alcoholic fatty liver disease, osteoporosis and diabetes. (Giovanni Musso, et al., 2013) Kumar and Roger are researchers who salute the emerging field of **osteoimmunology**, which is being more closely examined for its connection to osteoporosis, periodontitis, osteomyelitis, septic arthritis, and bone infections. They state that, *"After a decade of research, it seems that almost all immune cells are capable of communicating with bone cells and vice versa."* (Gaurav Kumar and Pierre-Marie Roger, 2019) Jin Shao et al. have labeled it an endocrine organ due to its role in glucose metabolism and regulation.

The kidneys maintain a direct connection to bones throughout life. They affect bone development, remodeling, and repair by regulating calcium and phosphate homeo-stasis, producing cytokines, and clearing bone regulators.

> According to Chinese Medicine, the kidneys are the *"most fundamental organ system of your body, which holds the genetic blueprint of your inherent body constitution and how healthy you will be."*

Some say that kidneys need to be protected from the cold, and that wintertime is the season for them to be rested and recharged. (EuYanSang.com, 2022)

Aubrey Lewis states that vital energy is stored in the kidneys to be used in time of illness or stress, but that the **jing/essence** of kidneys can become depleted with trauma, illness, injury, fear, and frustration. Lewis states, *"The kidneys are also responsible for the production of marrow, which in Chinese Medicine consists of bones, bone marrow, brain, and spinal cord. Therefore, a person's growth, maturation, and aging process are governed by the kidneys."* [132](Aubrey Lewis, 2021) My osteopathic teachers, Barral and Croibier, also emphasized the importance of regularly attending to the kidneys; the left one in particular due to its relationship to vitality and urogenital functions.

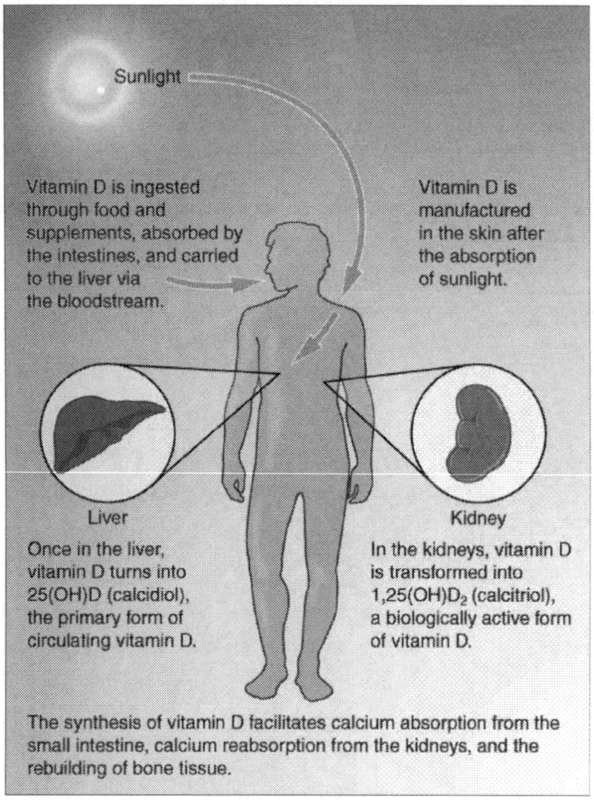

Sunlight
Vitamin D is ingested through food and supplements, absorbed by the intestines, and carried to the liver via the bloodstream.
Vitamin D is manufactured in the skin after the absorption of sunlight.
Liver
Once in the liver, vitamin D turns into 25(OH)D (calcidiol), the primary form of circulating vitamin D.
Kidney
In the kidneys, vitamin D is transformed into 1,25(OH)D$_2$ (calcitriol), a biologically active form of vitamin D.
The synthesis of vitamin D facilitates calcium absorption from the small intestine, calcium reabsorption from the kidneys, and the rebuilding of bone tissue.

Fig.7.1 – How the body uses sunlight through the kidneys and liver to produce a viable form of vitamin D

Too little or too much free calcium in the blood create unpleasant symptoms which may not readily be associated with calcium levels. Too little or too much vitamin D can also cause issues, but most come from too little. When **ultraviolet B rays** from the sun touch our skin, a precursor to **vitamin D3** (7-dehydrocholesterol) in the skin absorbs it and sends it to the liver, then the kidneys, where it becomes a biologically active form known as **calcitrol**. (Fig7.1)

The 25-hydroxyvitamin D is the circulating form, and 1,25-dihydroxyvitamin D is the **biologically active form of D**, which reaches the receptors of the many cells and organs in the body that use it for a variety of purposes. It also plays a major role in regulating calcium and phosphate metabolism for maintenance of metabolic functions and skeletal health. (Wacker and Holick, 2013) Xiao-Qin Wang and his team of researchers offered a blend between Eastern and Western views of the kidneys.

They report, *"Calcitrol and parathyroid hormone (PTH) provide tight control of plasma calcium levels through a negative feedback loop that regulates three pathways: intestinal uptake, renal reabsorption, and skeletal release of calcium and phosphate resulting in mineralization of the skeleton and greater bone density.*

In Chinese Medicine, kidney Qi Deficiency, or poor kidney function, leads to pathologically low calcitrol levels, leading to osteoporosis and osteomalacia." [133] (Xiao-Qin Wang, et al., 2016)

The authors list several Chinese herbal medicines as being helpful to tonify, detox, and improve renal function. Wang emphasizes that a disturbance in the yin/yang balance of kidney essence can accelerate the aging process and influence the progression of chronic disease. From an Eastern perspective, kidney essence can nourish bone marrow and strengthen the skeleton. He also mentions that among patients being treated for bone fractures, those using Chinese herbs as part of their recovery process healed faster, with reduced medical expenses. The herbal medicine group also had fewer cardiovascular complications, and reduced incidence of diabetes, stroke, and chronic obstructive pulmonary disease.

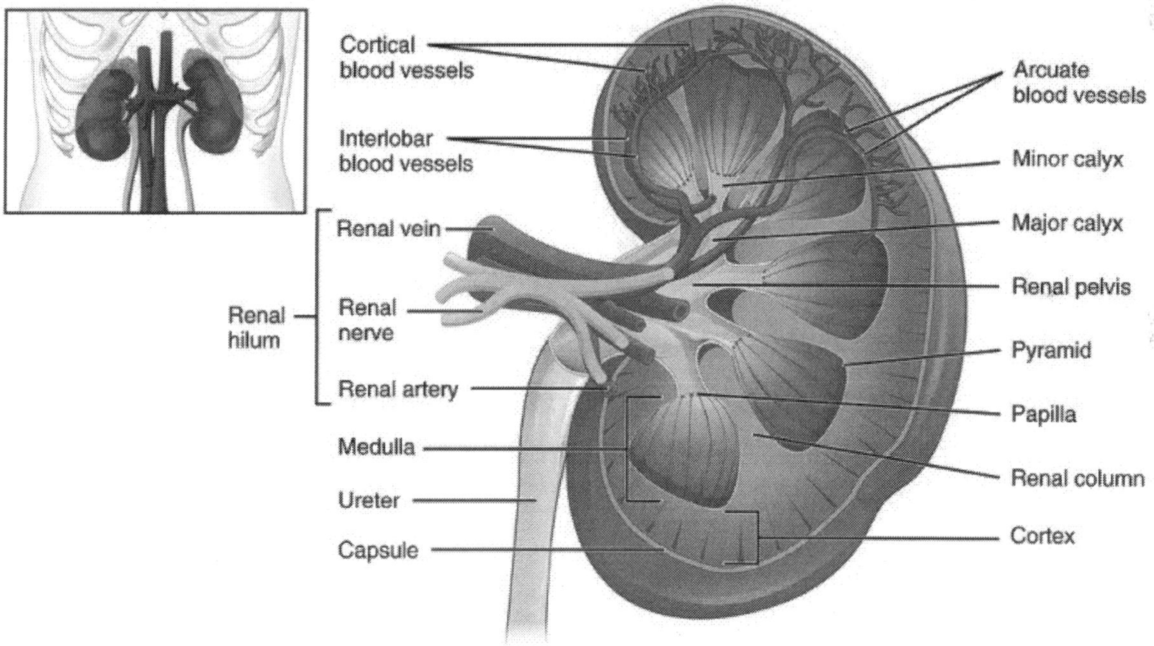

Fig.7.2 – Illustration of kidney anatomy

Image Courtesy of OpenStax CC BY 4.0 via Wikimedia Commons

Klotho is an FGF23 (fibroblast growth factor 23) co-factor, also considered to be an anti-aging protein, that plays a role in calcium-phosphate homeostasis. It is mainly expressed in the choroid plexus of the brain, the parathyroid gland, and the kidneys, and is secreted by osteoblasts and osteocytes. Wang states that, "*The **bone-kidney axis**, based on the bone-secreted FGF23 and the kidney expressed Klotho, plays a crucial role in calcium/phosphate metabolism and vitamin D regulation.*" This researcher links the presence of Klotho as the potential molecular equivalent of Kidney Essence that generates Kidney Qi, having the ability to offset signs of aging.

Apparently some studies have shown those having low levels of Klotho to be correlated with cardiovascular issues, fatigue, back pain, and pain or weakness in the knees, and diabetes due to inefficient glucose metabolism which involves both bones and kidneys. Although results vary and can even be contradictory in humans, in animals, higher levels of Klotho with lower levels of IGF-1 (insulin-like growth factor) represented longer life spans and stable or increased insulin resistance. (Vitale, 2019)

The renal hormone mentioned earlier, EPO (erythropoietin), gives even more credence to the importance of the kidneys in overall health. EPO is also related to the health of intervertebral discs and nerves in a protective role. *(Grosso et al. 2017, Vitale, 2019, Gorio, 2002)*

EPO also serves endochondral ossification, chondrogenesis and differentiation, and VEGF-mediated (vascular endothelial growth factor) angiogenesis during fractures. (Wan, et al., 2014) Researcher, Patricia Kimáková, also labeled EPO as a hematopoietic hormone, cytokine, and pleiotropic growth factor that "exhibits growth stimulation and cell/tissue protection on numerous cells and tissues." (Kimáková, et al., 2017)

The intricate relationship between bones and kidneys is so impactful, that Kai Wei's researchers recommend looking for kidney disease as the underlying cause when there are disturbances in bone, such as osteodystrophy. {113}{Wei et al., 2016} The liver has an additional relationship with bone metabolism, in that IGFBP1 (insulin growth factor binding protein 1), which stimulates osteoclast activity and plays a role in muscle building or growth (C.P. Velloso, 2008), is abundantly expressed in the liver. **IGF1** (insulin-like growth factor) stimulates osteoblast/bone building activity, (Fig.7.4) and has been shown to be at lower levels while there is liver disease. (Chung and Insogna, 2016) There is also some evidence revealing that **BMP9** can be helpful in regenerating the liver, but can also cause problems if it's out of balance.

Tuo Ji and his team of researchers found that **BMP 2, 4, and 7** are active in regulating epithelial cell proliferation and differentiation in the intestines, while BMP4 is particularly responsive to tissue issues and inflammation in the intestines. (Ji et al., 2016) On the other hand, injury and damage can interfere with BMP4 signaling and promote inflammation in the belly. I want to emphasize again and again the importance of conceiving of and correcting the impacts of injuries, infections, toxins, obesity, traumas, or surgeries/scar tissue at the level of how it influences cellular communication. Once the effects of an incident or series of experiences are no longer painful, are managed by medications or adapted to, we don't consider the micro environment that is still working with them on another level where there may still be imbalances. In this realm, even the macro environment is still pretty tiny.

Realizing that everything is processed at the cellular level throughout this intricate network of soft, hard, and fluid tissues, the idea of working with the systems that bear the most responsibility for regulating the others might make more sense. We have access to these cells! Bone serves multiple purposes in our

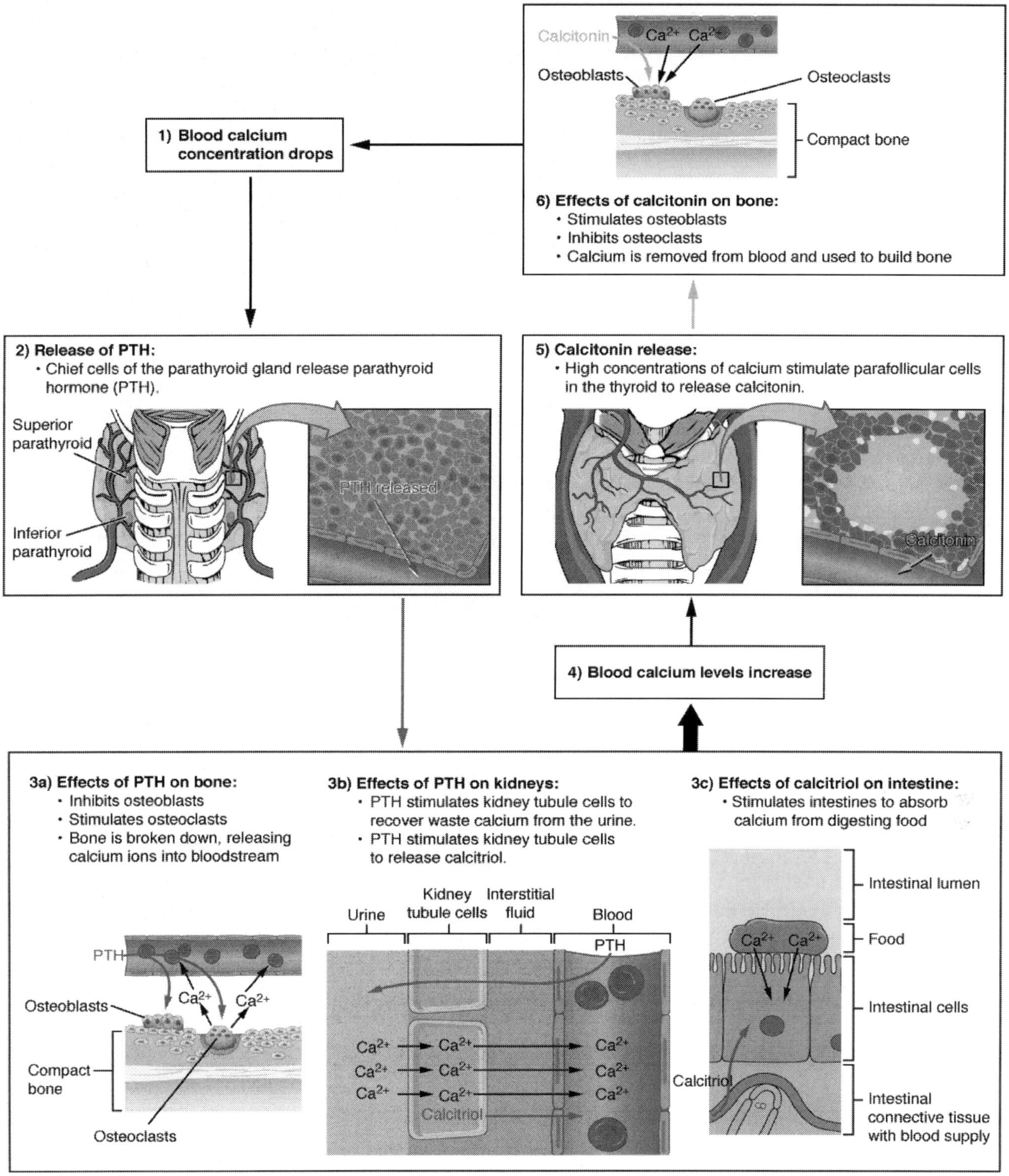

Calcitonin
Ca2+ Ca2+
Osteoblasts
Osteoclasts
Compact bone
6) Effects of calcitonin on bone:
• Stimulates osteoblasts
• Inhibits osteoclasts
• Calcium is removed from blood and used to build bone
1) Blood calcium concentration drops
2) Release of PTH:
• Chief cells of the parathyroid gland release parathyroid hormone (PTH).
Superior parathyroid
Inferior parathyroid
PTH released
5) Calcitonin release:
• High concentrations of calcium stimulate parafollicular cells in the thyroid to release calcitonin.
Calcitonin
4) Blood calcium levels increase
3a) Effects of PTH on bone:
• Inhibits osteoblasts
• Stimulates osteoclasts
• Bone is broken down, releasing calcium ions into bloodstream
PTH
Ca2+ Ca2+
Osteoblasts
Compact bone
Osteoclasts
3b) Effects of PTH on kidneys:
• PTH stimulates kidney tubule cells to recover waste calcium from the urine.
• PTH stimulates kidney tubule cells to release calcitriol.
Urine
Kidney tubule cells
Interstitial fluid
Blood
PTH
Ca2+ Ca2+ Ca2+
Calcitriol
3c) Effects of calcitriol on intestine:
• Stimulates intestines to absorb calcium from digesting food
Intestinal lumen
Food
Ca2+ Ca2+
Intestinal cells
Calcitriol
Intestinal connective tissue with blood supply

Fig. 7.3 – Illustration of the relationship between the parathyroid, kidneys and bones

When the parathyroid senses that calcium levels in the blood are low, it signals osteoclasts in bone to release calcium, then signals the kidneys to reabsorb rather than excrete calcium. It then increases the extraction of calcium from food in the intestines by stimulating calcitriol, which is made in the kidneys from vitamin D3. When free calcium levels rise, the parathyroid releases PTH, which signals the osteoclasts to stop dissolving bone, and signals the kidneys to excrete excess calcium in the urine, while the thyroid releases calcitonin which signals osteoblasts to use circulating calcium in the blood to build bone.

bodies, many of which have not reached the public en masse, which is why it is a focus of this book. There is hardly any system in the body that bones don't influence or share communication with. What might change when there's been a break, strain, bruise or compression?

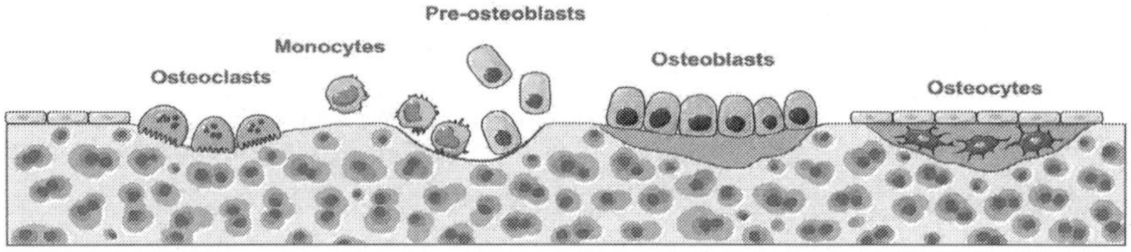

Fig.7.4 - Bone remodeling process

Image courtesy of OpenStax College CC BY 3.0 via Wikimedia Commons

Osteocalcin (OCN), a hormone secreted by bone, promotes proliferation of β cells in addition to targeting them in the pancreas, liver, and muscles. Osteocalcin also promotes insulin secretion and insulin sensitivity, and regulates fat cells as well as male gonad activity through the production of testosterone.

> According to geneticist, Gérard Karsenty, osteocalcin keeps blood sugar in check, burns fat, maintains brain functions, can restore memory, and trigger a fight/flight response and the release of adrenaline in the face of perceived danger. *(Emily Underwood, 2019)*

Sclerostin is a hormone produced predominately by osteocytes that activates osteoblast/osteoclast activity on the bone surface, but also helps to regulate adipocytes, energy homeostasis, and mineral metabolism in the kidney. [134](Wang, Mazur, and Wein, March 2021) The kidneys help to clear excess sclerostin, which preserves bone density. Wang and his team report that FGF-23, also produced by osteoblasts and osteocytes, have a more local influence by regulating phosphate homeostasis, while the hormone **lipocalin 2** in bone helps to "regulate glucose tolerance, insulin sensitivity, and insulin secretion to maintain glucose homeostasis."

There is also some evidence that circulating, bioactive (OCS) communicates with muscle fibers during exercise by the release of **interlueukin-6**. Interleukin-6 promotes adaptation to aerobic workouts, and triggers the uptake of nutrients. (Mera et al., 2016) IL-6 also has anti-inflammatory properties during exercise, plays a role in reducing fat cells, as well as in the insulin-stimulated glucose uptake in muscle fibers (Severinsin, 2020).

BONE CROSSTALK WITH MUSCLE

Severinsin and Pedersen have also named muscle to be an endocrine organ, because it, "*secretes hundreds of **myokines** (Fig.7.5) that exert their influence in an autocrine, paracrine, or endocrine manner.*

Recent advances show that skeletal muscle procures myokines in response to exercise, which allow for crosstalk between the muscle and other organs - including brain, adipose tissue, bone, liver, gut, pancreas, vascular bed, and skin, as well as communication within the muscle itself."

Although only a few myokines have been allocated to a specific function in humans, it has been identified that the biological roles of myokines include effects on — for example — cognition, lipid and glucose metabolism, browning of white fat, bone formation, endothelial cell function, hypertrophy, skin structure, and tumor growth."

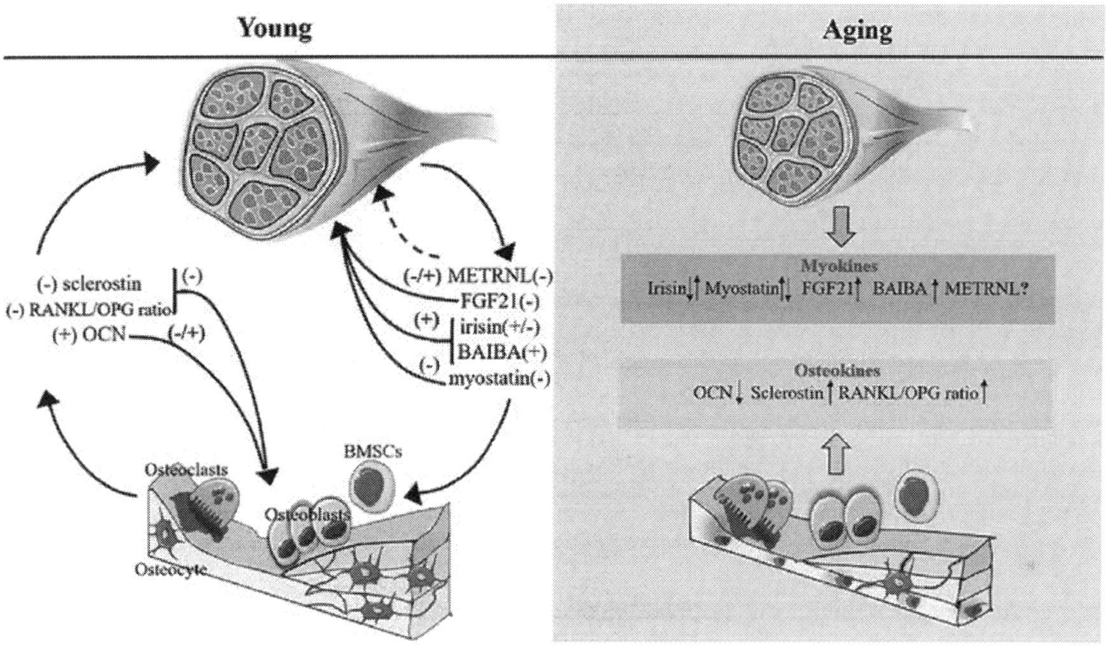

Fig.7.5 - As muscles age and fatigue, the secretion of myokines is reduced, along with their signaling to bone so that the osteokines that favors osteoclast production increases over the production of osteoblasts.

Apparently, hundreds of **peptides** are produced and released by muscle fibers when they contract, (Fig.7.6) but very few have been classified. So a world of new information on their function is on the horizon. Muscles are beginning to receive acknowledgment of their own domain, labeled by some as a 'myokinome'. Exercise-induced factors, such as peptides and nucleic acids, are released into exosomes in the extracellular matrix that already contain microRNA, mRNA and mitochondrial DNA, along with nucleic acids and peptides. The exosomes act as transport for the crosstalk that happens between muscles and other organs during exercise.

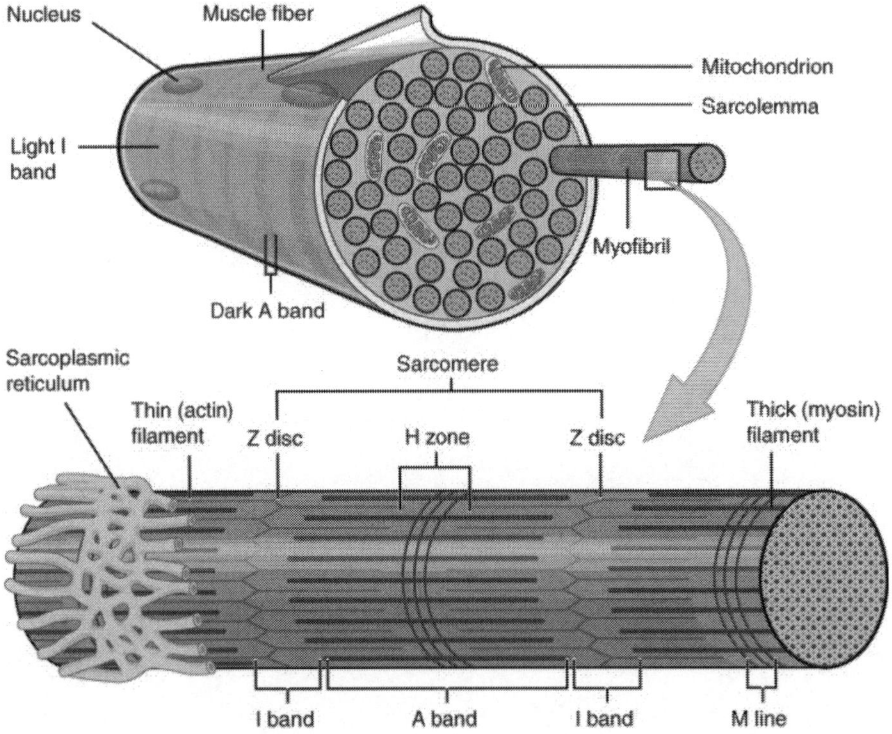

Fig.7.6 - The dark and light bands in the muscle fibers produce the striated look to the muscles that are able to contract by the sliding of the actin and myosin filaments that are inside the sarcomeres. Myokines, including irisin, are produced in response to muscle contractions.

Courtesy of OpenStax CC BY 4.0 via Wikimedia Commons

However, myokines are active in muscle proliferation, differentiation, and regeneration without exercise. Over 600 myokines have been discovered, although each function is still being uncovered. Some myokines are concerned with myogenesis and muscle mass as part of the TGF-β family, while others, like **musclin**, help alleviate muscle atrophy in cancer and promotes 'skeletal muscle mitochondrial biogenesis.' [135] (Severensin and Pedersen, 2020)

These researchers emphasize that the cognitive benefits from BDNF (brain-derived neurotrophic factor) expressed during exercise was not found to be circulating in the blood, but directly secreted by muscles, which have crosstalk with the brain.

In addition, the size of the hippocampus was shown to increase after 3 months of aerobic exercise. Studies by researchers at Harvard Medical School have found the specific receptor on osteocytes for the hormone **irisin,** which triggers sclerostin and subsequently bone remodeling. (Bruce Spiegelman et al., 2018) In rats, irisin has slowed muscle atrophy as well as increased bone mass. (Colaianni, et al., 2015,

2017; Morgan, et al., 2021) In the future, they hope to be able to apply irisin treatments for osteoporosis and neurodegenerative conditions. (Richard Altus, Harvard Gazette, 2018)

Hyeonwoo Kim and his team discovered that the aV class of receptors on osteocytes and adipose tissues enabled **integrins** to transduce messaging by physical activity. Ruiz-Ojeda et al. discovered that integrin signaling regulates white adipocyte insulin action and systemic metabolism, which may be how exercise benefits glucose levels. (Francisco Javier Ruiz-Ojeda et al., 2021) Apparently, there is still conflicting evidence regarding bone loss and exercise in the elderly. Some studies showed no change or even reduced bone mass in endurance training, and no benefit to the lumbar spine in resistance training. (Hyeonwoo Kim et al., 2018)

However, these researchers concur that numerous studies confirm the benefit for bone mass by injecting the irisin, one of the myokines released during exercise. Findings about the benefits for bone mass using exercise depend upon what the study is looking for. (Newsroom, 2019) The Cleveland Clinic reports that high intensity exercise benefits heart function for seniors, which can counteract the findings of Yang discussed earlier, who found heart and blood cells were among those that reflected age-related decline first.

The National Council on Aging lists numerous benefits of **exercise** in the over 60 category, including increased mental and emotional well-being, less pain, less bone loss (if not greater gains), a boost for the immune system, and fewer chronic diseases. ("Exercise and Fitness for Older Adults," August 2021) Increased balance, strength, cognitive function, and reduced expenditures on medical visits are among other advantages to a regular exercise regime for seniors.

There may be individual or age-related differences we're still learning about in terms of which exercises to recommend to which population. There could be differences in terms of the patient's history, current condition, levels of inflammation, or type of injury that would influence where the focus might be in a manual therapy session or somatic movement sequence. After looking more closely at how the biomechanics of communication function in the next chapter, ways to apply what we know so far about embryogenesis, transcription factors, and treatment will be covered.

Wnt Signaling and Skin/Bone Interactions

CONNECTIONS BETWEEN SKIN LAYERS AND BONE CELLS

Since bones and skin have widespread influence in maintaining our health and preventing many serious illnesses, it would be useful to understand the process a little more. Ross and Christiano talk about skin this way: "*The skin and its many appendages are responsible for functions as diverse as epidermal barrier and defense, immune surveillance, UV protection, thermoregulation, sweating, lubrication, pigmentation, the sensations of pain and touch, and, importantly, the protection of various stem cell niches in the skin.*

While in the adult vertebrate organism, bone and skin spend much of their time as separate entities with vastly different agendas, the skin dermis and the bone originate from a common primordial mesenchyme." [136](F. Patrick Ross and Angela M. Christiano, 2006)

The skin is also home to an array of vascular and neural networks, along with lymphatic vessels that reside in the dermis. (Fig.7.7) The researchers go on to describe the skin as "a highly specialized and meticulously regulated organ system populated by numerous different cell types that each contribute uniquely to its multitude of functions." Embryologically, the skin (ectoderm) and bone shared the same cells and signaling pathways as the initial limb buds were being formed. Both Wnt (Wingless int1, aka 'wingless-related integration site') signaling pathways and BMPs are involved in the morphogenesis of skin and bone.

Houschyar and his team declared that,

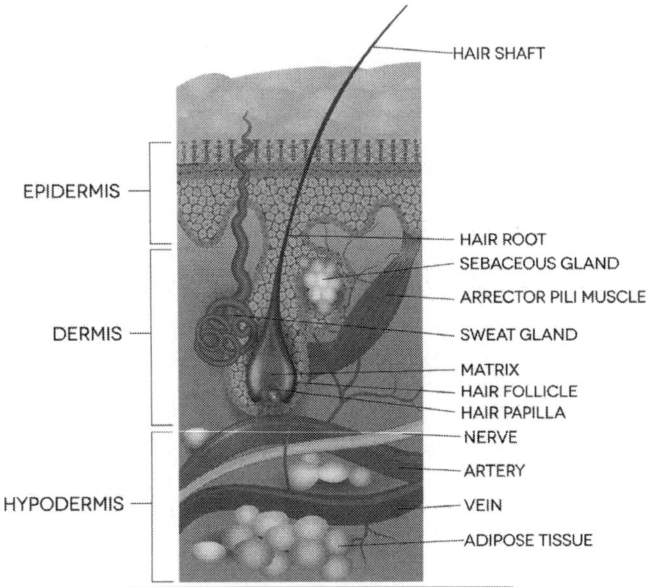

Fig.7.7 – Layers and components of skin

> *"Wnt signaling continues to play a critical role in adult osteogenic differentiation of mesenchymal stem cells. Disruptions in this highly-conserved and complex system lead to various pathological conditions, including impaired bone healing, autoimmune diseases, and malignant degeneration." [137] (Houschyar et al., 2019)*

This may be a place to look in cases of non-union bone fractures. Houschyar describes some of the post-natal functions this type of signaling is involved with. They report that,

"The Wnt ligands bind receptors on the cell surface of recipient cells to activate the Wnt pathway by triggering intracellular signaling cascades, which orchestrate numerous cell, biological, and developmental processes important in many physiological settings." (Fig.7.8) The same strict spatial, temporal parameters of the process modulated by antagonists remain a feature of the Wnt signaling in adults like it was during embryogenesis. Besides its essential involvement in bone remodeling, it is also central for tissue homeostasis. Steinhart and Angers reiterate the findings that disruptions in Wnt signaling often results in cancer and other diseases. [138](Steinhart and Angers, 2018)

Wnt signaling was central to the development of our skin. Lim and Nusse state that,

> *"It is increasingly apparent that many morphogenetic pathways with key roles in development are also important in regulating skin biology.*

Of these, Wnt signaling has emerged as the ***dominant pathway*** *controlling the patterning of skin and influencing the decisions of embryonic and adult stem cells to adapt the various cell lineages of the skin and its appendages, as well as subsequently controlling the function of differentiated skin cells."* [139] (Xinhong Lim and Roel Nusse, 2013)

It is, according to these researchers, the Wnt signaling from the epidermis that is involved in somitogenesis and the formation of the mesoderm and its derivatives. An intricate interplay between Wnt and other proteins facilitates the establishment of the keratinocytes in the skin's appendages, such as the sweat glands, hair follicles and shaft, and melanocytes. (Fig.7.7) Keratinocytes are a common skin cell type that are involved in migration, proliferation and differentiation in the repair process, and are also involved in killing pathogens at a wound site. (Minna Piipponen et al., 2020) Epidermal regeneration is fueled by epidermal stem cells located in the basal layer of the interfollicular epidermal cells and the outer layer of the bulge in the hair follicle. (Veltri, Lang, and Lien, 2017)

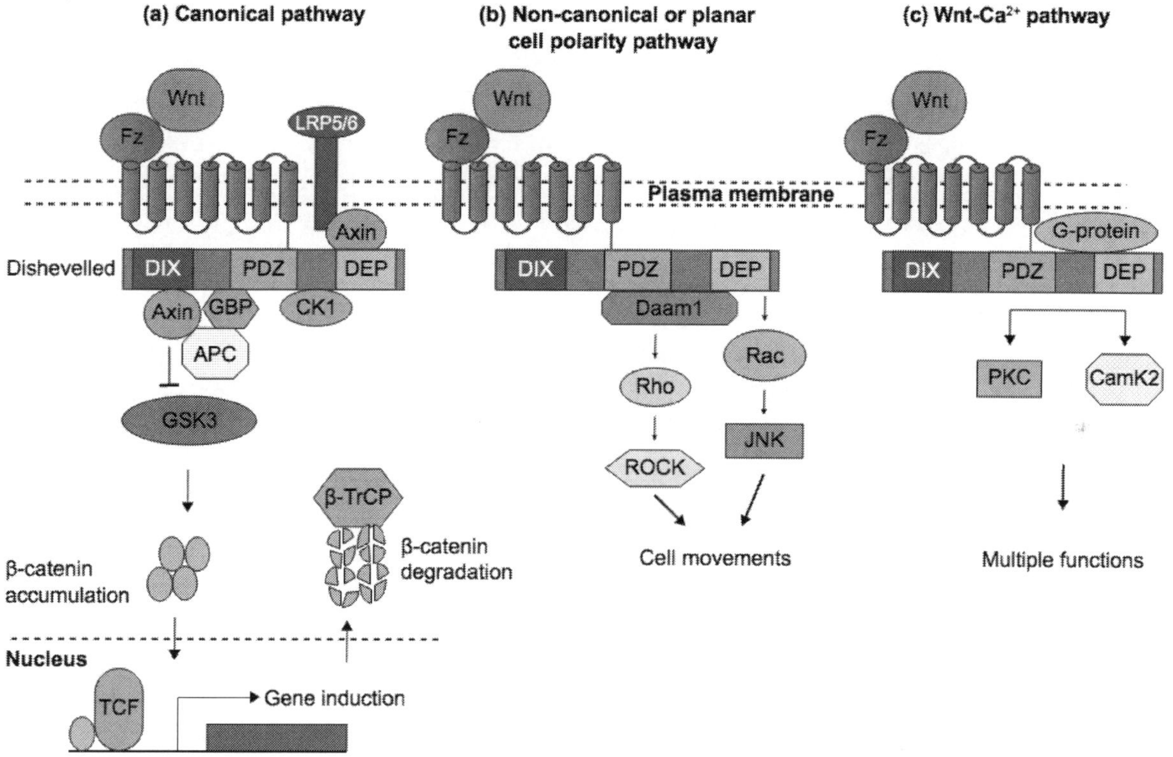

Fig.7.8 – Example of Wnt signaling - Wnt signaling happens in three ways: the canonical pathway whereby there is an accumulation of β-catenin which results in its translocation to the nucleus, the non-canonical pathway where that process is bypassed, AKA the planar cell polarity (PCP) pathway, which is mostly active during embryogenesis when it is integrating cellular, asymmetric, spatial/directional/orienting cues during tissue organization. (Ackers and Malgor, 2017) Ackers reports that non-canonical signaling tends to promote adipose tissue as well as the negative regulation of insulin signaling in white adipose tissue, implicating this pathway in Type 2 diabetes. The Ca2+ pathway is less understood, as is true in general of non-canonical pathways, but has been found to be involved in hippocampal neurogenesis in adults. (Arredondo et al., 2020) The non-canonical pathways often act as antagonists to the canonical/β-catenin activation, since over-stimulation of the Wnt protein secretion is implicated in the diseases indicated earlier.

There seems to be some agreement that **the hair cycle** involves this signaling as well. Xinhong Lim reports, "*Wnt/β-catenin signaling is known to play a critical role at multiple stages of the hair cycle, from the earliest stages at the transition from rest to growth, to influencing lineage decisions during hair follicle differentiation... High-Wnt signaling instructs keratinocytes to form hair, whereas intermediate to low levels of Wnt signaling specify the sebocyte and interfollicular epidermis lineages. When this delicate balance of Wnt/β-catenin signaling is upset, skin cells are driven excessively to form particular lineages, leading to developmental defects or cancer.*" Although Lim mentions the possibility that mechanical forces may play a role in the efficacy of this signaling pathway, there is an admission of limited research in this area. [139](Lim and Nusse, 2103)

EXTRA-CELLULAR MATRIX SIGNALING

In 2016, Jing Du and his team declared that, "*We observed that a stiff ECM (extra-cellular matrix) significantly enhanced the expression level of several members of the Wnt/β-catenin pathway in both bone marrow mesenchymal stem cells and primary chondrocytes. It has become increasingly apparent that each tissue has a characteristic 'stiffness phenotype.'*

> ECM stiffness, being a mechanical property, exerts its effects on a variety of cell behaviors such as proliferation, differentiation, apoptosis, organization and migration. The mechanical cues of ECM stiffness sensed by the cell are propagated, amplified and transduced into signaling cascades that lead to transient, sustained cellular responses. *[140](Jin Du et al., 2016)*

This is a significant finding, in that there seems to be a direct correlation between the disruption of mechanical cues in soft tissue fields and joint damage. Manual medicine may offer a better solution in these instances, as it can be more precise in locating and releasing restrictions. Extracellular matrix stiffness has been associated with tumor development, as its functions are so intricately related to immunity and the metabolic reprogramming of cells. (Heming Ge, et al., 2021) Ge and a team of researchers examined the possible role of metabolic irregularities stemming from ECM stiffness being a factor in consequent cell mutations when energy needs aren't being met.

They state that, "The ECM is mainly composed of collagen, fibronectin, laminin, elastin, and thrombospondin (a family of glycoproteins that regulate cellular migration, attachment, and invasion). (Fig.7.9) Previous studies have shown that increase in deposition and cross-linking of collagen as well as hyaluronan acid contents increase ECM's stiffness. In addition, this stiffness can transfer physical signals from the ECM to intracellular matrix through mechanical conduction, thereby changing the biological behavior of the cell." The metabolism of glucose, lipids, and amino acids is greatly influenced by signals resulting from the stiffness of the ECM, as is the invasion and proliferation of tumor cells. [141](Heming Ge, et al., 2021) Stiffening of this matrix can contribute to fibrotic conditions in the arteries, the heart, the lungs, kidneys, and just about anywhere in the body as it alters cellular processes and their communication pathways that are vital to health. Many research articles report that fibrotic or stiffening ECM is a bad sign. Marsha Lampi states,

"Extracellular matrix stiffness is emerging as a prominent mechanical cue that precedes disease and drives its progression by altering cellular behaviors. Targeting extracellular matrix mechanics by preventing or reversing tissue stiffening or interrupting the cellular response is a therapeutic approach with clinical potential." (Marsha C. Lampi and Cynthia A. Reinhart-King, 2018)

Else Frohlich and Joseph Charest reported that over-cross-linking of ECM protein molecules can lead to impaired kidney function, altered structure, and kidney disease. They described the delicate interactions like this:

"Cell response to matrix stiffness is a feedback loop that involves cell-exerted forces and the degree of substrate elasticity. In vivo, adherent cells reside in a solid microenvironment that can range from stiff and rigid to soft and elastic. Healthy tissue cells push and pull at their surroundings, thereby transmitting forces to substrates via adhesion molecules, such as integrins and cadherins. In turn, the degree of resistance of the substrate dictates the extent to which a cell can contract and migrate, causing the cell to respond through adhesion adjustment and cytoskeletal reorganization. The mechanisms that allow cells to communicate and probe their microenvironment are complex and allow cells to be sensitive to changes in substrate stiffness." [142](Frohlich and Charest, 2013)

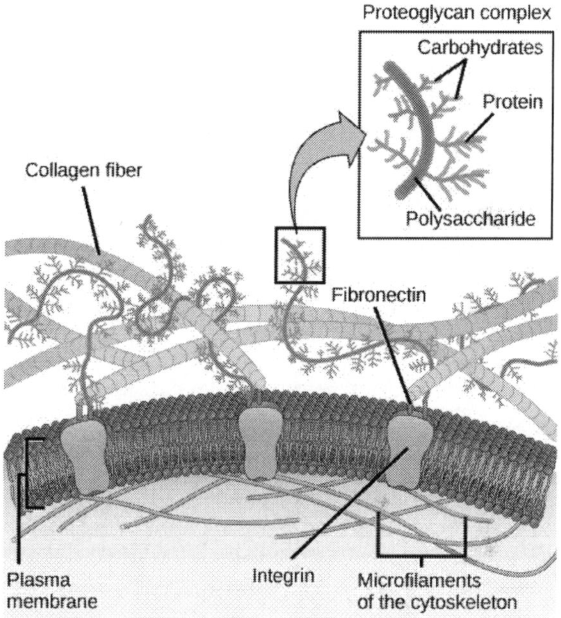

Fig.7.9 – Components of an Extracellular Matrix

CNX Open Stax CC 4.0 via Wikimedia Commons

Injury, surgery, infection, and trauma can all impact the stiffness of the ECM. All of these, in addition to lack of mobility can create sticky fascia. Integrins enable cells to perceive the chemical makeup as well as the physical properties of the matrix. Its elasticity or stiffness regulate the ability of the cells to develop forces using their actomyosin cytoskeleton for the sensing and transmission of forces. In certain cases, biochemical activity alone can signal alterations in the matrix without input from integrins. The whole of the process is very complex, involving a cascade of interwoven biochemical and biomechanical responses that occur within the matrix.

The 'pulsing' technique through the soma that happens in a Hanna Somatic Education session is one way of assessing the capacity of the tissue field to transmit mechanical input from one end of the body to the other. Fluid dynamics in the vascular or Biodynamic Cranial systems, and energy flow through meridians in acupuncture or acupressure are all ways to monitor where possible restrictions in the matrix may be located. Myofascial methods are an excellent way to palpate and resolve imbalances in the tissue field at varying depths.

At the micro and nanomolecular level, the structure and function of every cell, as well as its surround are interconnected and interdependent. From this perspective, the most useful way to approach preventative maintenance, and even recovery in some instances, is to build upon the health of the systems that have the most impact on all the others via multiple modes of communication. The skin via the Wnt signaling pathways appear to be one of the most effective ways to sense into and rebalance several other systems, including organs, the nervous system, the brain by way of fluid and solid connective tissue, and bones.

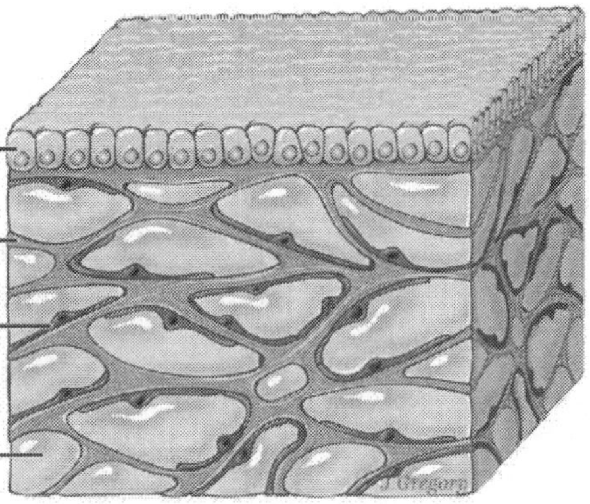

Fig.7.10 – Illustration of perforating quality of the interstitium

Courtesy of Pau0500 CC BY-SA via Wikimedia Commons

INTERSTITIUM

We are, according to physicists, 99% space and are also an average of 60% water or fluids. Apparently, a new structure called the **interstitium**, previously thought to be connective tissue, has recently been discovered Interstitial fluid contains sugars, fatty acids, amino acids, coenzymes, hormones, neurotransmitters, metabolic waste products, and minerals. As it accumulates between cells, it is picked up by lymph vessels and returned to the blood. (NIH, 2022) (Fig.7.10)(Dr. Neil Theise, New York University School of Medicine, 2018) Similar to the perineural system, it is currently thought to be a shock absorber, but as deeper investigations ensue, we may discover other functions and roles in communication this structure has. Fluids are responsible for a great deal of the mechanical sensing in our bodies, and as this layer permeates the skin, surrounds all arteries, nerves, organs, muscles, digestive, lung, and urinary tracts, it most likely is also directly involved in signaling.

What used to be considered a wall of collagen, according to Theise, is now known to be an "open, fluid-filled highway" that is supported by a lattice of thick collagen bundles. They were previously missed under a microscope because the dye and preparation process caused them to collapse so the fluid was missed. This system does connect with and drain into the lymphatic system, and is under study to clarify its potential role in the spread of certain cancers. [143](Rachel Rettner, 2018)

According to author and instructor, Tom Meyers, the interstitium is also a, "body wide communicating system for the push and pull of mechanical information." He finds that the viscosity of the fluid is able to dissipate forces and protect organs and delicate tissues, while the elasticity enables the resultant deformation to resume its normal shape once the pressures subside. (Myers, 2018) Myers credits the interstitium with *"running a continuous mechanical linkage from the DNA through the nuclear membrane via the microtubules, to the cellular membrane through the trans-membranous proteins, to the glycocalyx (the first mucousy later outside the cell) to the interstitium, and on up to the more gross and dissectible fascial structures."*

Myers goes on to say that, *"The real excitement here is the mechanical continuity from cell to organism. The larger insight is that our 'biomechanics' – muscles working via tendons over joints restrained by ligaments – requires total re-think in terms of these new findings of mechanical continuity from molecular on up through cells, tissues, and the entire human being."*

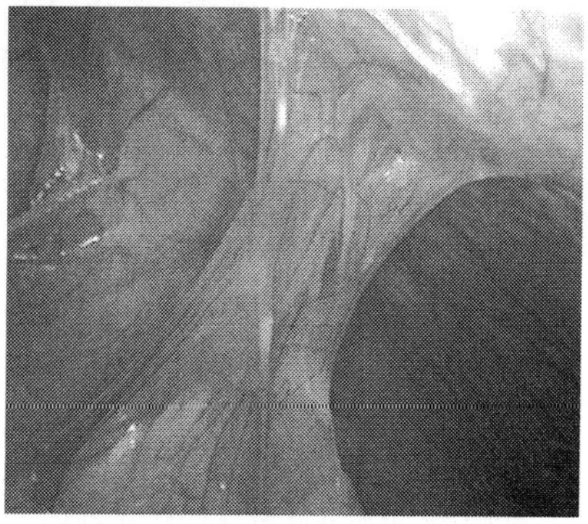

Example of adhesions

In addition to the fluid inside and surrounding each cell, it is transformative to realize that there are also structures that carry fluids throughout the fascial system, joints, bones, brain, lymphatic, and circulatory systems that are capable of sensing and transmitting signals. The interstitium (Fig.7.10) is responsive to the slightest change in its environment - including shear or pressure forces, tethering forces at cell-matrix connections, and hydraulic changes. (Huxley and Korthius, 2010)

Regarding the Wnt pathway, Diez-Ulloa is looking at the degree of mechanical stimulation needed to produce a response in the Wnt pathways. Diez-Ulloa states, *"It is known that: a) if there is repeated stimulation in time, it is more effective than an isolated spot; b) if there is some rest / recovery time from an hour and up to three (hours), there is a bigger effect afterwards; c) forces can vary from tension to compression, but above all, uni- or biaxial deformation generated Wnt activation."* [144](Máximo-Alberto Díez-Ulloa and Ramiro Couceiro-Otero, 2016) There is also evidence to support the crosstalk between skin, endocrine, bone, and organ systems through shared pathways. Ross and Christiano explain that, *"In the adult, Wnt signaling is reprised again during tissue homeostasis, and is a key regulator of the hair cycle as well as osteoblast and osteoclast regulation. Both skin and bone are home to specialized stem cell niches that provide a safe haven for their relevant progenitor cell populations. There are common transcriptional regulators of bone and skin, such as the vitamin D receptor, whose cascade of downstream effectors are clearly crucial in both tissues, since mutations in this gene cause profound effects in the form of irreversible alopecia as well as rickets.*

Given the anatomical proximity of the two tissues, it is not beyond the realm of possibility that a common adult mesenchymal progenitor cell population supports both the skin dermis and underlying bone." [145](F. Patrick Ross and Angela M. Christiano, 2006; Krausova & Korinek, 2014)

Some key questions remain in my mind related to the feedback between the signaling pathways, the extracellular matrix, and repair mechanisms for chondrocytes and connective tissue. We've heard for so long that the lack of blood supply is the reason that cartilage doesn't repair itself, yet when it comes to cellular signaling pathways, indications are that it can. There is some evidence to support the fact that the mechano-transduction processes can exchange input and stimulate chondrogenesis directly without using the circulatory system. What are we missing in the communication methods that could enhance that process manually or by using movement guided by the type of forces, frequency, length of time and so on that may be needed to trigger a repair response?

There is an abundance of research underway to discover either an injectable stimulant to repair cartilage utilizing the BMPs responsible for chondrogenesis, or by fabricating hydrogels or engineered tissue matrix replicas. Again, the natural process is extremely complex and interdependent in its signaling process, some of which will be altered when the tissue is damaged. At that point, certain steps in the process are inefficient, or hampered by continually being re-injured before the healing is complete. This is common for many joints and likely in most cases. Up to now the efforts to use transcription factors for regenerating cartilage has been limited due to the expense, short supply of volunteers for trials, side effects, drug delivery carrier safety, optimal dose, and effective scaffolds. (Z. H. Deng, et al., 2018)

Care for Skin and Bones

So far, the main disruptors of cellular signaling that researchers have focused on have been toxins. Avoiding the list of chemicals described earlier in the text that are added to cosmetics, lotions, hair dyes, deodorant, shampoo and conditioners, perfume, any added fragrance and cologne, toothpaste, laundry detergent, dry cleaning chemicals in our clothing, and soaps could make a big difference. Also avoiding chlorine, fluoride, and heavy metals in water that come into contact with our skin would be very helpful. Any of these can create disruptions in messaging and cell mutations. They also might not be among the suspects for conditions like cancer, birth defects, or reproductive issues that turn up later in your life when the system's ability to adapt has been spent.

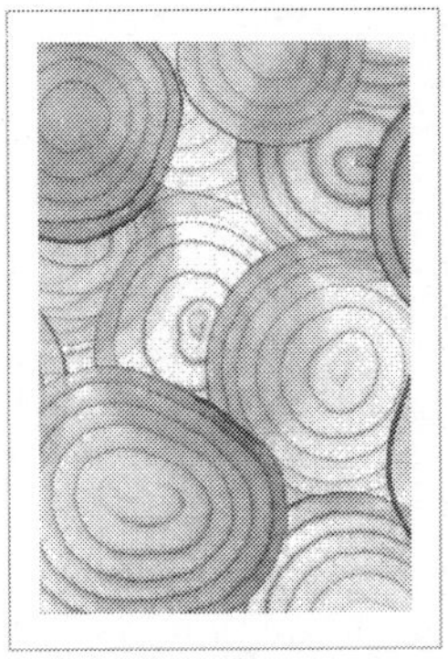

Taking care of our skin is pretty simple. Drinking clean water, sleeping well, using a cleanser and exfoliator, skin brushing, breathing clean air, using a sauna or some form of exercise that allows you to get your heart rate up, using a non-toxic moisturizer, and eating a healthy enough diet (with 'good' fats) are all very beneficial for the skin. UVB protection is important to avoid mutations in the skin. Red raspberry seed oil has an SPF of 25-50, and some say carrot seed oil ranges between 35-40 SPF. Avocado and hazelnut oils are at SPF 15 and coconut oil is at SPF8 for UVA rays that can age the skin. Tomato seed, Moringa, Maracuja, sesame seed, and prickly pear seed oils are all helpful for the short UVB rays that can burn the skin.

In addition, mango, illipe, shea, kokum and tucuma butters that also have protective and nourishing qualities would be good carriers for the oils. Manual/myofascial therapy to reduce adhesions and unlock sticky places from wear, stagnation, or trauma would also be advisable. Adhesions very much impact the flow of communication through the fascial fields, neural networks, vascular and other fluid sources of input, as well as the delivery of force vector information to bones. Bones receive a lot of their information from force vectors and mechanical loads, which will be covered more fully in the next chapter.

There are also ways that diet can make a difference for the bones. Dietary sources of calcium and vitamin D are helpful, along with a few other nutrients. The reason that **prunes** are beneficial and have been shown to increase bone density, is due to the high vitamin K content which works synergistically with vitamin D in the calcification and mineralization process. They are also high in potassium and magnesium, and have trace amounts of boron which supports the excretion of extra calcium. (Leigh Merotto, 2019)

In addition, prunes enhance the expression of BMP2, which participates in bone remodeling. (Jennifer Graef, et al., May 2018)

Onions are a superfood for bones. Studies show an increase in bone density and decrease in hip fractures in women over 50 who consume onions regularly. (Menopause, July-Aug, 2009) Vivian Goldschmidt mentioned in her article on the subject that, *"The high sulfur content in onions has a direct effect on the formation of connective tissue such as tendon and cartilage... Onions are an excellent source of polyphenols, which has been shown to increase the production of osteoblasts."* Apparently, high levels of arginine in the system generate ammonia, which is toxic to Wnt signaling and can cause it damage, whereas intermittent fasting and correct levels of **iron** help to regulate Wnt signaling. (Chesner & Korenblit, 2019; Austin Armstrong et al., 2021) Many nuts and particularly the white meat in turkey have high amounts of arginine, but in moderation it is favorable to bone density. Wnt signaling continues to play a critical role in adult osteogenic differentiation of mesenchymal stem cells. It is also a factor is healing bones after trauma. (Khosrow S. Houschyar, et al. 2019)

According to Dr. Susan Brown, onions contain flavonoids like quercetin, which reduce inflammation caused by oxidation that signals osteoclasts to break down bone. They also contain sulfur compounds that stimulate the production of glutathione, which is a *"major intercellular antioxidant that prevents excessive homocysteine accumulation which damages collagen in the bones and arteries." (Goldschmidt, Better Bones, 2016)*

There has been conflicting evidence for quite some time regarding the amount of **calcium** to consume in supplement form. Some studies suggest that the body can't absorb more than 500 mg. at a time, and if more is taken, it should be spread out. Apparently, while 95% of most supplements are dissolved in the stomach, not much more than 30% is absorbed by the small intestine, regardless of the form, and about half that unless vitamin D is available. Vitamin K2 is an important nutrient to ensure that calcium is delivered to the bones, but there's more. The bones are a mixture of calcium hydroxyapatite and collagen, which lends to suppleness. Over-mineralization could make bones more brittle.

Recent data is emerging that suggests overloading the system with calcium can overload and/or weaken the calcium-cAMP signaling, cause inflammation and neuronal atrophy resulting in cognitive deficits. (Amy F. T. Arnsten, et al., 2021) A long-term analysis of 10 studies involving over 75,000 subjects taking calcium channel blockers, over half of which were female, showed a 44% reduction in risk of dementia for elderly hypertensive patients. (Salman Hussain, et al., 2018)

Johns Hopkins reports that calcium supplements do nothing to prevent bone fractures in seniors, and may lead to calcium buildup in the arteries.

Erin Michos, MD stated that "A nutrient in pill form isn't processed in the body the same way as it is when ingested from a food source. Furthermore, people believe that the proof that calcium supplements bones is more robust than it really is." (Health, Johns Hopkins Medicine, 2022)

It has been shown to be particularly beneficial for colon cancer. Studies have also linked this pathway to neurogenesis, particularly in hippocampal cells. Regarding this connection, down-regulation of Wnt signaling is associated with amyloid β neurotoxicity and an increase in senescent cells. Some forms of Chi Kung, like Iron Shirt and Bone Marrow Chi Kung, help to build, strengthen, and cleanse the bones. Percussive techniques in manual therapy as well as inductive methods that release intraosseous compression and vector forces can help surrounding tissue fields as well as bones.

Taking care of **joints** is equally important, as micro tears and strains can lead to arthritic changes that are challenging to reverse. **Hyaluronic acid** helps to keep joints lubricated, and taking it in 80-150mg doses daily for 3 months showed significant improvement in pain and muscle strength in a variety of studies internationally. After certain intestinal bacteria break down the HA, it is more easily absorbed by the small intestine so it can be utilized by the body. Although the joints have the largest quantity of HA, it is also found in connective tissue, skin, blood vessels, brain, heart valves, and more. (Mariko, Oe et al., 2016) It can also increase elasticity in the skin and decrease wrinkles. (Wong, 2021)

Food sources of hyaluronic acid include bone broth, and it is increased indirectly by foods with magnesium like almonds, kale, and sweet potatoes. These foods support the uptake and production of HA, as well as tofu and edamame that have phytoestrogens that can also increase the production of HA. The vitamin C in citrus also helps to stimulate the production of collagen.

Oranges and grapefruit contain naringenin, which blocks the enzyme hyaluronidase that breaks down HA in the body and helps to maintain higher levels. *(Rachel Link, MS, RD 2021)*

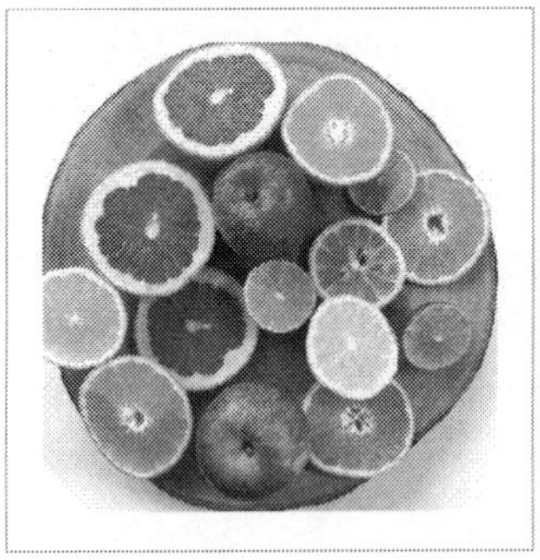

Hydrolyzed collagen supplements have been shown to improve the elasticity of the skin (Choi, et al., 2019) Type I collagen is found in the skin, tendons, internal organs, and parts of bone, whereas Type II is found in cartilage. Chicken collagen contains both glucosamine and chondroitin, but studies yield mixed results on the benefits of these popular supplements as well as collagen on joints. (Mali Schantz-Feld, 2021) The dosage needs to be above 950 mg. for there to be a measurable effect with hydrolyzed collagen, so the amount in food sources may not be enough. Industry-sponsored studies may not be the best measure of the efficacy of any supplement, and placebo effects have shown great results using belief alone. It could be that movement medicine and manual medicine are the best routes for joint protection.

Glucosamine sulfate is an amino sugar that is a major constituent of extracellular matrix macromolecules and is also found in large quantities in articular cartilage, but is also in intervertebral discs and synovial fluid. Studies have shown 25% of glucosamine is utilized when taken orally, but given its potential impact on blood sugar and interactions with warfarin, it is no longer recommended for long term use by some doctors. (Michael A. Gropper, MD, 2020) Glucosamine sulfate appears to act as an anti-inflammatory along with enhancing proteoglycan synthesis, which is impaired with osteoarthritis. (Ramesh C. Gupta, 2016)

Glucosamine can be sourced from lobster, crab, and shrimp shells, but there are no food options other than animal bones and gristle, and some fungi. Consuming foods like spinach and raw parsley that contain glutamine may help stimulate the body's production of it, (Maier, 2007) but most researchers find the evidence for it being effective inconclusive. Glucosamine and **chondroitin sulfate** seem to act as anti-inflammatories and may slow the breakdown of cartilage in hip and knee joints. Chondroitin is often used in solutions that help dry, irritated eyes and to reduce post-surgical complications after cataract surgery. (Daniel Preiato, RD, 2021) Chondroitin is found in the connective tissue of animals, fish, shark, and birds.

As a rule, these supplements appear to be safer than long term use of NSAIDS, (non-steroidal anti-inflammatories), and some people seem to benefit from PRP (plasma replacement therapy) and prolotherapy. Nonetheless, there can often be additional benefit from using mechanoreceptors as a doorway to stimulating integral changes in joints that have sustained damage. There are many stories of those who have bone-on bone levels of deterioration in joints who have no pain, making it worthwhile to explore movement and manual therapy options where long-term drug use may not be advisable.

Ancient methods like t'ai chi and chi kung are helpful for almost anyone, but of particular use to those who may not be able to sustain load-bearing activity very easily. Bones absorb and transmit thousands of tons of force on a daily basis so can be a source of great relief and rebalance on many levels. These gentle movements can help to redistribute and balance those forces. Professional athletes who have rarely given their bodies time to recover from the strain of a practice much less a game or an injury, could do well to consider including more subtle cellular signaling methods to help reset their systems and reduce cumulative damage.

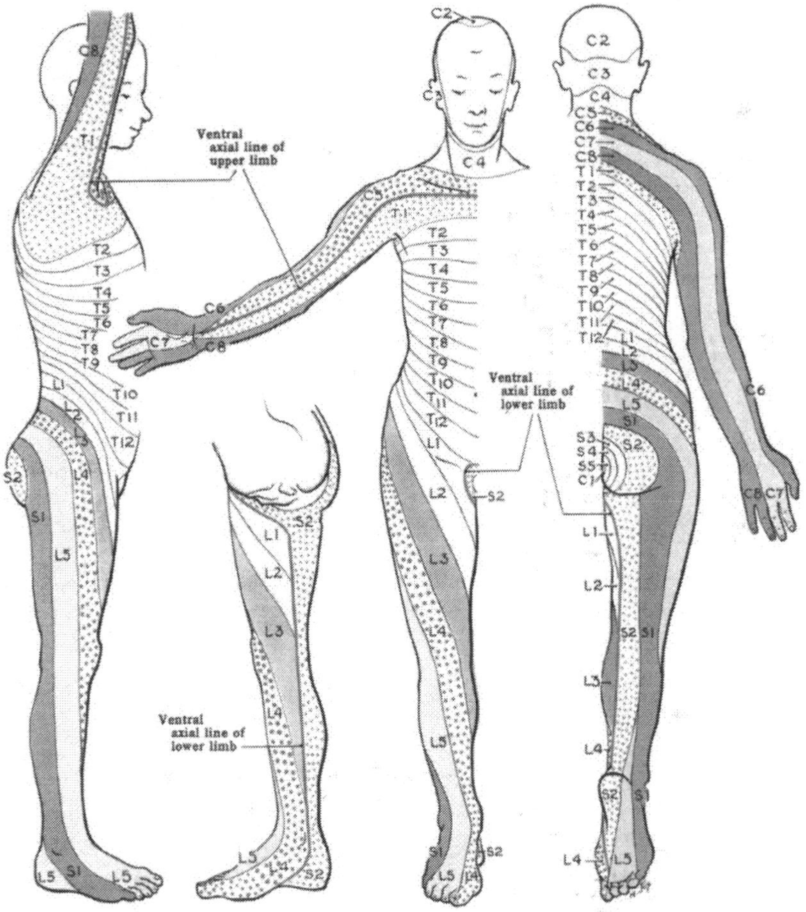

Fig.7.11 – Dermatomes

Pain referral regions associated with each vertebrae

Pain referral is common with organ and nerve (dermatome) (Fig.7.11) or ligament (sclerotome) referral patterns, where, perhaps through shared signaling pathways, the pain is reflected in the dermis.

Cumulative forces are also shared and distributed along connective tissue or energetic pathways, including fluids and bone. There have been countless instances where, for example, the level of tension in the anterior or posterior tibialis muscles in a client were resistant to release until the forces in the tibia were reorganized or discharged. In other instances there was compression at the fibular head that was applying pressure laterally on the knee but was being expressed medially.

It is probable that pain in the bone becomes expressed in neighboring tissue and vice-versa; in my experience it is true. It is not often that someone will report that their bones hurt, but when you go to touch it – for example, the bones of the arch in the foot — they will be very tender. For the client day-to-day, the pain will be expressed in adjacent tissue in the small muscles of the feet or further up the leg. Decompress the bone and the soft tissue no longer carries tension or sensation. One can learn to release intra-osseous compression and torsion for themselves; it's pretty easy and empowering.

In Chinese medicine, it is believed that kidney issues are expressed in back pain. Western approaches have some correlations on the subject as well, in terms of cross-talk and referral patterns. Once the correct source is identified, the reaction in adjacent structures leaves almost immediately and further strain on the joints and functionality can be spared. In many instances where there was tenderness and seemingly raised, tight muscles above the kidney, it was often the kidney being squeezed between the psoas and the quadratus lumborum. Each time, facilitating the glide of the kidney along its normal path of excursion released the sensation, the raised muscle tension, and tenderness.

When we're looking for causality in the expression of uncomfortable symptoms in the body, viewing the source of the issue as a signaling problem changes how the body responds. Efficiency of inter- and intra-cellular communication is, in my opinion, an important perspective to consider as part of the solution. The primary restriction may not be in the same place the symptoms express themselves, as our Somatic pioneers attest. To me, it makes sense to give priority to midline systems, skin elasticity, and balanced bones for maximum therapeutic benefit.

I'm voting for the key regulators and the global signaling potential found in the skin and bones for number one. Number two would be the midline structures with embryological significance like the gut tube, the heart and aorta, spine, and central nervous system. Addressing these key signaling systems using the biomechanical 'language' that optimizes the potential for correcting dysfunction at the cellular level will be the focus of the next chapters of this book.

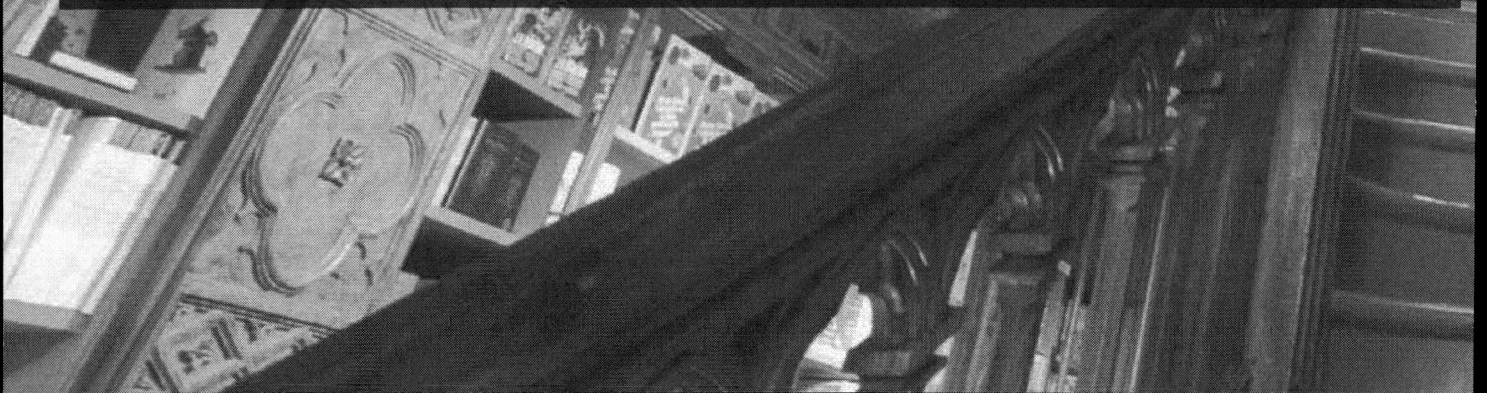

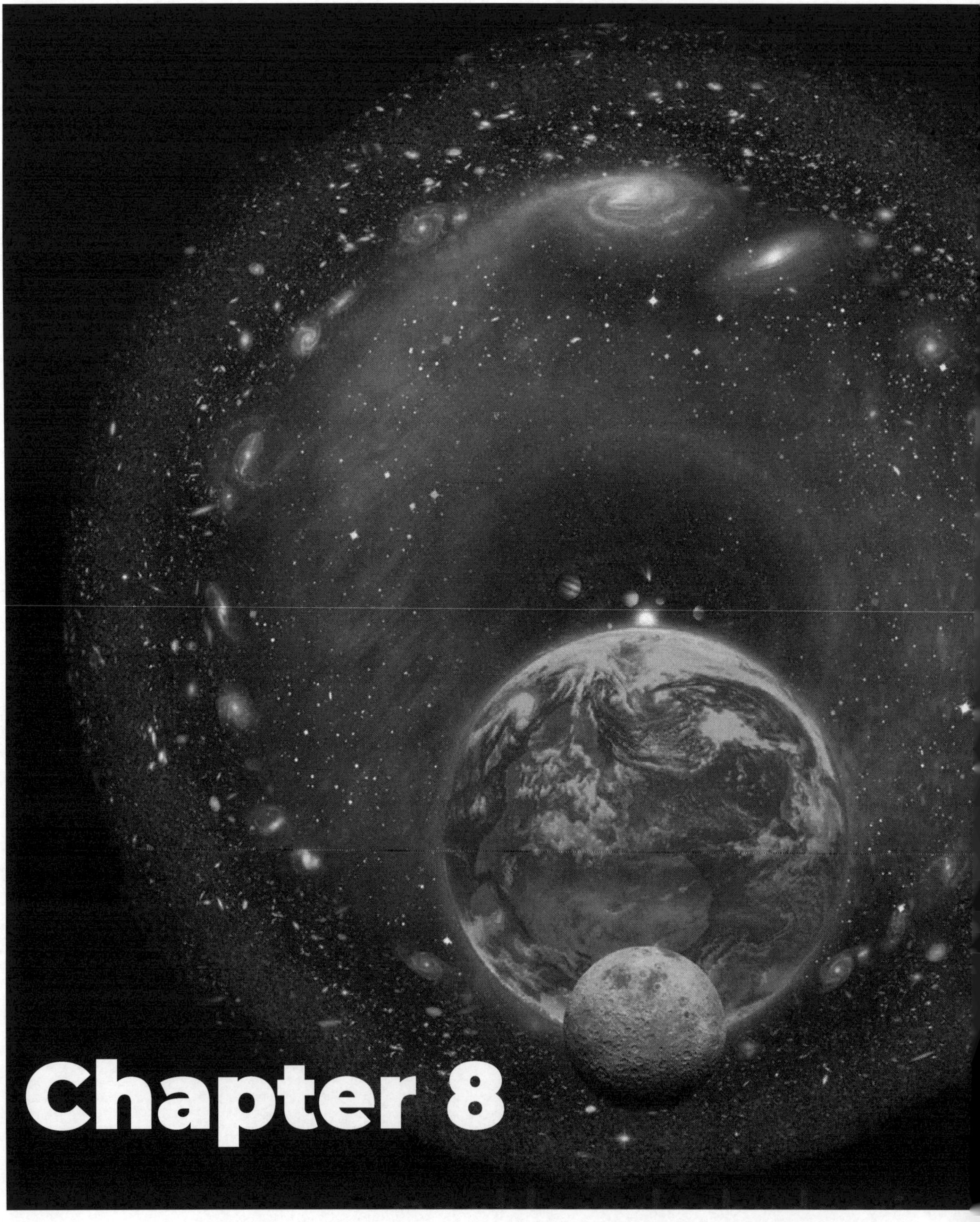

Chapter 8

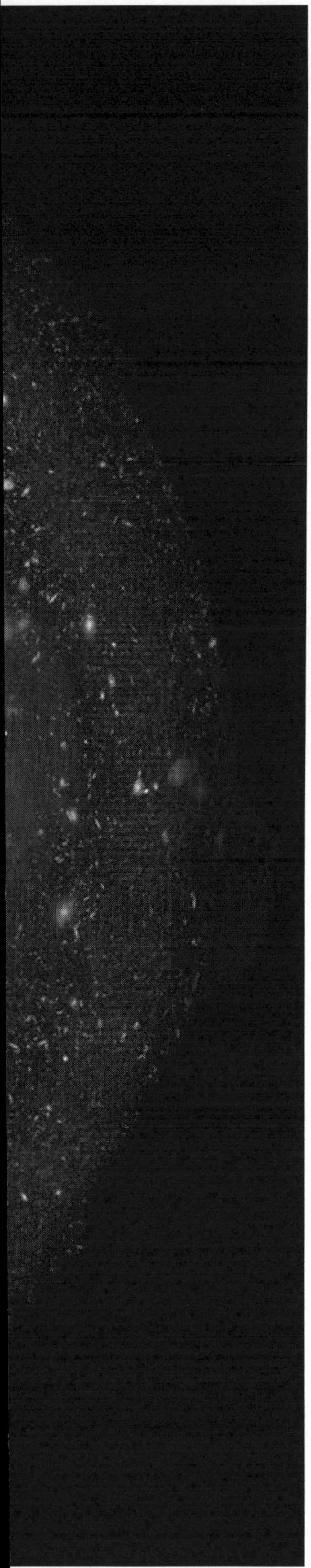

Mechanotransduction

Communicative forces

Mechanotransduction has been defined as the process by which physical forces are transduced into biochemical signals, often resulting in cellular responses that have the potential to affect gene expression. Mechanoreceptors are located along nerves, in skin, muscle, joints, bone, ears, epithelial layers of vessels, the extra-cellular matrix, the cell membrane and cell nucleus. The types of forces being sensed, interpreted, and transmitted by the body include: gravity, weight, compression, vibration, stretch, shear stress, bending, torsion, touch, osmotic and hydraulic pressures, electrical potentials, and sound waves. Force transmission often uses the transforming growth factor (TGF-β/Smad) pathway, calcium ion, MAPK (mitogen-activating protein kinase) and G protein, Wnt/β-catenin, tumor necrosis factor TNF-a/NF-kB, and interleukin pathways. (R. Ogawa, 2016, Geoffrey C. Gurtner, MD 2018)

Mechanotransduction happens in both smooth and striated muscles, in both passive and active conditions. Mechanosensory feedback "modulates cellular functions as diverse as migration, proliferation, differentiation, cell repair, and apoptosis" as it did during development, but these functions continue as a part of regular homeostasis and regulation of the cell cycle. (Jaalouk and Lammerding, 2009) All cells need mechanosensory feedback to be able to respond and adapt to their environment. The subject is ripe for deeper investigations into the therapeutic possibilities involving imbalances that are both bio-chemical and bio-mechanical in nature, since both are interwoven aspects of cellular signaling. Some studies have already been underway, yet more are needed to help determine which types of mechanical input, targeting which types of receptors, could provide the optimum rebalancing for key tissue fields.

Dobner, et al. reported in 2012 that,

> *"While increased mechanical load is an important extrinsic contributor to cardiac disease, the importance of mechanotransduction in the adaptation to biomechanical stress is underscored by evidence that malfunctioning intrinsic components such as defective sensing, transmission, integration, and adaptation to mechanical stress likewise lead to cardiac failure."*

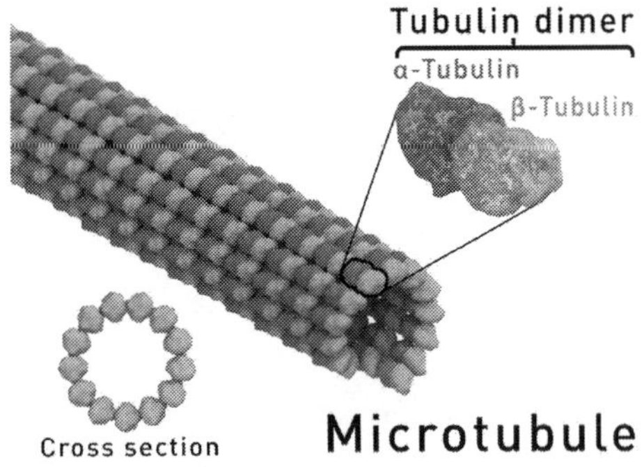

Fig.8.1 – Illustration of the microtubule's structure
Courtesy of Thomas Splettstoesser (www.scistyle.com) CC BY-SA 4.0 via Wikimedia Commons

Every tissue field is related to each other, so developing methods that target the signaling systems that have the farthest reach and the greatest influence peaks my interest. Addressing layers of skin, bone, and connective tissue that release pressures on the pericardium, whether proximal or distal, could yield promising outcomes in this field of growing concern: heart disease. One of the exciting aspects of realizing how these types of interconnections interact – i.e. epidermis, bones, and organs - is that assessment and reeducation modalities can be individualized according to the way the body responds best to specific input. Mechanotransduction has enormous preventative as well as rehab potential. As a midline structure that has been shown to be the first to express signs of aging, balancing tissue fields in and around the vascular system may be a key area to support signaling in most therapeutic modalities.

Dunn and Olmedo report on the subject that,

> *"The application of these (mechanotransduction) technologies to a physical therapist practice may hold answers to some age-old questions, while creating new avenues for our profession to optimize movement for societal health. Embracing this science as foundational to our profession will allow us to be valuable scientific collaborators with distinctive knowledge of the effects of loading." [146](Sharon L. Dunn, Margaret L. Olmedo, 2016)*

Microtubules–transporters for the mind of the body?

MICROTUBULES AND NEUROGENESIS

Microtubules (MTs) are structures within structures than are highly active in the transmission of information. They are one of the three types of filaments (actin, intermediate filaments, and microtubules) that make up the cytoskeleton of a cell. They form from the centrosome, which is adjacent to the nucleus and considered to be a microtubule organizing center (MTOC). They play a significant role in cell division, cell motility, maintenance of the cell's shape, and intracellular transport.

MTs interact with the extracellular matrix surrounding the cells which is sensitive to protein (signal) type, amount, and stiffness. Many of their functions are related to the generation of mechanical forces, but their function can be inhibited by an opposing force. (Kent and Lele, 2016) There is also some evidence that microtubules help to evenly disperse incoming forces to minimize the compression of the actin cytoskeleton and maintain balance in the tissue field at large. (Baas & Hamad, 2001)

Craddock and Tuszynski describe MTs as being "composed of tubulin dimers, which are globular protein subunits." (Fig.8.1)Dimers are two molecules that are connected, either with two that are the same (monodimers) or with two different molecules (heterodimers). The alpha/beta heterodimers that form the microtubules in our neurons use the long distance chains, or filaments called 'tubulins' that are globular, or spherical in shape. Many neurodegenerative diseases have been identified as being related to over-activity in the process of modifying the tubulins for transport.

A microtubule is about 25 nanometers wide, with the wall being approximately 5 nm thick. A human hair is on average 80,000 nm thick, so you have a framework for comparison. You can imagine how precise the timing and amount of the addition or removal of any substance on one of these tiny structures would have to be to avoid a mishap. Rapid response changes in the structure led some researchers to the conclusion that microtubules are loaded with signaling information. [147](Erik W. Dent & Peter W. Baas, 2014) Dent & Bass also posit that the interactions of microtubules with other proteins within the neuron influence its plasticity.

Microtubules (MT) are a superfast method of communication that is not only in the brain, but has the capabilities of operating as a major type of mechanotransduction throughout the body. (Friesen, et al., 2014) They are involved in whatever we do. Since MTs are quite small, they may respond best to doses of input that are much lighter that we've previously imagined in some cases. The level of force for draining lymph would be different than that for reducing gluteal tone, and modified again for the wall of an artery or targeting a microtubule within a nerve.

> Dunn and Olmedo go on to state, *"The correct dosage of mechanical stimuli applied during the correct phase of healing may have a profound impact on our therapeutic outcomes. They ask, "Which types of force are most effective? Which dose is optimal?"*

In countless studies where a positive outcome resulted from intervention with a natural supplement, the results were dose dependent. Every signaling pathway is sensitive to under or over-expression, so learning to tune in a bit more to listen for the system's response during the session could make a significant difference. The same consideration would apply to movements or exercises we explore on our own. For example, listening to subtle indications the body expresses during rehab could mean the difference between progress and exacerbation; opening and releasing, versus straining and closing. There are ways for both practitioner and patients to allow the body to guide, if not lead the process.

We now know that there is a direct line of communication between the most exterior and most interior layers of any cell, tissue field and the organs they surround. This means that each therapeutic input has the potential to influence gene expression in a positive way. We are part of that sensitized, highly conserved feedback loop, so our conscious participation and full of embodied listening may be a tremendous support for the system modifying things in a coherent direction.

There are so many factors involved in the ways that cells respond to loads and forces applied at different rates, researchers have not yet agreed upon which approach most effectively reaches a target threshold to generate a response. Some say that response depends upon the energy/heat expended, or the rate that the pressure is applied. Some claim it's the amount of distortion in the cell, or the stiffness in the ECM, the changes in fluids, or ion channels opening, or the accumulation of adhesion proteins on the cell membrane as the best measure of response.

There are sensors continually monitoring all of the above, so, like the story with several people having their hands on a different part of the elephant and describing things from that perspective, each outcome only reflects a portion of the whole picture. The cell may be taking all of it into consideration and making decisions based upon conditions of the whole in that instance. Sensors from different regions are intimately involved in both structure and function, so it could be the simplest test would be to initially use the least amount of pressure in the system and in the direction that elicits the most coherent response. Pairing different systems manually or in movement is often a good way to confirm paired associations or co-activations and reach a deeper integration. Examples of this concept will be presented in detail in Volume 9 of this series.

Currently, much of the research about a therapeutic approach with microtubules concerns neurogenesis and cognition, so let's look at that in a little more detail. The science behind the influence or crosstalk between the 'mind' and the rest of the system is still being scrutinized and explored, but for now, the current thinking is that microtubules inside the neurons are the receivers and transmitters of information or substances, and for some researchers, MTs help to transmit the essentials of cognition, memory, and learning.

To that end, they may necessarily be involved in the breakdown of cognitive functioning if their structures become dysfunctional. Right now, science seems to be indicating that movement and cognition are related, and very influenced by bone health. Dr. Jon Lieff says that, "*Microtubules are large, complex scaffolding molecules that work closely with the two other rapidly changing structural molecules, actin and intermediary filaments, to provide structure for the entire cell, including the spatial placement of organelles.*

> *"In neurons, microtubules respond instantly to mental events and constantly take down elaborate structures for the rapidly changing axons and dendrites of the synapses. They are highways for long distance transport of materials and organelles. They control the signaling at local regions of the extremely long axon." [148](Jon Lieff, MD, 2015)*

The way microtubules function, according to Lieff, suggests that a thought or intention can influence the way systems operate anywhere in the body. It could be looked at as a response to a desired action being planned, or it could be interpreted in a wider context if emotions are involved. Microtubules are able to adapt and change shape along the way, becoming the framework for the shafts of axons and dendrites. (Flynn and Bradke, 2020) So they are laying down the tracks they'll be traveling upon as they go.

ACTIN

Actin is a protein that forms filaments essential to the cytoskeleton of every cell, including neurons. They move or '**walk cargo**' towards the head (+) or tail (-) of the chain it is producing that either continues to quickly deliver input to the cell nucleus as it participates in the cycle of the cell, or by constructing towards the slow-growing end. (Fig.8.2) Actin is complementary to microtubules, and intermediate

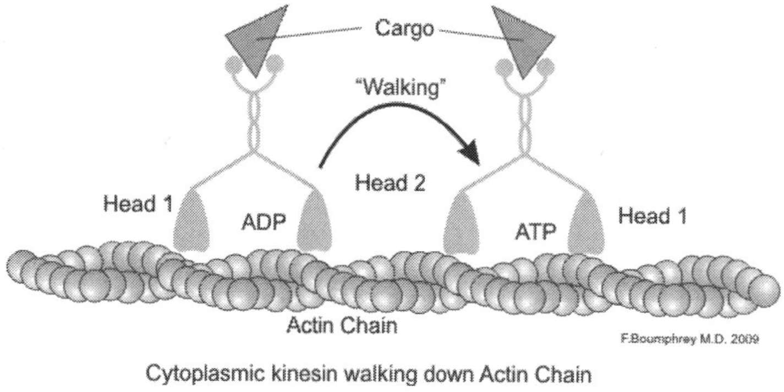

Fig. 8.2 – Illustration of how actin carries substances across a distance

Courtesy of OpenStax CC BY 4.0 via Wikimedia Commons

filaments are cytoskeletal polymers that help small molecules bind together. Researcher, Thomas D. Pollard describes it this way:

"Actin contributes to biological processes such as sensing environmental forces, internalizing membrane vesicles, and moving over surfaces ... as it provides internal mechanical support, tracks for the movement of intracellular materials, and supplies forces to drive movement. Actin is essential for the survival of most cells." [149] (Pollard and Cooper, 2009) Although initially discovered in muscle cells in 1940, a couple decades later, actin was found to be in all cells. In general, cells become more elastic under light pressure, and stiffer under stronger pressure, rapidly changing shape and density according to loading signals from the surface. Lieff maintains that the control is distributed throughout the axon, is complex and highly regulated, and that a dysfunction could lead to brain disease.

In fact, he finds that disruptions in the transport within the axon is associated with ALS, Alzheimer's and MS. Pascale Barbier and several other researchers wanted to better understand the role of **tau**, which is considered to be a 'microtubule associated protein' (**MAP**) that is found in numerous places in the axon where it helps to stabilize microtubule bundles. These researchers explain that, *"Tau plays a central role in MT dynamics by regulating assembly, dynamic behavior and the spatial organization of microtubules."* They explain that there are other MAPs binding to MTs that also have a role in its regulation, where some missteps could occur. [150](Barbier, et al., 2019)

FAULTY FUNCTION ALTERS STRUCTURES IN THE BRAIN

There may be mutations in the tau protein itself that contribute to its aggregation in places where the transport is inhibited. However, in October 2020, Japanese researchers from Tokyo Metropolitan University discovered that a mutation to the enzyme responsible for breaking up the aggregations may play a significant role. They found that mutations in **MARK4** (microtubule affinity-regulating kinase 4) changed the properties of **tau**, making it both more likely to aggregate and more difficult to dissolve.

> Under normal conditions, MARK4 helps tau to detach from the arms of the cytoskeleton that the microtubules are building and disassembling, but when this enzyme goes rogue, the tau is misformed.

Associate Professor Ando noticed that, *"This mutant form of MARK4 makes changes to the tau protein, creating a pathological form of tau. Not only did this 'bad' tau have an excess of certain chemical groups that caused it to misfold, they found that it aggregated much more easily and was no longer soluble in detergents. This made it easier for tau to form the tangled clumps that cause neurons to degenerate."*

MARK4 dysfunction has been named in a number of other diseases. [151](Toshiya Oba et al., 2020; Kane Ando, et al., 2020)

The body doesn't seem to process information in a straight line of cause and effect. It is responsive and adaptive moment to moment and making choices based upon the environmental stimuli at the time, along with prevalent patterns and conscious input. Given the same extent of plaques and **tau tangles** (Fig 8.3), two different people may have very different expressions of 'symptoms' or none at all. Alzheimer's expert, Thomas Grabowski, says, "**Amyloid** isn't as toxic to some people as it is to others." Some scientists believe there that there is a 'cognitive reserve' which the brain can draw upon when neurons are becoming dysfunctional or are dying in significant numbers. In some brains it has been observed that protective mechanisms become deployed that either break down the plaque or prevent it from forming. (Begley, 2020)

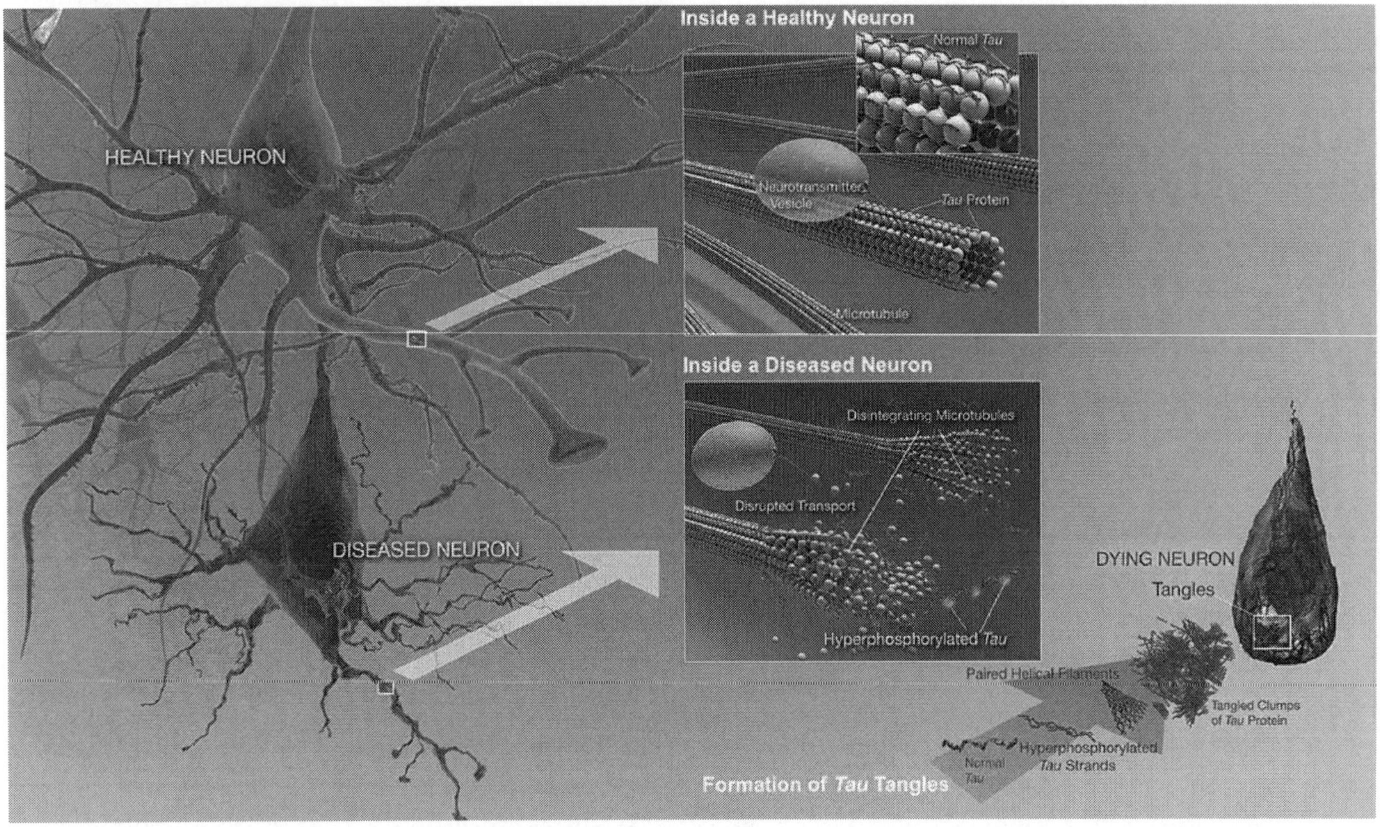

Fig.8.3 – Illustration of the changes that happen in the tau protein inside a microtubule of a neuron as it becomes toxic and diseased

Courtesy of Health and Human Services Department, National Institutes of Health, National Institute on Aging, pg. 24(1) Public Domain via Wikimedia Commons

High amounts of heavy metals can become toxic in the aging brain. Copper, lead, cadmium, manganese, and iron – some of which under normal conditions would be naturally occurring - have been found in the tau tangles of Alzheimer's patients. Heavy metals are more difficult to expel in an aging brain, and contribute to oxidation, inflammation, cell death, and brain shrinkage. They can hijack transport mechanisms, gain entry into the brain, and wind up in the cerebral spinal fluid via the choroid plexus. There are a few known remedies for this type of toxicity. Zinc competes for binding sites of cadmium and lead, so can help the body eliminate them, and selenium has been reported to be protective of cell damage from heavy metals.

Deficiencies in C, B1 and B6 vitamins can increase sensitivity to heavy metal accumulation, whereas adding them in supplements has been shown to reduce levels of lead in the liver, kidneys, bones, and blood. Garlic, ginger, green tea, grapes and curry leaves are all protective against cell damage from exposure and promote excretion. Tomatoes have proven to "significantly reduce accumulation of cadmium, lead, and iron in the liver of rats." [152] (Qixiao Zhai, et al., 2015)

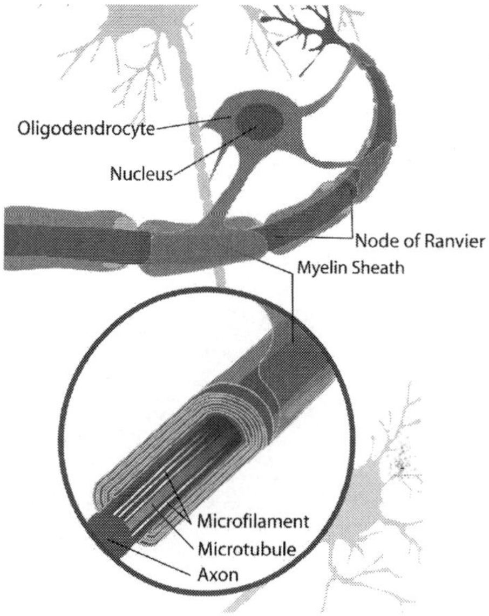

Fig. 8.4 – Illustration of oligodendrites surrounding the nerve cell

Lead by itself discovered in blood samples has not been shown to have a strong association with AD (Alzheimer's Disease), but lead found in the tibia was related to cognitive deficits. Lead found in the tibia, patella, and blood was associated with ALS and Parkinson's, but not necessarily AD or dementia unless exposed early in life. (Bakulski, et al., 2020) **Manganese** toxicity is implicated in both AD and Parkinson's. Industrial exposures and smoking are the most common ways for neurotoxic levels of manganese to occur, as the body tightly regulates the levels absorbed from food.

It isn't recommended for those over 50 to take vitamins with **iron** unless anemic, and the use of cast iron cookware may be risky. A study in 2013 by UCLA determined that perineural **oligodendrites** (Fig.8.4) and the myelin sheath surrounding nerve cells can be damaged by iron, creating oxidation, tissue damage, and disrupted communication with tau buildup due to structural compromise in the fatty tissue. (Wheeler, 2013) On the other hand, being low in iron also isn't ideal.

There has been some controversy over whether amalgam fillings are a key contributor to cognitive deficits, but **mercury** in the brain is a problem for neurodegeneration and Cerebral Small Vessel Diseases (CSVD). Mercury may be implicated in up to 45% of dementia cases. (Patwa and Flora, 2020) These researchers suggest that chelation therapy is a plausible remedy for heavy metal toxicity and possible relief for the resultant diseases, but other researchers have found that chelation can present its own issues, which then also need resolution.

POTENTIAL REMEDIES FOR INJURED BRAIN TISSUE

In 2017, a group led by Kaustubh Chaudhari investigated earlier studies that Brahmi, an Ayurvedic **nootropic** herb that has been able to avert free radical damage, protects cells in the hippocampus, striatum, and prefrontal cortex from cytotoxicity and DNA damage. It was also proven to reduce hippocampal β-amyloid deposits and stress-induced damage of the hippocampus. Jatamansi, Vacha, and Shankapushpi are other Ayurvedic herbs that support cognitive function. In addition, Chinese club moss, CoQ10, phosphatidylcholine, acetyl-l-carnitine, Gotu Kola, DHA, Malkangni seed oil, and numerous other herbs and supplements have been shown to be **neuroprotective** and supportive of brain function.

Maintenance of the delivery system and the energy it requires to transport the goods through the system are as important as the 'package' being delivered. Avoidance of toxicity, inflammation, and oxidation that lead to cell damage and death is paramount for cellular communication to be accurate. Supporting the homeostasis, repair, and detox of the cells while providing proper nourishment, activity, and exercise, is the best approach for both physical and brain health. The brain is as much a transceiver as a controller of the body's experience. It is beholden to the accuracy or efficiency of the information coming to it, and is therefore limited by its ability to produce a current, balancing response rather than a patterned, habitual response.

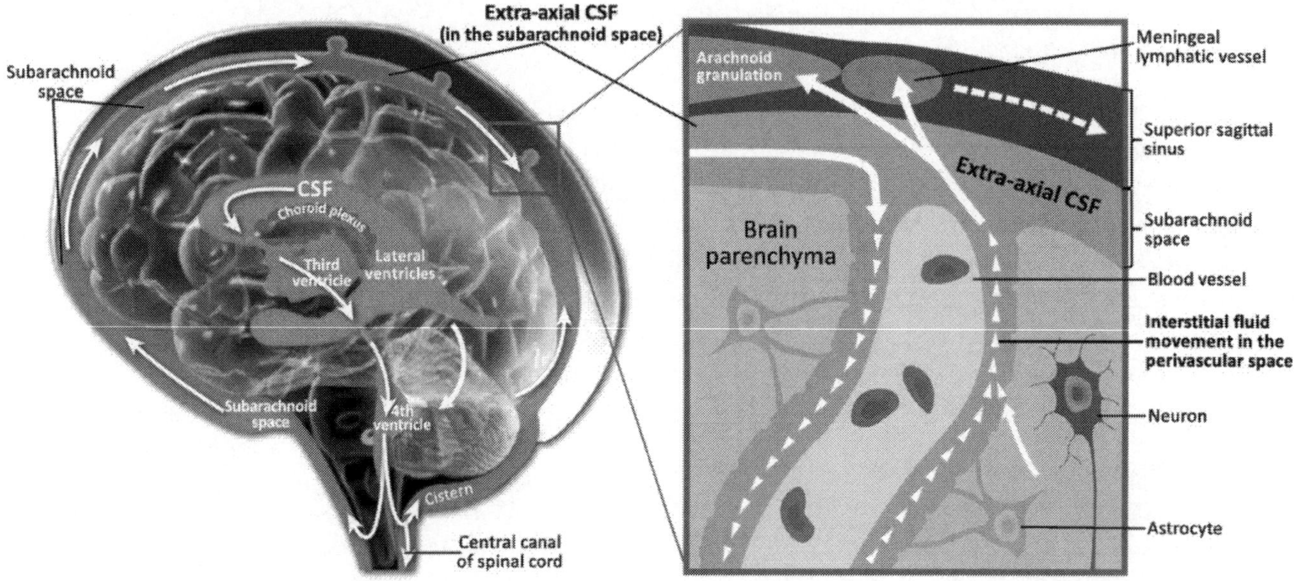

Fig.8.5 – Direction of the flow of CSF from the lateral ventricles across to the Foramen of Monroe to the third ventricle, down through the Aqueduct of Sylvius to the fourth ventricle where it bifurcates to proceed around the lateral aperture (foramen of Lushka not shown) and up through the subarachnoid space where it is taken up by arachnoid granules and absorbed into the dural venous sinuses and internal jugular system. There is some evidence that it proceeds downward through the spinal cord, cervical lymphatics, and forward through the cribriform plate where it is absorbed by the olfactory mucosa, certain cranial nerves, spinal nerve sheaths, and into the lymphatic system again.

The **glymphatic** system (Fig.8.5) in the brain is a key delivery system. It's designed to do a systematic cleanse daily, particularly during the parasympathetic phase while sleeping. Our cerebral spinal fluid (CSF), that we now know also carries BMPs associated with neurogenesis and spinal cord repair, is involved in numerous key brain functions. Zappaterra and Lehtinen reported in 2012 that both Wnt and Shh signaling are expressed in the CSF.

They found that CSF is 99% water and the rest is "proteins, ions, lipids, hormones, cholesterol, glucose, and many other molecules and metabolites," including growth factors, insulin, and melatonin, that are currently being studied for their influence in injury, sleep/arousal, and appetite. Zappaterra states that, *"Taken together, CSF-distributed factors play an active role in many aspects of normal adult brain activity, setting the stage for investigating how the CSF may dynamically regulate development as well as disease."* [153](Zappaterra and Lehtinen, 2012)

Fluid systems, including the CSF, are increasingly found to be participating in a wider variety of roles than originally believed. In addition to protection, increased mobility, nutritive, repair and maintenance aspects, fluids are revealing their integral roles in signaling. Cells are meant to interpret incoming forces in order to regulate cellular responses and adapt, whether it be to muscle contraction, loading of bones, blood flow, digestion, pathogens, or trauma. Embryologically and functionally, fluids are considered to be connective tissue, and are a major source of mechanical sensing and feedback. The role of fluids has profound implications for manual and movement practices. They should top the list of those we consider including among the communication systems that are the most pervasive and efficient for prevention or recovery.

ROLE OF THE CYTOSKELETON – THE MICRO SUPPORT AND TRANSDUCTION SYSTEM

Within each cell, including those that provide support for fluids as well as the fluids themselves, is a cytoskeleton. It is just a few nanometers in size, but carries substantial responsibility for the architecture and shape of the cell, as well as for the means to transmit information and substances. The Georgia Institute of Technology finds that:

"In the cytoskeleton of nearly all cells, ***actin*** *forms dynamic microfilaments that provide structure and sustain forces. (Fig.8.6) Actin is fundamental to how cells accomplish most of their functions and processes. A cell's ability to assemble and disassemble actin allows it to rapidly move or change shape in response to the environment. For the first time we have shown that mechanical force can directly regulate how actin is assembled and disassembled."* [154](John Toon, 2013)

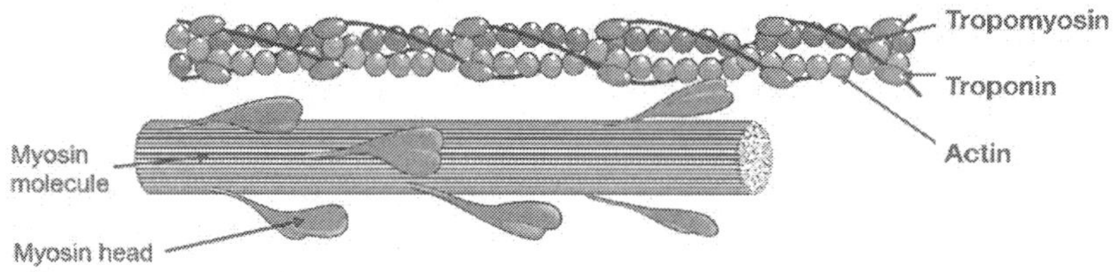

Fig. 8.6 – Illustration of troponin binding calcium within the actin/ tropomyosin filaments generating an ATPase reaction that causes the muscle contraction

Courtesy of Jeff16 CC BY-SA 4.0 via Wikimedia Commons

Integrins are cell regulators related to their proliferation, repair, signaling, angiogenesis, migration, cytokine activation and apoptosis, serving as receptors that bridge the actin-cytoskeleton of the cell interior with the world outside. *(Mezu-Ndubuisi and Maheshwari, 2021)*

The way that the interior cytoskeleton of a cell receives information about external (outside the cell membrane) forces is through the mechanosensors in the gel-like external matrix facilitated by adhesion proteins. A series of complex interactions between the adaptive conformational responses to stretch, bending, or compression expressed through macro molecules, become decoded at the nano-molecular level.

This is the level where focal adhesions and other cell surface molecules act as 'information handling machines or mechanosensors'. (Mechanobiology, ref: Geiger, 2009, Ingber, 2008) This same article cites a study by Cheng Zhu, a professor in the Coulter Department of Biomechanical Engineering who stated,

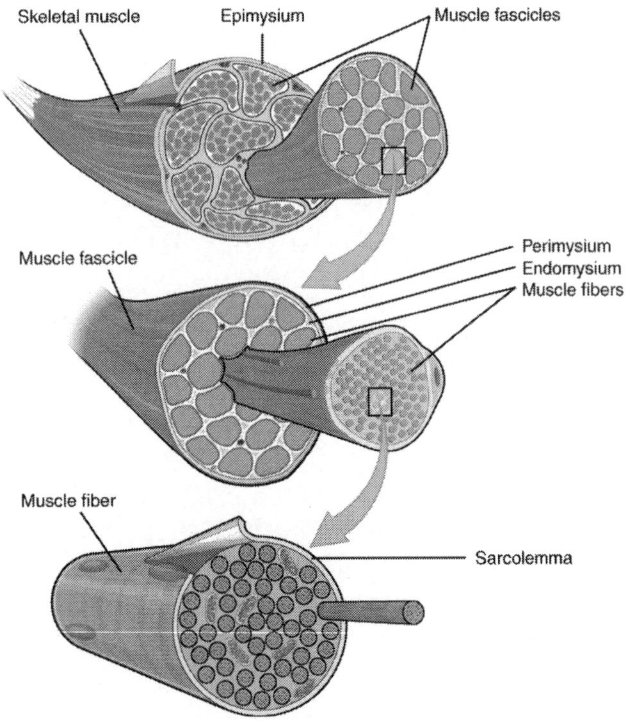

Fig.8.7 – Illustration of perimysium, endomysium and epimysium layers of muscle fibers

Courtesy of OpenStax CC BY 4.0 via Wikimedia Commons

> *"We found that when you apply force, the force induces additional interactions at the atomic scale. When you apply force, you find that residues that had previously not been making contact are now interacting. These are force-induced interactions.*

Previously, it was thought that sensory molecules at the cell surface were required to convert the mechanical cues into biochemical signals before the actin cytoskeleton could be altered. The mechanism we describe can bypass the cellular signaling mechanisms because actin bears the force in the cell."

On a macro level, the connective tissue network around (**epimysium**) and within muscle fibers (**endomysium**) form an interconnected web that serves to transmit length, shape, and force changes in each muscle fiber (**perimysium**). (Fig.8.7) These fibers will be passing current status information in both active and passive therapeutic conditions. Actin is involved in cellular processes at the level of genetic transcription, not just at the level where it interacts with myosin to create a contraction in the muscle.

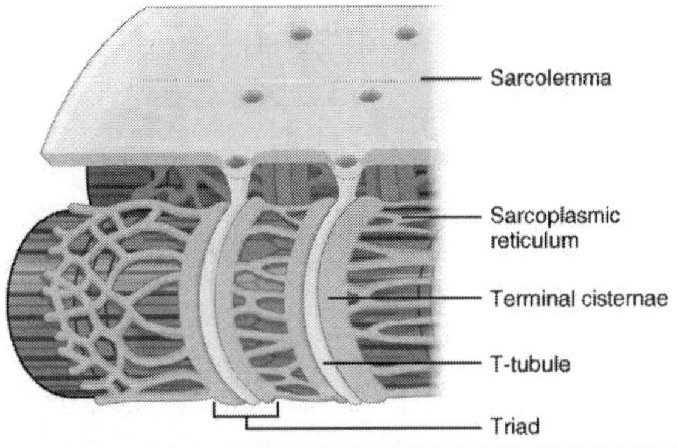

Fig. 8.8 - T-tubule sunken into the sarcomere as a signal transmitter into the muscle fiber

Image Courtesy of OpenStax CC BY 4.0 via Wikimedia Commons

Bin Zheng et al. reported in 2009 that, "Recent investigations suggest that nuclear actin plays a role in gene transcription associated with three main entities: a) components of the three RNA polymerases, b) ATP-dependent chromatin remodeling complexes, and c) RNP particles in the eukaryotic cell nucleus. Nuclear actin is required for transcription of all three RNA polymerases." RNA polymerases are enzymes that copy a DNA sequence into an RNA sequence. Zheng goes on to say that Hoffman et al. found in 2006 that "actin is associated with actively transcribed genes, and plays an essential role in transcriptional activation." [155](Zheng, et al., 2009)

Actin is mostly known for its role inside muscle fibers as it provides the sliding mechanism for myosin inside the sarcomere as the muscle contracts. As the action potential reaches the sarcomere, an extension of the cell membrane — called the **T-tubule** — transmits the signal, whereby the tight calcium regulator, **Troponin**, binds the Ca2+. (Fig.8.8) This creates structural changes throughout the actin-tropomyosin filaments, activating ATPase activity and subsequent muscle contraction. (Fig.8.9) Muscle contraction is not a superficial event. In fact, it is a major activator of cellular responses right down to the cell nucleus that can trigger gene transcription for cellular homeostasis. Shama Iyer and his team recently addressed the process this way:

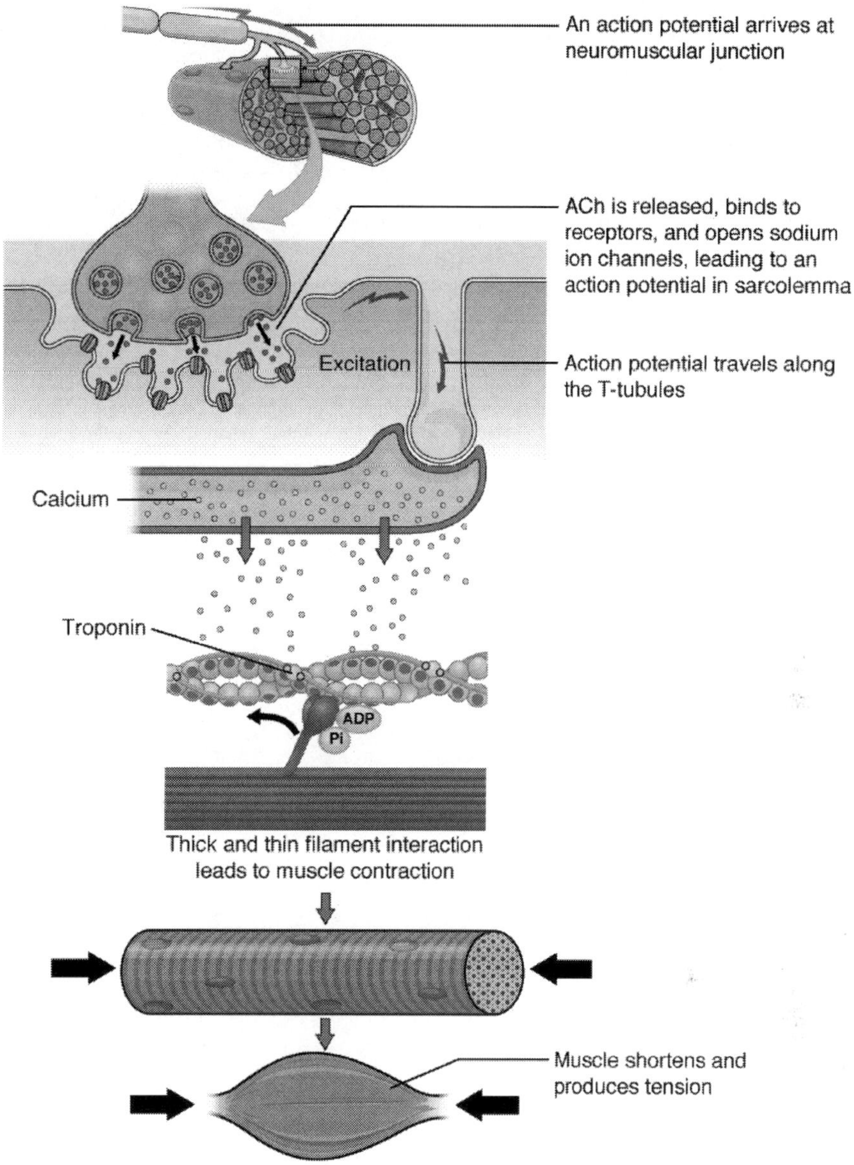

Fig. 8.9 – Action at the cellular level after Ca+ and Troponin trigger filaments that generate a contraction in the muscle

Image Courtesy of CNX OpenStax 4.0 via Wikimedia Commons

"Mechanical forces also act on the nuclear cytoskeleton, which is integrated with the myofiber cytoskeleton by the linker of the nucleoskeleton and cytoskeleton complexes. Thus, the nucleus serves as the endpoint for the transmission of force through the cell.

"The nuclear lamina, a dense meshwork of lamin Ifs *(*intermediate filaments*) between the nuclear envelope and underlying chromatin, plays a crucial role in responding to mechanical input. Myofibers constantly respond to mechanical perturbation via signaling pathways by activation of specific genes." [156](*Sham R. Iyer, et al., 2021) (Fig.8.10)

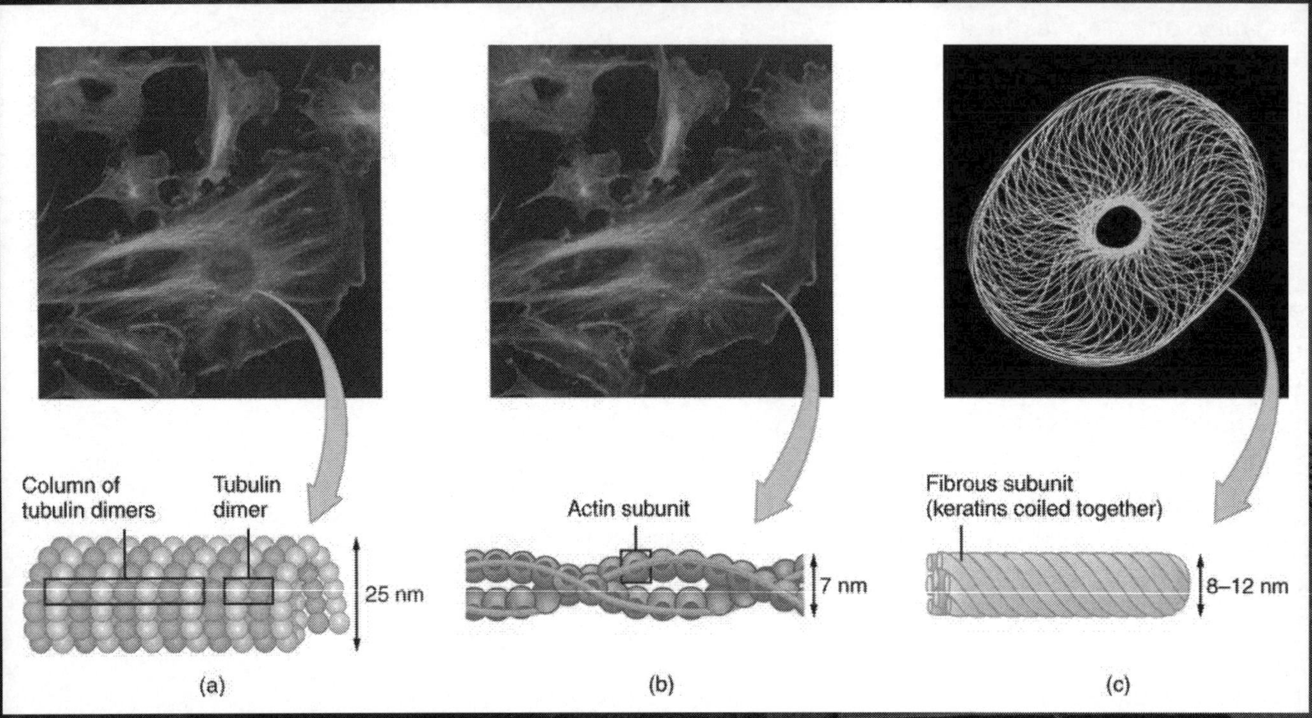

Fig. 8.10 - The tubulin dimers (a) of microtubules provide structure for the cell and are approximately 25 nm wide. They have 'dynamic instability' which enables them to form and disassemble very quickly according to what is needed. They protect the cell from compression. The actin subunits/filaments (b) can be used as tracks for transport, which can also assemble and disassemble as they promote cell migration, such as immune cells. The fibrous subunits (intermediate filaments) (c) are more permanent structures and are only 7-10 nm wide. They help to maintain the shape of the cell and anchor certain organelles as well as the nucleus in place. (Khan Academy, 2021)

(Image courtesy of OpenStax CC BY 4.0 via Wikimedia Commons)

According to Iyer, there are a variety of proteins in the cell that are about 7-10 nm in size, that link **myofibrils** to one another and transmit both active and passive forces while helping to stabilize the shape of the cell. Muscle fibers are somewhat unique in that they are multinucleated. There are nuclei "evenly positioned along the cell periphery to minimize transport distances and to assume local responsibility for the regulation of a particular volume of muscle fibers." (Hall and Ralston, 1989) In these instances, each nucleus also functions as a mechano-sensor for the cell. (Cho et al., 2017) Of interest to researchers currently, is how the nuclei interpret stress to alter gene expression in a way that can contribute to aging and disease or not, since it is directly connected to cell behavior.

This emerging field of mechanotransduction is producing more and more interest in how to intervene in some of these communication processes in order to correct or minimize the progression of disease. The inseparability of structure and function opens many doorways of perception into how to correct both simultaneously. Improving structure by signaling with discreet forces in key locations can vastly improve functioning, which will ultimately lead to more balanced biochemistry and more optimal signaling. Signaling requires adequate structures that can send and receive messaging, so it may be a better place to start in some cases before adding chemicals that may be landing in damaged transport systems.

The opportunity here, whether approaching balance from a manual or movement direction, is to continue to refine our sensory awareness and listening to somatic signals. When we can easily perceive increased restrictions, increased density or compression, and malalignments, we can also employ our sensory awareness and listening to somatic feedback to regain elasticity and integrated functioning. The manual methods or movements needed to return to balance will become a familiar language both to our bodies and to ourselves.

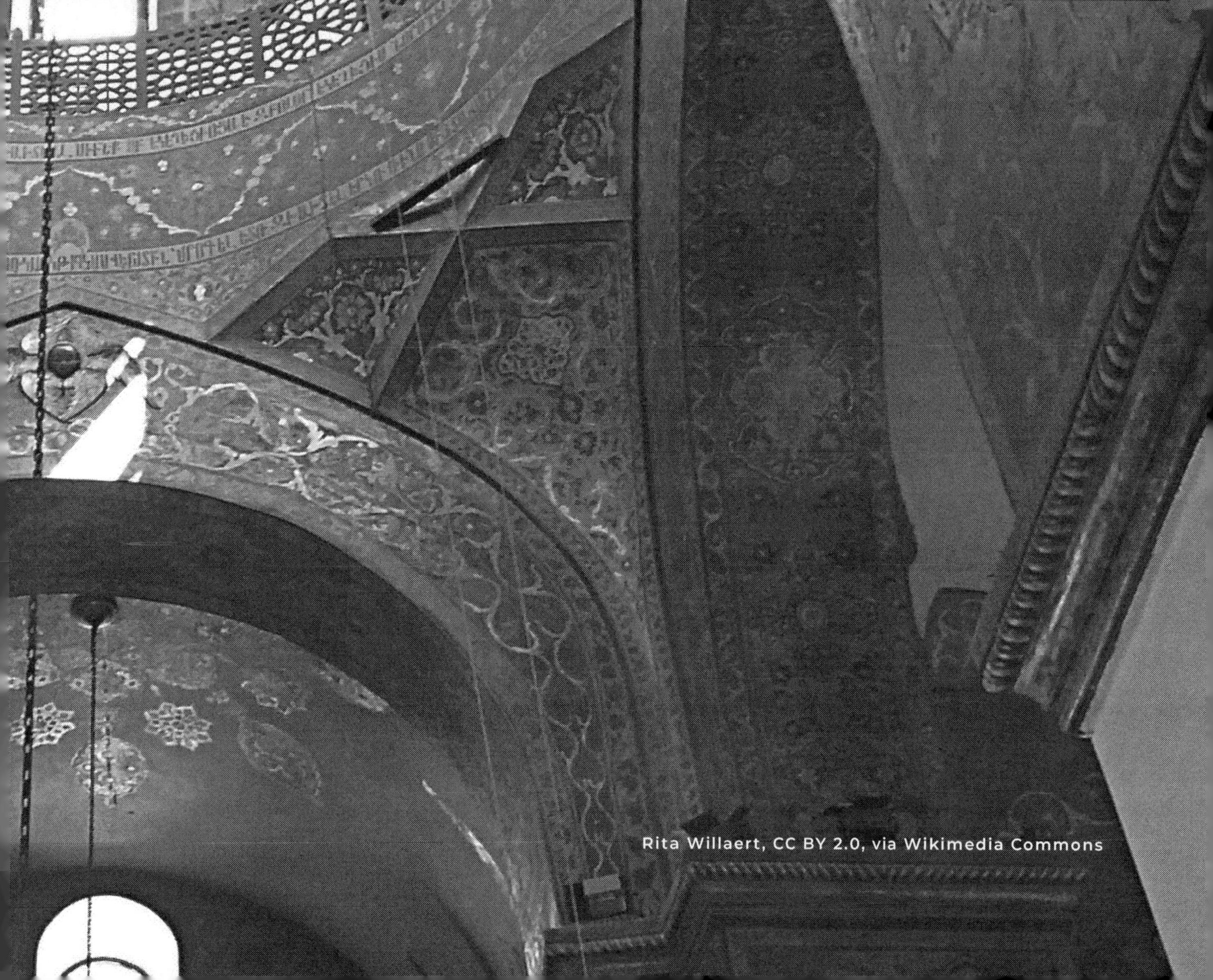

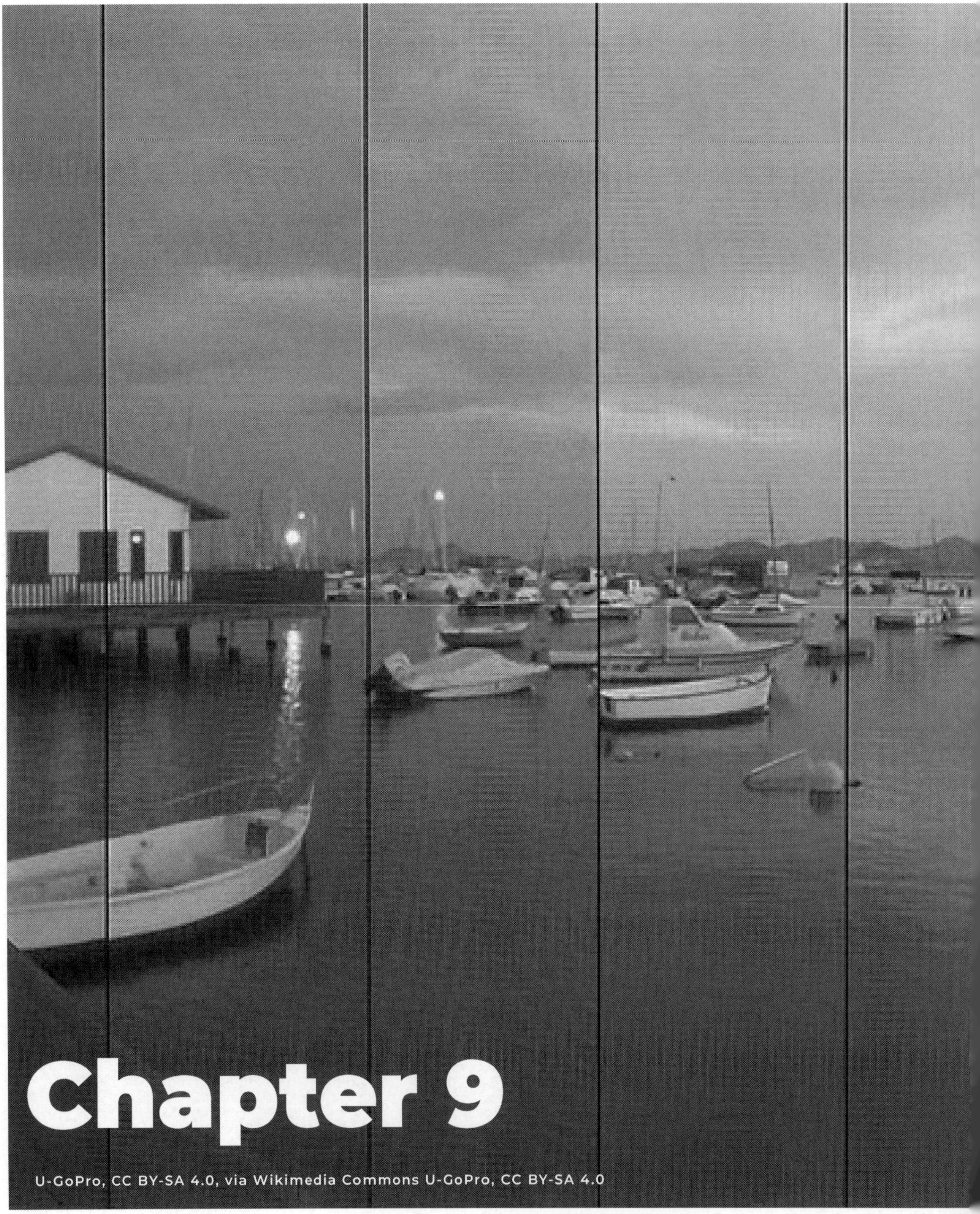

Chapter 9

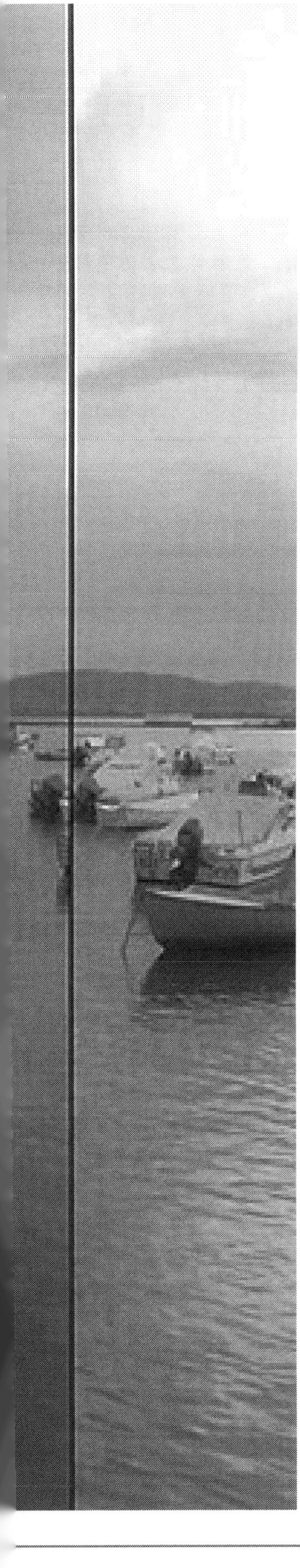

Addressing the Challenges of Time

Role of the Extracellular Matrix and the Skin in Mechanotransduction

IMPACTS OF ADHESIONS FOR SIGNALING

"The extracellular matrix has many functions," according to Meilang Xue and Christopher J. Jackson, *"including: providing structure, organization, and orientation to cells and tissues; controlling morphogenesis and cellular metabolism by acting as a template for cell migration, proliferation, apoptosis, differentiation, and adhesion; regulating cell activity and function via directly binding to integrins and other cell surface receptors; acting as a reservoir for growth factors and regulating their bioavailability."* 157](Xue and Jackson, 2015)

One of the main physical interruptions to optimum cell signaling through the matrix is going to be scar tissue. (Fig.9.1) Xue and Jackson list the components of the ECM as being, *"structural proteins such as collagens, elastins, laminins and fibronectins for flexibility; proteoglycans and hyaluronan to stabilize growth factors and the three-dimensional space using water-binding ability, and glycoproteins like integrins to regulate cell adhesion and signaling between cells."* Collagen is the most abundant protein in the ECM and is the most responsible for scarring.

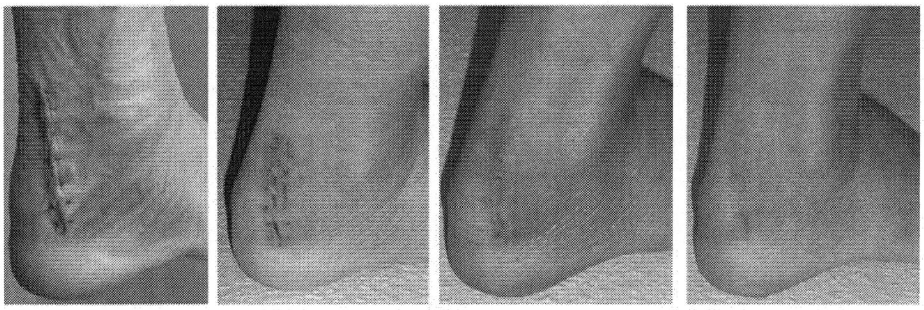

Fig. 9.1 - Progression of post-surgery scar tissue from 5 days to 6 months

Image courtesy of Kaspar 1892 CC BY 3.0 via Wikimedia Commons

The role of collagens is significant including cell adhesion, cell migration, tissue morphogenesis, tissue scaffolding, and tissue repair along with regulating the inflammatory response. There are apparently over two dozen types of collagen in the skin layers, although each function has not yet been determined. Type I is involved with the skin, bone, connective tissues, and their elasticity and strength, whereas type II is commonly found in cartilage for cartilage formation stability or integrity, as well as for an anti-inflammatory. (E. Makareeva, 2014; Von Der Mark, 2006; Åkesson, 2006; Xue, 2015; Kamal Patel, 2022).

Type III is commonly in hollow organs, the uterus, bowel, and large blood vessels, is implicated in the vascular form of Ehlers Danlos syndrome, and is an important wound healing signaling molecule, along with playing a role in structural integrity. (Kuivaniemi and Tromp, 2019) The first three types are most often found in supplements in the hydrolyzed form, whereby the amino acids are broken down into smaller particles, which may alter some of their functions. According to Xue and Jackson, up to 85% of the dermis layer of the skin is composed of collagen, where the ECM is the most prominent.

Scarring of the skin can create a more fragile area in the matrix and may take up to a year to fully heal. Although the ECM is intimately involved in tissue repair, even without issues, the repair process is imperfect. It may involve prolonged inflammation, impaired vascularization or enzyme activation, and cumulative fibrillary collagen retained as scar tissue. (Fig.9.1) Researcher Sachiko Koyama from the University of Indiana found that the beta-caryophyllene in certain essential oils like Melissa and Copaiba can stimulate genetic expression for the renewal of skin cells. (Koyama, 2019, Johnson et al., 2020) Systemic enzymes can also reduce inflammation, speed healing, and reduce scarring.

If the inflammation, proliferation, or remodeling phases of healing are disrupted, which can easily happen with most burns, infections, injuries, or surgeries, it prolongs the process and may increase chances of hypertrophic scarring that will have several times more collagen fibers.

Aging and active disease processes like diabetes and artherosclerosis can further impair wound healing. Changes in remodeling of the matrix, cell shape, or integrity will alter cellular communication and potentially generate other types of dysfunction down the road. Currently, research is pointing to the finding that interrupting certain types of signaling, such as FAK (focal adhesion kinase), and GJIC inhibition (Gap junction intercellular communication) during wound healing shows promising outcomes for reduced scarring during tissue regeneration. (Chen et al., 2021; Erhlich, 2013)

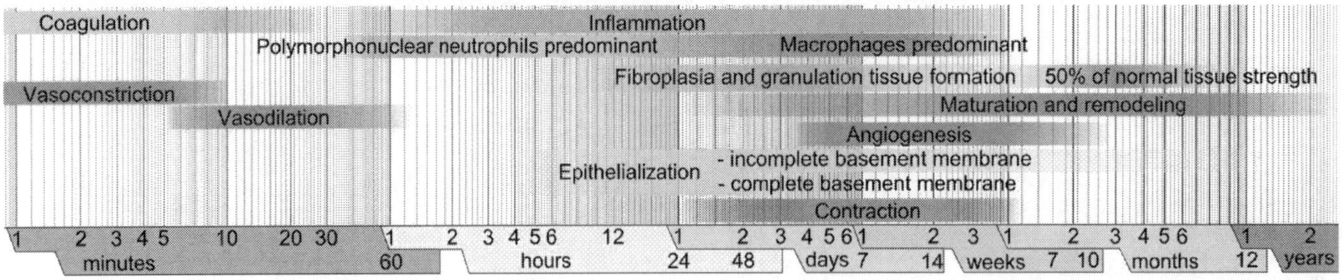

Fig. 9.2 - Timing for the stages of wound healing

Courtesy of Mikäel Haggström, used with permission, Public domain via Wikimedia Commons

Mechanical forces trigger many intercellular forms of communication, so, according to Potekaev and his team of researchers, limiting the types of forces, particularly during the proliferation phase of the healing process, would be most helpful. Between 2-3 weeks into the healing process, a major coordinated effort happens with several components of the process. (Fig.9.2) Disruption during this phase could prolong the inflammation stage, create more irregularities in the organization and density of the scar, and cause improperly regulated signaling. [158](Potekaev et al., 2021)

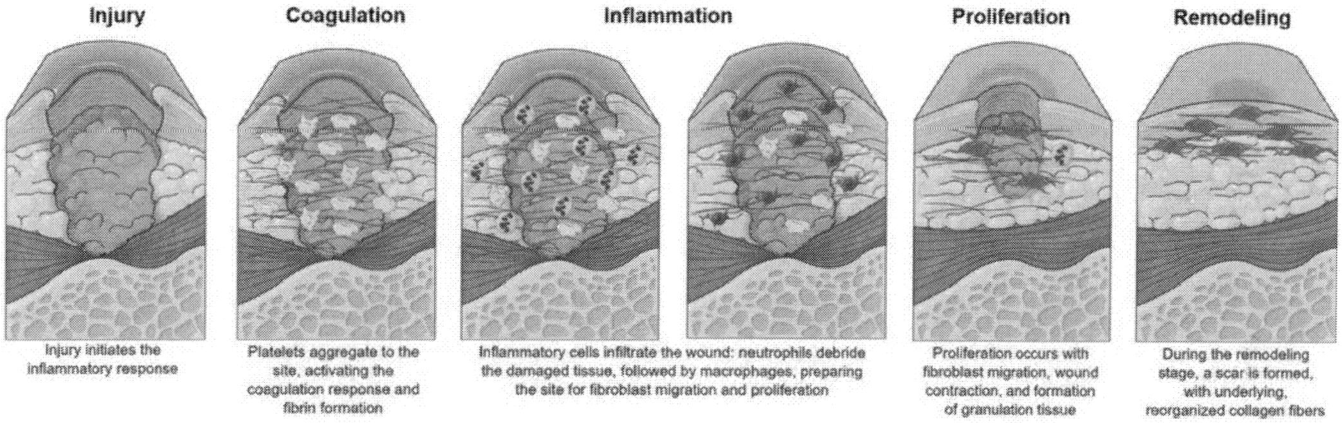

Fig. 9.3 – Phases of wound healing in the tissue: Hemostatis / blood clotting, inflammation stage that triggers the immune system; the proliferation phase when new cells are generated and old cells, then the remodeling phase where some scar tissue forms

Courtesy of Reveal Biosciences

In 2018, Martino and her team of researchers reported that, *"Local changes in ECM (Extracellular Matrix) composition and mechanics are driven by a feed forward interplay between the cell and the matrix itself, with the first depositing ECM proteins that in turn will impact on the surrounding cells. As such, these changes occur regularly during tissue development and are a hallmark of the pathologies of aging. Only lately though, has the importance of mechanical cues in controlling cell function been acknowledged."* [159](Fabiana Martino et al., 2018)

She quotes other studies to emphasize the predictive behaviors of these micro alterations in the fields of communication that interpret and transmit forces: *"The nanostructure and the composition of the ECM are strictly controlled in a tissue-specific fashion during development and in adulthood in order to favor cell and organ function."* (Smith et al., 2017)

Changes in ECM composition and mechanics have been encountered during the progression of all degenerative diseases as the result of aging or as a compensatory attempt of the tissue to preserve its function. *(Kim et al., 2000; Parker et al., 2011; Klaas et al., 2016)*

Proprioception reduces with age, and a great deal of position sense comes from signaling of the skin which is also age-impaired. (Proske and Gandevia, 2009)

Plasticity, the ability for cells to regenerate themselves, can be facilitated when given the attention the system — in this case the skin — that needs to function more efficiently. The method I'll be proposing has worked as well on clients in their 70s and 80s as it has on those in their 20s and 30s. I have experienced many instances with clients, as well as with my own body, whereby light traction over the skin of a tight muscle releases easily with gentle traction. Particularly for muscles that may not respond well to deep pressure – like the masseter – respond well to this method. Vertical traction over the muscle belly in a cranial direction softens the masseter in seconds, but patient listening is needed. Gentle horizontal contact of the skin at the bony origin of the masseter at the zygomatic arch also signals a softening response in the muscle by including the tendon and bone as messengers.

Fabiana Martino discusses the fact that science has only recently opened to the discovery of the various ways that mechanical forces impact cellular, biochemical, and transcription-related processes.

She cites four main ways that this happens: *"Cells perceive mechanical stimuli through diverse mechanosensitive molecules at the cell membrane including integrins, stretch-activated ion channels, G-protein coupled receptors, and growth factor receptors, activating different mechano-transduction pathways." (Fig.9.4) (Martinac, 2014; Luis Alonso and Goldmann, 2016)*

When the process becomes disrupted and ion channels are no longer opening reliably in response to mechanical stimuli that trigger biochemical signals, a wide variety of diseases, such as hearing loss, artherosclerosis, heart disease, muscular dystrophy, or cancer can result.

Along the same lines, several biomechanical dysfunctions can also be generated by poor signaling. The causative relationship is becoming clearer now that researchers are aware that "mechanotransduction signaling has a critical role in the maintenance of many mechanically stressed tissues, such as muscle, bone, cartilage, and blood vessels. Consequently, research has expanded to diverse cell types such as myocytes, endothelial cells, and vascular smooth muscle cells. (Jaalouk and Lammerding, 2009)

As the slowed-down, altered functioning that accompanies aging teams up with dysregulation of the ECM homeostasis due to scarring and compromised communication, pathogens, infections, skin eruptions, and even cancer cells can more easily express themselves. *(Karin Pfisterer, et al., 2021)*

Timing details are often confusing for patients and clients who don't understand that phases of the healing process are still underway after the initial pain and outer symptoms of the wound or injury has passed. "Don't do more right when you begin to feel better," has been a constant refrain of mine over the years in order to help clients avoid setbacks, but the temptation is usually too great. Pain had been such an inhibitor of activity that when it lessens or goes away as a result of the reeducation process they immediately want to do some of the things they couldn't do before. This urgency will tend to create more issues in the future, as the stages of healing need to start over from the beginning. Studies suggest that the consequences can lead to more serious issues down the road.

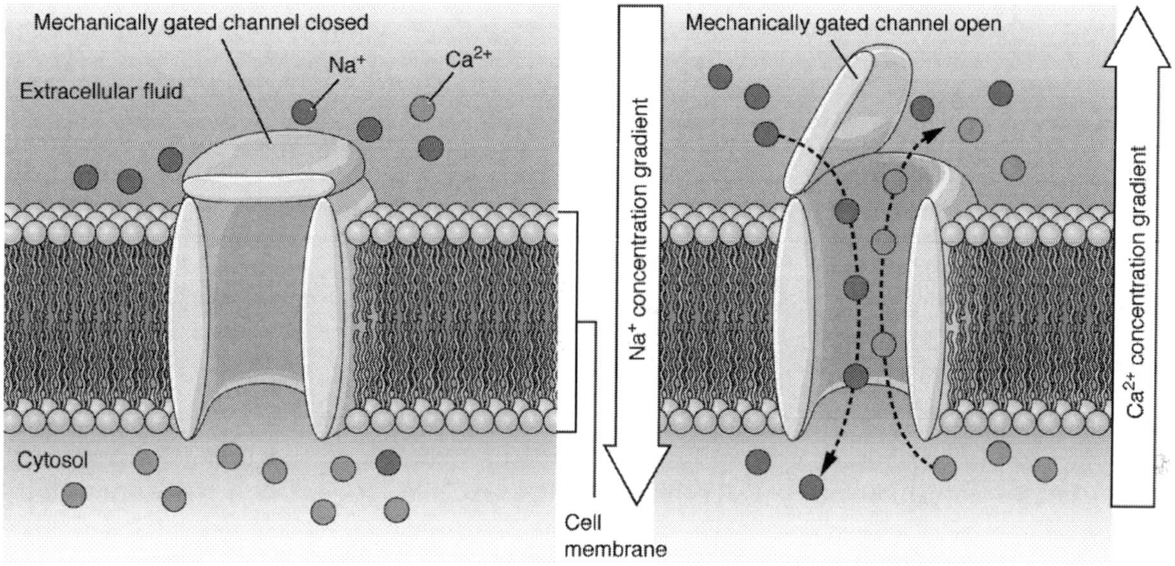

Fig. 9.4 – Example of ion gates opening in response to mechanical stimuli
Image courtesy of OpenStax CC BY 4.0 via Wikimedia Commons

INFLAMMATION IS A TWO-SIDED COIN

Offering gentle movements as homework seems to provide the type of input that cells can immediately use to return to balanced functioning. Muscle energy, PNF (proprioceptive neuromuscular facilitation) and pandiculation help reduce swelling, minimize scarring, and help to retain full articulation of the joint involved in a sprain/strain injury. This is perhaps due to the myokines produced in response to muscle contractions whether or not there is an additional load on the muscle using a weight or therabands. This may be a safer way to go for rehabilitating an injury during critical phases of repair. Whatever methods employed should be on a case-by-case basis using sensory awareness and somatic feedback as a guide.

Jenny Kwon and her team found that IL-6 (interleukin-6), a signaling cytokine from immune cells, is secreted during muscle contraction. This is one side of the coin. It has several helpful functions during an injury or intense exercise related to tissue repair, and in general during prolonged exercise. [160](Kwon, 2020) During prolonged or intense exercise, IL-6 helps to build muscle and coordinates with other organs to regulate glucose metabolism so the workout has fuel. (Steensberg, 2003, Hennigar, et al., 2017) Aging arteries tend to have higher circulating levels of IL-6 and adhesion molecules which can promote the expression of artherosclerosis. (Song et al., 2011) This represents the other side of the coin.

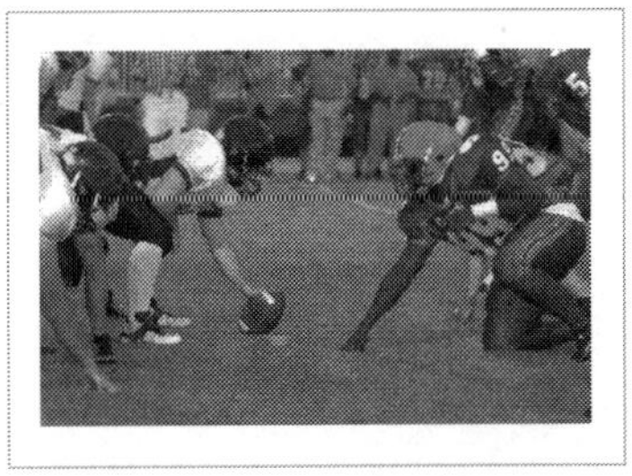

Researcher, Jeffrey Woods, says that chronic, low-grade inflammation is unavoidable in the elderly, which increases their vulnerability for disease. He concurs that regular exercise that increases muscle mass is the best strategy to reduce inflammatory markers and avoid health complications that would otherwise set the stage for increasing dysfunction. Woods lists some common offshoots of chronic inflammation as obesity, heart disease, diabetes, kidney disease, osteoarthritis, and Alzheimer's. [161](Woods, 2012) These studies could raise valuable questions as to which type and duration of exercise should be given to seniors, or for ex-athletes for that matter, and maybe how to approach educational programs aimed at preventative measures.

EXERCISE AND INFLAMMATION

Kwon also observed that anaerobic and aerobic exercise stimulate different categories of myokines from muscles in the aging population. Over a dozen myokines decrease as one ages, while IL-6 and myostatin increase. Myostatin is down-regulated during exercise, protecting muscle growth. Aerobic exercise upregulates apelin, β-aminobutyric acid, IL-15, IL-6, irisin, stromal cell-derived factor-1, sestrin, secreted protein acidic rich in cysteine (SPARC), and vascular endothelial growth factor-A (VEGF-A). Whereas, anaerobic exercise upregulates BMP-7, decorin, IGF-1, IL-15, IL-6, and VEGF-A. Therefore, developing movement programs would also need to consider a person's history and how it may have impacted the aging process in their system along with injury or health status.

To put 'aging' in a slightly different perspective, in the mind of many scientists, muscle mass, strength and stamina begin to fade at age 30 for males, and a little later for females who don't have as much of it. (Dan Brennan, MD; 2021) Apparently muscles have a faster metabolism, which ages tissue faster than fat. Some evidence suggests that a faster metabolism can cause a higher rate of mutations in the cells each year, which can shorten a lifespan. (Sarah Knaptom, 2022) In any case, many professional athletes will retire before the age of 35, and most before the age of 30. Placing those types of demand on the body makes it clear when the strength and stamina can no longer keep up. Those who played high school and college sports fare worse in their overall health, than those who take up exercise later in life. (McMahan, 2017)

Injuries sustained early in life in basketball, baseball, hockey, volleyball, football, diving, soccer, and so on, whether male or female, lead to chronic pain and inflammation for a large percentage of athletes. They then have reduced ability to exercise later in life, and increased risk for heart disease, diabetes, and post-concussion syndrome. Quite a few sustain injuries that never fully healed, and that's where this research comes in. It is probable that a different approach to training, timing, injury prevention and rehab strategies, along with athlete education about their bodies could make a tremendous difference for the rest of their lives. Employing methods that take advantage of inherent cellular epigenetic potential through mechanotransduction could be highly beneficial.

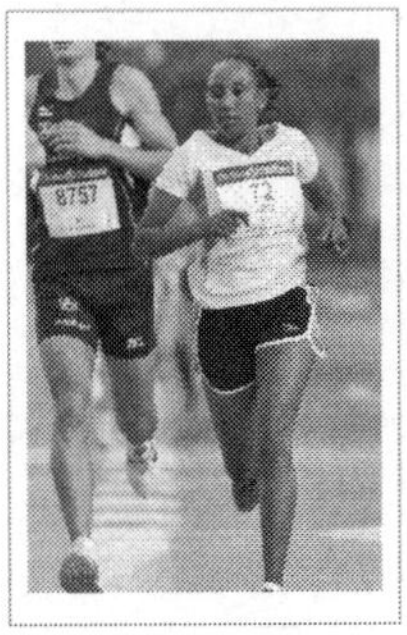

Studies show that 20 minutes of an aerobic exercise like dance, swimming, walking, a bike ride, or even a virtual reality sport reduces inflammation. (Molly Triffin, May, 2021) Certain types of yoga workouts have been able to reduce circulating levels of

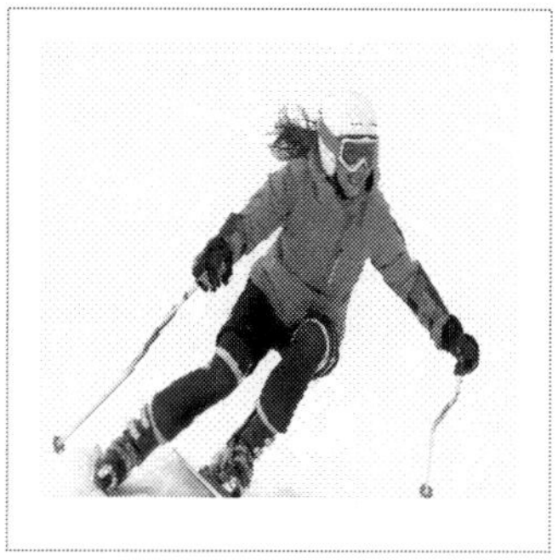

IL6, TNF-α, and C-reactive protein. Like with most therapeutic interventions, optimal results are dose dependent, as well as measures of intensity, and inclusion of breathing and/or meditation. [162](Dilarom M. Djalilova, et al., 2019) In my experience, those who rely on walking, biking, or swimming as their sole form of exercise create tension patterns from repetitive strain that may in fact build onto inherent imbalances. Including approaches that include restoring a balanced, neutral tone and sensory awareness would be an optimal addition to aerobic workouts.

By middle age, the body's immune functions are slowing down, oxidative reactive species are increasing (Woods et al., 2011), work and family rearrange physical activity levels, and toxic exposures have most likely accumulated in the system. That's why even those who haven't had major injuries may be subject to higher levels of inflammation, and a pro-active approach is encouraged. Remember that bones and kidneys work together to regulate glucose metabolism, and have powerful signaling potential to all other systems. Finding some sort of movement workout that loads the bones, involves stretch receptors, builds sensory awareness, and increases the heart rate a few times per week could potentially be the best combination for preventative maintenance.

Physical activity reduces the risk of cardiovascular mortality by 35%, and all causes of (premature) death by 33%, along with protecting against the development of type 2 diabetes. (Brandt and Pederson, 2010) Bone and muscle loss due to aging or inactivity also impacts cognition, as does glucose sensitivity. A combined Finnish and U.S. study for participants having some glucose tolerance issues implemented lifestyle and diet changes and followed them for nearly three years. The researchers concluded that those who stayed with the recommended diet and 150 minutes of exercise per week reduced their risk for diabetes by 58%, a level that is better than the group who were given metformin - a drug to help balance blood sugar.

Brandt and Pederson also investigated the impacts of TNF-α and IL6, which are helpful myokines released by muscle contraction under balanced conditions, but create problems if not balanced. TNF-α (tumor necrosis factor-α) is now thought to be a causative factor in insulin resistance after discovering that healthy humans developed insulin resistance after TNF-α was injected into skeletal muscle, and it also has been shown to have an inhibitory effect on insulin signaling. (B.K. Pederson, 2008) Although TNF-α has a role of repressing the growth and proliferation of tumors, it can also switch roles and *"stimulate the proliferation, survival, migration, and angiogenesis in most cancer cells that are resistant to TNF-induced cytotoxicity."* (Xia Wang and Yong Lin, 2008) It can also make auto-immune conditions worse when used as an anti-inflammatory, when it somehow decides to act as pro-inflammatory.

TNF-α has also been linked to arthritis and rheumatoid arthritis, ulcerative colitis, and Crohn's disease. (Barrell, 2019) Chronic inflammation is unfortunately very common and many don't realize they have it. According to Lilli Link, MD, approximately 133 million people in America were living with chronic disease in 2019, most likely caused by inflammation. Since psychological stress is one of the causative factors, no one is immune to it.

Furman and his research group list cardiovascular disease, cancer, diabetes mellitus, chronic kidney disease, non-alcoholic fatty liver disease, and autoimmune and neurodegenerative disorders all as outcomes of systemic, chronic inflammation. *[163](Furman, et al., 2019)*

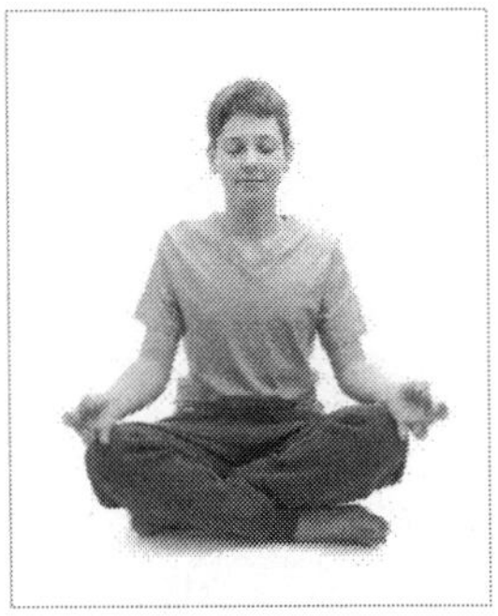

The right type and degree of exercise can reduce those numbers. There are several myokines released by muscles during exercise that are epigenetic. Brandt and Pederson reported that BDNF (brain-derived neurotrophic factor) is released from muscles although its benefits are neuroprotective. It plays a role in learning and memory, and some patients tested for BDNF levels with Alzheimer's, depression, obesity, and type 2 diabetes were found to have low plasma or serum levels. Exercise has also been shown in separate studies to release: epinephrine, cortisol, growth hormone, prolactin, IL-8, IL-15, and LIF, in addition to IL-1, IL-1ra, IL-1β, FGF21, IL-10, and Follistatin-like-1. (Leal, 2018; Hennigar, 2017) Most of these are in response to injury and inflammation, for tissue protection and homeostasis.

Stephen Hennigar and his team find that nutrition intake before exercise helps to maintain muscle glucose levels and reduces the chance of the over-expression of IL-6.

A common way to induce chronic inflammation and breakdown of muscle is with extended workouts and inadequate rest in between, which are counter-productive in that they can impair nutrient absorption and the muscles' ability to adapt to the work they're being given. [164](Stephen R. Hennigar, et al., 2017) The intake of carbohydrates and protein before a workout along with fatty acid and antioxidant supplement afterwards could "mitigate IL-6 response during recovery" according to Hennigar.

He goes on to explain that exercise-induced IL-6 has also been found to decrease minerals, such as iron and zinc while also reducing their ability to be replenished and absorbed due to the release of the hormone hepcidin. Depleted iron and zinc in the system also impair cognitive functioning, physical performance, and present risk to the cardio-respiratory system. Exercise that remained under two hours did not create an elevation in IL-6 that remained elevated, but instead attenuated at a regular rate, as did the levels of marathon runners who used a carbohydrate beverage during their run. These researchers were a part of a military investigation into how to better train soldiers and find the balance for optimum fitness without diminishing returns.

There are many ways that we can, through understanding how the body functions at these micro-cellular levels, improve ease of function and well-being even if we're not professional athletes, dancers, or 'weekend warriors.' Under-use of the body is probably just as unhealthy as overuse or imbalanced use. Certain factors are inevitable with age, yet imbalanced, under- or over-use can age the entire system prematurely and unnecessarily. The message in our physical experiences is verified by many scientific studies. Many beneficial, regulatory myokines decrease with age, are changed by inflammation, and chronic, low-grade inflammation that is responsible for a plethora of disease conditions is epidemic in the population.

MOVEMENT OFFERS A LONG-TERM, PROMISING OPPORTUNITY FOR WELL-BEING

It is also abundantly clear that movement is the medicine of choice to upregulate many helpful cytokines, stimulate regulatory cellular functions, improve health outcomes, and avoid medical interventions that have lasting side effects. Since cellular oxidation, toxicity, and inflammation are built into most lifestyles, incorporating some of the foods and supplements mentioned earlier that combat these outcomes and support homeostasis would be a great choice. Modifying dietary options before and after workouts could also be helpful in preserving muscle mass, muscle strength, and avoiding inflammatory responses. Proteolytic (systemic) enzymes are beneficial for many inflammatory conditions and may help limit the production of scar tissue. There are many variations worth looking into regarding fat, protein, carbohydrate intake, and the duration and intensity of exercise that produce different results in the regulation of myokines.

The right combination could be optimal for recovery as well, but would need to be individualized, which is why knowing your system is possibly the best medicine. Testing or assessing the 'waters' (fluid systems or connective tissue) gently while listening and waiting for the system to respond has great potential. It has been shown that individuals respond differently to the same form of exercise, even when young and healthy. So prescribing the same exercises for a similar injury or pain pattern may not be the best thing. How a person's body responded to what they've already tried can give a good indication of where to start. Responses to diet, supplements, or movement choices will change over time, so staying current with how the body is behaving is a key component to having a successful outcome.

As a rule of thumb, whether using a manual or movement approach on yourself or your client, there will usually be 4 to 7 different restrictions that are sending forces into the location where the symptom is expressing itself. The restrictions may be coming from different layers in the system; one may be skeletal compression or mal-alignment, another could easily be vascular or lymphatic restrictions, fascial adhesions, organ distress, energetic restrictions, posture or gait issues, or compensatory patterns from old traumas, stuck memories, old or fresh injuries, illnesses, or surgeries. Restrictions mean that messaging isn't getting through efficiently and motion will be suppressed in fluid systems. Finding the path to a neutral point in the system that brings down the tension and neurological 'noise' is a great beginning for the body to consider opening to a reset.

If there is still dynamism and responsiveness in a system, it can learn to improve. If a person learns to self-sense and alter how they use their body based upon sensory information, the improvement will be even greater. One client who was using a walker and dragging the leg most affected by polio as a child, was pleased to see the swelling go down in that foot and ankle she believed to be paralyzed. Her ability to sense that leg and move her foot continued to increase using somatic reeducation and lymphatic drainage. I've also noticed therapeutic benefits on clients with cerebral palsy and MS.

In 2021, Stephan Kröger and Bridgette Watkins remarked in their article on muscle spindles that targeting functional reeducation using proprioception in neuromuscular diseases could be a promising therapeutic option. There have already been somatic practitioners who have focused on this population, but there are very few studies to verify their results. They are practitioners and not researchers, but it is indeed an area of study that is under-represented. We don't know yet if there are limits to what cellular signaling and sensory awareness/awakened-ness can accomplish in healing.

In the 1950s, an osteopath named Parnall Bradbury was working alone in a clinic that suddenly became swamped with flu patients. Under time pressure, he was inspired to find the key lesion as quickly as possible. He noticed similarities in restrictions along the spine, and after a few light adjustments, to his amazement, "The clinical results were astounding." Specific cervical and upper thoracic vertebrae were relieved of their force vectors, along with the sacrum, spawning a method further developed and termed, Specific Adjustment Technique by Tom Dummer, D.O. He saw the artery as primary, which has subsequently been shown to be the first system to 'age'. (Highland Chronic Pain Center, U.K.) Dummer, along with others of his peers, perceived that structure governs function, even though most would also agree that form follows function.

Roca-Cusachs, from the University of Barcelona, declares that cells, "can detect the position of molecules (or ligands) in their surroundings with a nanometer precision." Their study in 2017 confirmed that, "*Depending on the cell force distribution, it can affect the activation of genetic transcription, a phenomenon that determines which genes are expressed.*" [165](Pere Roca Cusachs et al., 2017) Realizing that a tiny adjustment in local tension patterns can open cascades of signal restoration is a significant principle to use in practice. Less can be more in many instances, and the body can respond to it even if you can't feel it.

The method of 'induction' that is employed by osteopaths and cranial sacral therapists demonstrates that the actin fibers everywhere are intelligently responding to the new input and creating changes across the field of influence. Sensitive hands can feel the tissue changes within seconds of offering a manual stimulus. The recognition and reorganization is immediate, waking up the local environment, and initiating cross-talk among several layers in the body. It is also probable that adding a conscious movement will be helpful to facilitate the recognition and retrieval of the changes by the brain.

The molecular processes that are continually streaming through our systems are supremely complex and intricate in their precision. We leave the micro details of that process to the intelligence of the soma. Nonetheless, the degree to which we are specific in what we're attempting to target is perhaps the degree to which the system's response will target the same thing. In each case there is an inclusion of the whole in our awareness while focusing on the part. Ideally, we would return — manually or in movement — to check the improved function and integration of the whole after releasing restrictions in a particular spot or area. A major aspect of the therapeutic value is in becoming a conscious part of that interaction, whereby the observer and the observed become one in a palpable way.

PROTECTING CARTILAGE, CONNECTIVE TISSUE, AND BONES

Bones receive and transmit thousands of tons of pressure during an average day without doing anything special, like a dance performance or running a marathon. There are bound to be some cumulative compressive forces, whether it be in a long bone, flat, or irregular bone, depending upon your activities. (Fig.9.6) A certain percentage of the captured forces will generate intraosseous compression that eventually alters the shape of the surrounding muscles and connective tissue as the bone begins to spiral under the pressure rather than absorb it straight on.

Long bones tend to spiral, whereas flat bones and irregular bones can generate a myriad of subtle distortions in shape. This change in shape can be palpated with sensitive hands when our sensory awareness is attuned to the body's feedback during exploratory light touch. As mentioned earlier, there are fluids in the small canaliculi and lacunae of bones (Fig.9.5) which are very sensitive to any type of perturbation. These fluids are able to transmit that mechanical information to the appropriate receptors in order to adapt to the forces and coordinate changes in the tissue field. We can use this sensitized signaling capability to our advantage.

In the same way that it is important to load bones and contract muscles in order for their signaling processes to engage regulatory processes, it is also important to unload the cumulative work and compensatory patterns in order for those signaling cascades to remain efficient and effective. It will be easy to tell whether there is intra-osseous compression once contact is made, but it may be even easier after adjacent forces are removed. If the femur or tibia have compressed and spiraled, there will be additional forces exerted upon the fibular attachment, and the tibia and femur may very well have spiraled in opposite directions.

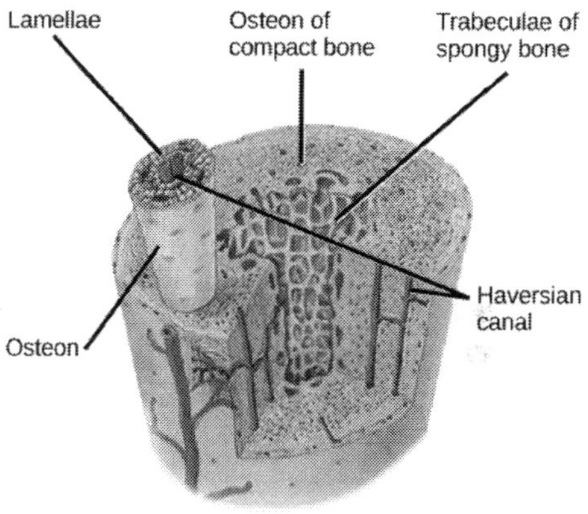

Fig. 9.5 – Interior of long bones that contain fluid-filled canals in the microscopic canaliculi between the lamellae capable of transmitting mechanical force information

Courtesy of CNX OpenStax CC BY 4.0 via WikiMedia Commons

In each case, the pressures upon the articular surfaces and ligaments of the knee will struggle to maintain balance. If physical exertion continues without resolving these opposing forces and compression, the joint will eventually show wear. Damaged tissue will have a more difficult time recruiting the repair mechanisms, which is already more challenging for the joints. Chondrocytes that might be able to repair damaged cartilage could continue the progression into forming bone (hypertrophy), and develop into arthritic changes if these forces aren't resolved. (van der Kraan and van den Berg, 2011; Rita Dreier, 2010; Ripmeester, 2018)

In a review of 28 studies involving over 3100 patients, it was reported that the majority of those studies for use of the micro-fracturing technique in articular cartilage repair of the knee saw significant improvement. There was conflicting evidence in terms of the durability of the benefits in a follow-up study after an average of five years, but all reported improved function in the next two years. (Kai Mithoefer, et al., 2009) Goyal, et al. observed in a review of fifteen studies that long-term outcomes were poor, and led to osteoarthitis of the knee. (Deepak Goyal, et al. 2013) In his article in 2020, orthopedic surgeon, Kevin R. Stone, MD, explained the issue this way, "The data from multiple studies in athletes [i],[ii],[iii],[iv],[v] shows that the repair tissue breaks down over a few years, leaving exposed bone and causing more pain. Microfracture fails because the body loses the race between durable healing and repeated injury from weight-bearing." Stanford University researchers have developed a process using micro-fracturing,

BMP2, and VEGF (Vascular endothelial growth factor) that also stimulated the regrowth of cartilage, which may produce longer-lasting benefits. [166](Vaughan, 2020)

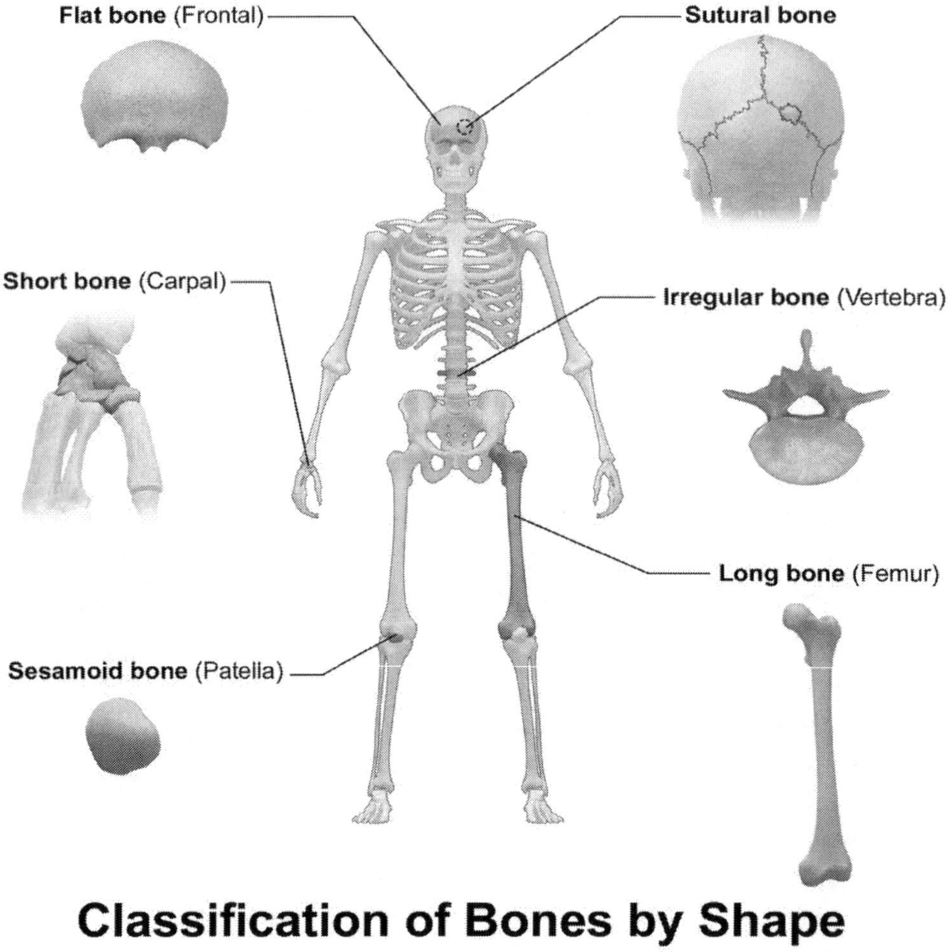

Fig. 9.6 – Illustration of the varied types and shapes of bones

Courtesy of CNX OpenStax CC BY 4.0 via WikiMedia Commons

According to Sergio Ammendola, chondrocytes, the cells responsible for replacing cartilage as it ages or becomes injured, makes up only 1-2% of the total volume in cartilage and have a very slow metabolism and turnover rate. (Fig.9.7) The rest consists of proteoglycans, type II collagen, small amounts of collagen types I, IV, V VI, IX, and XI, with a significant percentage being water. The water contains ions such as sodium, calcium, chloride, and potassium, and helps to lubricate and distribute the nutrients to the chondrocytes as it flows around the articular surface. The pressurized fluid helps the cartilage to withstand the enormous amounts of pressure it receives regularly. Being an avascular tissue, Ammendola says that chondrocytes must rely upon intracellular survival activities to maintain themselves physiologically, and he also believes that the anti-inflammation qualities of the Mediterranean diet can help preserve cartilage. (Sergio Ammendola and Ann Scotto d'Abrusco, 2020)

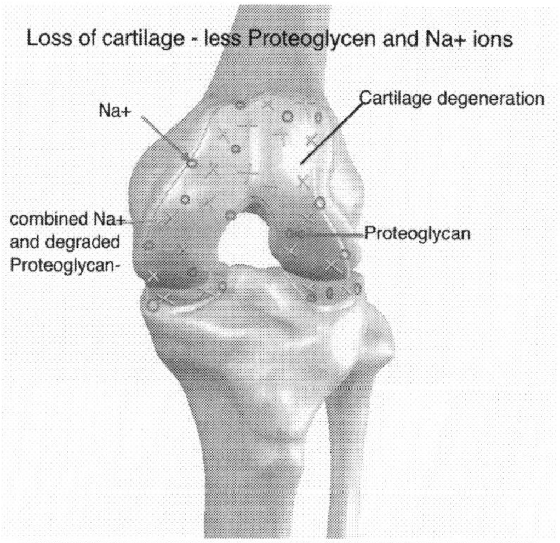

Fig. 9.7 – Example of articular cartilage of the knee
Courtesy of BruceBlaus CC BY 3.0 via Wikimedia Commons

Mehdi Shakibaei found that curcumin protects chondrocytes from the degradation effects of IL-1beta pro-inflammatory cytokine. (Shakibaei, et al., 2005) In 2018, Chi Zhang's team of researchers discovered that chrysin, a flavonoid found in honey, propolis and many fruits such as noni juice, has several actions that suppress inflammatory markers, including IL-1beta. (Zhang, et al., 2018; Shukla et al., 2019; Zheng, et al., 2017) Zhiquiang Chang reported that ascorbic acid acts as a powerful protector of chondrocytes against oxidative stress by "regulating multiple regulatory pathways." (Chang, et al., 2015)

Aggrecan is the proteoglycan that is most responsible for its ability to withstand pressure, as it contains several cross-linking, triple helix chains of chondroitin sulfate and keratin, and interacts with hyaluronic acid to produce osmotic properties. [167](Alice J. Sophia Fox, et al., 2009)

Chondrocytes repair and maintain their own ECM, mainly through the metabolic properties of secreted enzymes, and the propagation of the necessary proteoglycans. Inflammatory cytokines are the main disrupter of this enclosed regulatory process, which may render the ECM unable to protect the chondrocytes.

Fox reports that chondrocytes rarely participate in cell-to-cell contacts for direct signal transduction and communication between cells. *"They do, however, respond to a variety of stimuli, including growth factors, mechanical loads, piezoelectric forces, and hydrostatic pressures. Unfortunately, chondrocytes have limited potential for replication, a factor that contributes to the limited intrinsic healing capacity of cartilage in response to injury. Chondrocyte survival depends on an optimal chemical and mechanical environment."*

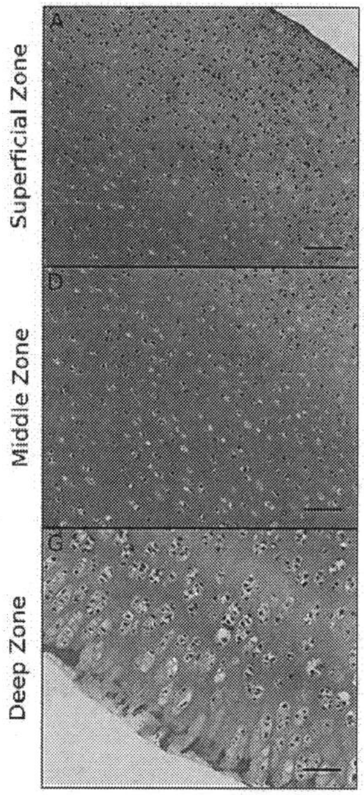

Fig. 9.8 – The 3 zones in cartilage approximating their variance in morphology

Cartilage has 3 zones, each with a slightly different cell morphology. The first, most superficial zone called the lamina splendens, contains flat, elongated chondrocytes comprised mainly of type II collagen. The second is the middle layer that has a higher proteoglycan content and thicker, more spherical chondrocytes that are arranged in an oblique, random distribution. (Fig.9.8) Zone 3 is the deep zone that contains calcified collagen fibrils along with high proteoglycan content running perpendicular to the surface layer's fibers. This layer can sustain the most force and is attached to the bone, holding the cartilage in place. (Hooi Yee Ng, et al. 2017)

Whereas the skeleton has been said to replace itself every 10 years, cartilage takes 25 years. According to Fox and her team, the total number of cells in the articular cartilage doesn't change, but their placement does. There are fewer cells in the first zone, and more in the other two zones. As time passes, the cells become less hydrated, and the matrix becomes stiffer in response. One brilliant adaptation is how the cartilage will remodel itself under steady pressure until it has equalized the deformation across the entire surface so that all areas can support the load evenly, effectively decreasing the focus of the force, just like a bed of nails. Goldman states that repair after injury may depend upon factors such as "genetics, joint site, depth of the cartilage lesion, age, and inflammation." He added that the joint's inability to recruit specific endogenous growth factors is a place to look for regenerative potentialities.

> Contrary to popular belief, articular cartilage has been shown to regenerate itself when the source of the abnormal mechanical stress has been removed, even when osteoarthritis has set in. *(Lee Goldman, MD, 2020)*

There are certain foods that are recommended to support cartilage regeneration —namely proteins — that help replenish cartilage. Vitamin C in oranges that stimulates the production of collagen is one option, pomegranate is a powerful antioxidant and anti-inflammatory, and green tea with its polyphenols and catechins that support cellular health could all be helpful. Brown rice, peanuts and tree nuts, bone broth, and pumpkin seeds contain, and also may stimulate the production of hyaluronic acid. Nuts and kale are a source of magnesium, and brussel sprouts or green veggies that provide vitamin K are capable of joint protection as well as joint nutrition.

There is a **matrix Gla protein** called MGP that depends upon **vitamin K** to help prevent cartilage calcification. As vitamin K is also associated with blood clotting, those who are on anti-coagulants are twice as likely to develop osteoarthritis. MGP, a calcification inhibitor, has been found to be involved in calcification of the arteries, as well as in joints. It is secreted by chondrocytes and vascular smooth muscle cells, but requires "post-translational modification by a γ-carboxylase, a vitamin K dependent protein, which is inhibited by (the drug) warfarin." (Shira G. Ziegler, et al., 2018)

> A longitudinal study in the Netherlands with 3400 participants confirmed the relationship between vitamin K and arthritis. *(BMJ blog, 2021)*

It is also activated in part by **vitamin D**, retinoic acid, and extracellular calcium ions, according to an article by Daniela Quaglino in 2020. Quaglino also described MGP's ability to protect vascular walls by binding to calcium crystals and inhibiting hydroxyapatite mineral formation as well as interfering with BMP-2 signaling. While PRP (plasma replacement) has been shown to improve cartilage wear and tear after two treatments, it has not yet been helpful for injuries to shoulder rotator cuff or Achilles tendons. Pulsed Electromagnetic Field (PEMF) treatments have had positive results in treating cartilage by reducing inflammation and stimulating the genesis of proteoglycan and chondrocytes. The benefits held up over a 3-year period in this study. [168](Kenneth Zaslav, et al., 2012)

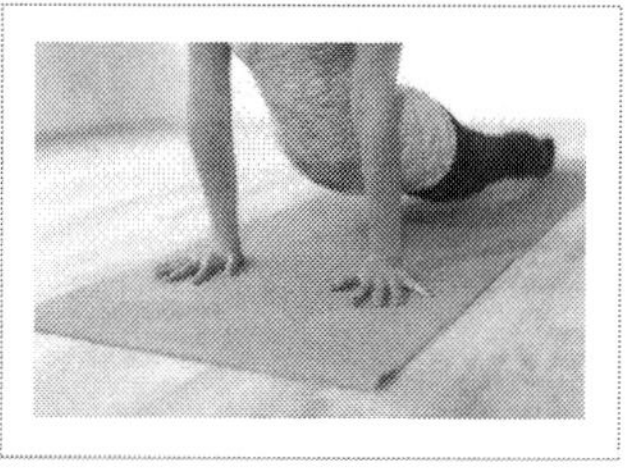

Movements or exercises that work and stretch the joints help to produce lubrication and nourishment that the synovial fluids provide. Keeping weight down is a prime way to protect the cartilage in joints, which happens to be more of an issue for women than in men. It could be that men have more muscle mass and do more strengthening exercises, and the shoes women wear that imbalance muscles and throw forces unevenly into the joints could also play a role in the differences.

Yoga or chi kung methods that run energy through bone, somatic education movements, and soft tissue mobilization by a manual therapist are possibilities to release forces adjacent to bones. Manual medicine can monitor the tissue fields to see if there is evidence of compression, change of position, or changes in shape. Very often a domino effect through the system is experienced when a prominent point of restriction is released while palpating the skeleton.Some osteopaths recognize that,

> *"Every tissue of the body creates a field of awareness that is palpable and recognizable as the field to which that tissue belongs. For instance, every bony cell in the body 'knows' that it belongs to the bony field, and in that belonging it behaves in harmony with every other bony cell wherever it may be found."* (Lamb, 2019)

ATTENDING TO TENDONS

Overuse injuries are common in **tendons**, (Fig.9.9) and evidence is beginning to surface that chronic inflammation in connective tissue can lead to arthritic joints. (Gracey, et al., 2020) Cashiers, hairdressers, carpenters, musicians, and mechanics are examples of work or hobby activities that require the same action to be repeated throughout the day making certain muscles prone to overuse. Falls onto the hip or shoulder are also very common ways to tear a tendon or ligament, and many people land on their shoulder and tear a rotator cuff. A fall is spontaneous and often difficult to avoid, but do check in with your practitioner to help release the trauma. Balancing the muscles attached to the most vulnerable tendons related to your line of work is a simple preventative measure. It's very easy to re-injure a tendon because it takes 4-12 months for it to fully heal, and most can't afford to take that much time off from work.

Icing and cross-fibering the tendon daily while using a topical anti-inflammatory and a brace during work hours can be very helpful and shorten the time it takes to heal. Author and educator, Mark Sisson, recommends a wide variety of movement throughout the day to keep the fluids pumping. He also suggests eccentric exercise, partial reps, explosive movement, explosive isometrics, intensity training, stretching out to the end range, massage, and myofascial bodywork.

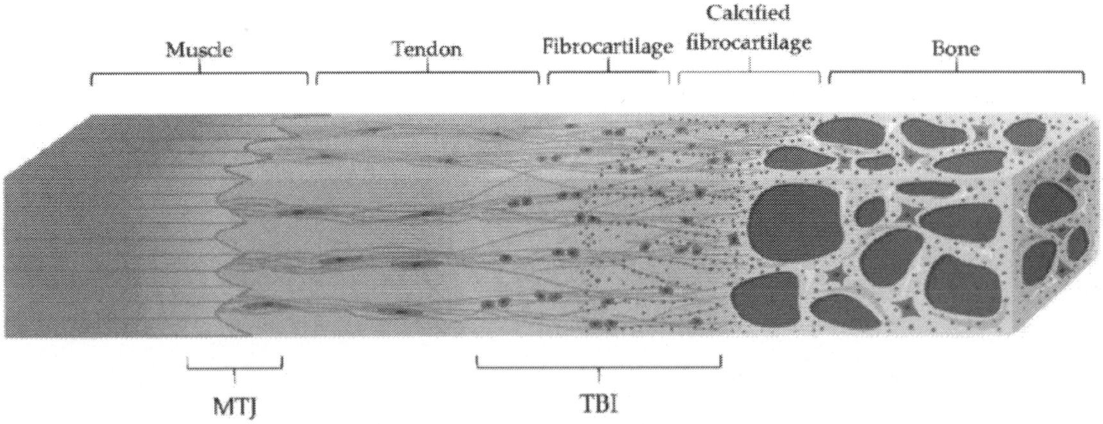

Fig. 9.9 – Illustration of bridge between muscle and bone known as the myotendinous junction

Image courtesy of Creative Commons International

Benjamin, Kaiser, and Milz analyzed the relationship of tendons to bones in varying parts of muscles at the cellular level, including the perimysium. They described that tendons can take a different shape and density depending upon where they are attaching to the muscle. For example, aponeurotic or flattened sheets of tendon can arise from a bony attachment and become more oval or rounded at the junction with the muscle. These aponeuroses can also appear as fibrous sheets of tissue within a muscle such as the soleus, or gluteus minimus, changing the texture and feel of the muscle, as well as its ability to compartmentalize. [169](Benjamin, et al., 2008)

There are ways to strengthen tendons, which also takes longer to accomplish than building muscle. Mature tendons, like cartilage, rely upon nourishment from components of synovial fluid rather than blood supply, and synovial fluid only circulates through movement.

These researchers report that tendons are vulnerable to compression and shearing forces, experiencing the strain of force transmission according to their location and orientation direction. Although they can withstand enormous physical loading, over-training or repetitive stretching can lead to injuries. Tenomodulin is a type II transmembrane glycoprotein that plays an essential role in stem progenitor cell proliferation, differentiation, and senescence. Pu Xu and his researchers report that the mechanosensitive collagen fibers in tendons, called tenocytes — during maturation or injury — "migrate to the damaged site and facilitate the repair process through the secretion of ECM, thereby making them key players in the tendon tissue regeneration and repair process." [170] (Xu, et al., 2021)

TISSUE FLUIDS AND HYDRATION IN SIGNALING

Citing tendon repair as a major concern of the orthopedic community, Yuang Li's group of researchers stated that, "It is more likely for injured tendons to be damaged again after repair which can lead to adhesions, tissue calcification, and degenerative changes in the tendon." (Li et al., 2021) Xu was able to confirm that even a 10% stretch in a tendon elicits a response from tenomodulin that increases migration of tenocytes. Xu's team summarized their findings as:

> *"Mechanical forces are crucial for tendon development, maturation and functional maintenance. Tenocytes are responsible for sending and translating biomechanical signals into biochemical signals. The translated biochemical signals alter tendon-related gene expression to induce cellular functions that enhance tissue maturation, remodeling, and/or repair."*

There are tendons that have a more positional function, along the long axis of a muscle, that share loads as they facilitate muscles moving the skeleton to a new position. Other tendons are more flexible, and store energy when stretched, are fatigue-resistant, but more prone to injury. (Fig.9.10) The more flexible tendons functions like springs that have the ability to recoil and regain energy in preparation for the next demand, such as the Achilles tendon. While running, the force this tendon processes is at least 12 times the body weight with each step. The energy stored during deceleration is released for acceleration. (Quigley, et al., 2018) There are micro levels of fascicles within fascicles that enable sliding and rebounding for maximum efficiency and adaptability. (Fig.9.11)

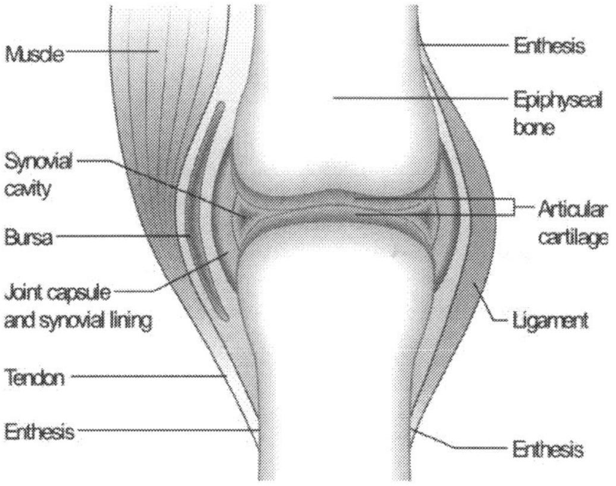

Fig. 9.10 – Illustration of a tendon as it attaches to the (enthesis) bone

Courtesy of Madhero88 CC BY-SA 3.0 via Wikimedia commons

According to Shoulder Doc, Lennard Funk, most tendons do heal, although not to the exact replication of how they were before injury. Finding the correct amount and type of exercise seems to be the key throughout the connective tissue aspect of designing a movement plan for prevention or rehabilitation. Heavier loads tend to stimulate more response from tenocytes, so tuning in to where that threshold is as 'just the right amount' to build strength without overdoing it, particularly for those past a certain age, will be important. Some tendon injuries, particularly the biceps tendon, are commonly torn in seniors due to dehydration.

The glycosaminoglycans (GAG) in the our connective tissue and ground substance are highly negatively charged, inflexible, long, sugar chains that act like a binding agent for the water needed by connective tissue. Hyaluronic acid is an example of a GAG, containing 25,000 disaccharide units. They draw water that we drink into the tissues. The ground substance is a gel-like substance in between the fibers of the extra-cellular matrix whose viscosity can vary. It contains proteoglycans and GAGs that, depending upon

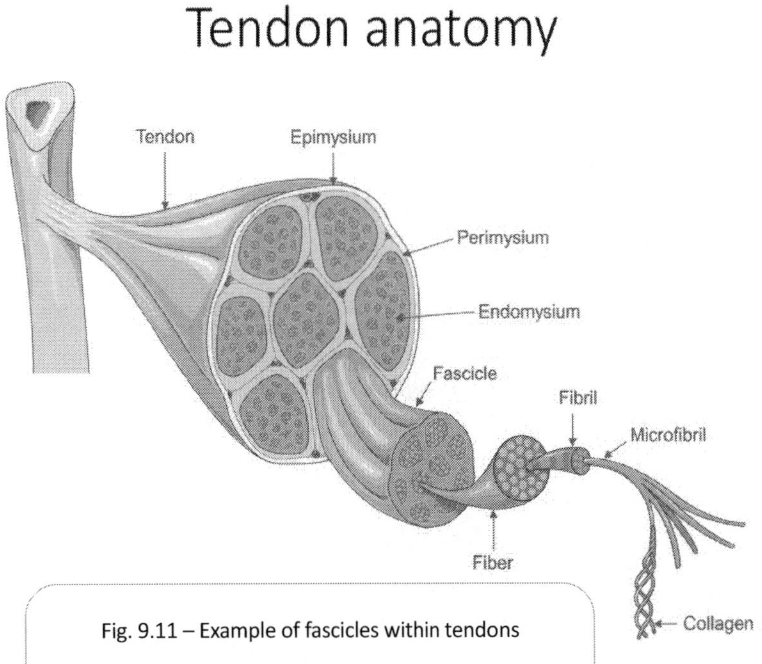

Fig. 9.11 – Example of fascicles within tendons

Courtesy of Laboratoires Servier CC BY-SA 3.0 via WikiMedia Commons

the permeability of the fibers in it, can transfer nutrients between cells as well as water to hydrate tendons.

Apparently, aging can cause there to be more fibers and less fluids in the ECM, creating more trapped toxins. Dehydrated tissue is more likely to become injured, as the water in our bodies also acts as a shock absorber along with facilitating the glide of connective tissue. Movement, and the muscles that have to contract in order to move, help to circulate fluids in our system. Fiber can help to absorb water which enables it to be absorbed by the small intestine and circulated through the system, so adding fruits and vegetables with more fiber supports hydration. (Depta, 2021)

Diane Cochrane wrote an article on the subject in 2018 where she stated, "*The importance of tissue fluid cannot be underestimated. Within the fluid of the tissues are platelets, white blood cells, plasma which is the liquid part of the blood that contains salts, glucose, amino acids, vitamins, urea, proteins, and fats.*

An exchange occurs between the cells and blood but also provides an environment for the cells to do their job at keeping the body functioning. Maintaining tissue fluid at an optimum level is necessary for internal homeostasis and balance."

There are some who have expressed that much of this country is chronically dehydrated. Dehydration can cause tight muscles and sticky, congested fascia, neither of which can absorb and transfer fluids. Once this condition occurs, it's likely that the tissue will need to be manually separated to be restored to its normal buoyancy and permeability. (Eric Owens, 2019) Owens goes on to say that,

---

"Research has shown that when fascia becomes dehydrated, fascial planes can adhere together preventing fluidity of movement and causing symptoms such as stiffness and pain.

The anatomy is now in an unfavorable state because water has more difficulty penetrating fascial planes that are stuck together. Even consuming large quantities of water is often ineffective because the tissue simply can't absorb it effectively."

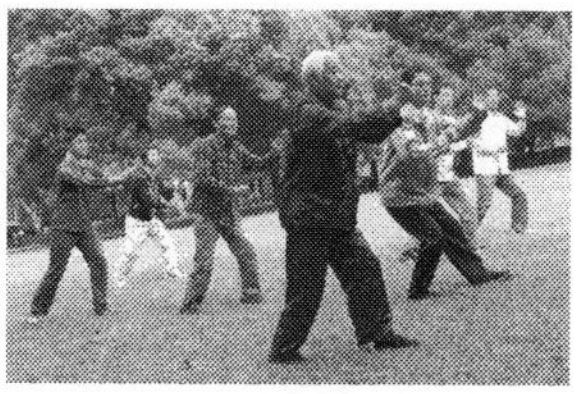

Seattletaijiquan, CC BY-SA 4.0, via Wikimedia Commons

A kidney specialist at Harvard Medical School, Dr. Julian Seifter, reports that the kidneys 'lose some ability to eliminate water as we age,' so eating foods that contain water is helpful to maintain hydration. (Leslie LaPlace, 2021) Inflammation and toxins are also counter to tissue health and cellular communication. Both water and movement help to reduce inflammation and eliminate toxins. Building in regular movement throughout the day by switching up activities could be as helpful as drinking more. Guzzling large amounts of water, particularly cold water, can also cause issues in the system, so do check in with your body and perhaps a health care professional if you're on medications that effect fluid levels in your body.

In summary

Movement is the key to resetting so many functions in the body by cellular signaling connected to epigenetic processes that retain homeostasis. Movement also helps protect against some of the most damaging impacts for tissue stability, elasticity, and signaling potential, such as inflammation, stagnation, toxicity, and dehydration. Developing gentle movements using your own self-awareness or by using a physical therapist or movement re-educator is one of the best prescriptions for prevention or restoration. Consider including activities on a regular basis that move your body in a wide variety of ways. Incorporating conscious movement that focuses on releasing restrictions along the midline would be optimal, along with those that target the systems that have the broadest cellular communication potential; namely, the skin and bones.

Diet is a huge factor in the health of the cellular membrane, cell signaling, and renewal. Foods that have antioxidants, that induce cellular renewal, that provide joint nutrition, support detoxification, and nourish the skin and bones will help insure great health, well-being, and cognitive capacity into old age. Including fats that protect the cell membrane, and excluding trans fats are extremely important. Finding ways to hydrate will help everything to run more efficiently, and clean fluids, movement, and manual medicine are all part of that scenario.

Taking care of little issues in tissue and joints early, and giving injuries time to fully heal sets the stage for continued use later in life. 'Aging' can happen at almost any age, depending upon how you respond to your body's experiences. Addressing bony compression and torsion can be relieving for joints, adjacent muscles, and connective tissue. It can make a difference in keeping all your original parts and avoiding arthritis. Consider using a manual therapist to periodically break up adhesions and balance overused and strained soft tissue before it gets worse and creates a chronic condition that may then require surgery to resolve. You can also learn how to do it yourself once you're familiar enough with where the issues are and your practitioner teaches you the appropriate technique.

Using a slight motion of the skin over tight tendons, stuck fascia, and bound ligaments can be very effective. Volume 9 in this series will go into great detail about these methods. Try not to rely on rollers and massage guns to get the pain down to be bearable; have a professional work it through for you, then carefully use those devices to help maintain it.

Finding ways to clear difficult 'undigested' experiences, whether they are physical, mental, emotional, or stressful situations that are still stored in your system, is healthy at any age. Consider using a perspective that includes how your body sees the world: as information to be processed by several different systems, just like food is. Appreciate that there is an immeasurable amount of data being processed at the nano-molecular level every millisecond, and that your body is listening to your thoughts and feelings as part of how it will be processed and whether it will be stored.

Employing ways to avoid and alleviate stress is as important as any of the other factors that contribute to health and well-being, but there are countless articles, blogs, books, and videos on that subject. That said, a great deal of stress and tension in the body can be released using somatic education movement sequences, t'ai chi, or chi kung, a good, old fashioned massage, and spending time in Nature. There have been many studies published on the benefits of meditation and visualization, but if sitting still doesn't come easily to you, many activities can become a meditation when the mind is quiet while doing them.

Making efforts to develop and refine your felt-sense (sensory awareness) is endlessly rewarding. It is a language that your body speaks and gets you in the conversation. Your body is intelligently responsive at the molecular level, so tiny, gentle movements are also helpful, whether or not you have pain. Almost all major diseases and conditions come from cellular dysfunctions that could have been prevented! Only 10-20% of conditions are actually genetic, and some of those could have been avoided based upon what mothers are exposed to or put in their bodies while pregnant.

There are a series of exercises at the back of Somatic Intelligence, Volume 5 that will be very helpful to get started with conscious movement using sensory awareness if you haven't already begun a practice. Some somatic adaptations to yoga postures are included there. Volume 4 contains a section that introduces exercises to increase sensory awareness and how to discern and contrast kinesthetic information if you're brand new to the concept or don't think you're good at it. Volume 4 also discusses in great detail most of the types of communication our body uses and discusses which systems are involved. It describes the multi-dimensional nature of its intelligence without going into the specifics of the molecular level of activity that this text focuses on. This text explains the science behind all those levels of communication.

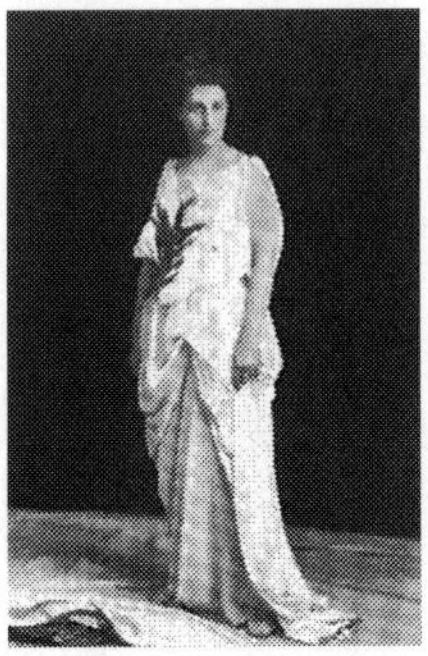

Genevieve Stebbins
1902

The discoveries in the power of movement started in the West a couple of centuries ago, each with a different motivation. Somatic Pioneers in the 1800s like François Delsarte and his star student, Genevieve Stebbins, were opening doorways into new freedoms of expression through the body and emotions in theater, particularly for women. The beginning of women's liberation explored a wider range of movement just by wearing clothing that allowed more fluidity. This initial exploration enabled harmonic gymnastics and modern dance to emerge in the early 1900s as the Ruth St. Denis couple and **Isadora Duncan** came into view. Taking the courage to dance without shoes after traveling and witnessing women in other cultures like Greece and Egypt was a big step in the process of opening the mind and body using dance.

Not long after that, Gerda Alexander began movement exploration (Eurythmy) for its own sake as a process of discovery in a scaled-down, gentle way to accommodate her frail body that had issues with myocarditis and residuals from rheumatic fever. By the 1930s and 40s Elsa Gindler was also exploring conscious movement and self-sensing, and was able to cure herself of tuberculosis. During that time she partnered with a music enthusiast and teacher, **Heinrich Jacoby**, who inserted sensory awareness and body consciousness to bring more life into music expression. Gindler had a wide influence on other pioneers who took the work in a more therapeutic direction, like **Moshe Feldenkrais**, Fritz Perls, Wilhelm Reich, and Charlotte Selver.

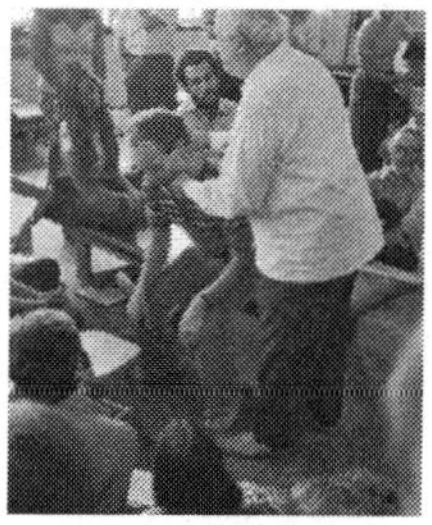
Moshe Feldenkrais

Of course, **Thomas Hanna** was my first teacher and ongoing inspiration for deepening in sensory awareness and the ongoing discovery for restoring balance and integration in the body. He also opened a curiosity for the scientific basis behind how the body shapes itself in response to its wiring as well as to experiences. The applications for the many benefits provided by the underlying science behind movement and sensory awareness are vast. Each application (i.e. adding breath, tuning into fascia, or fluids, or bones, or very slow, micro movements), each underlying principle (i.e. gentleness and safety, novelty, conscious/meditative movement, using cellular messaging structures, releasing cumulative forces) by itself can generate transformative experiences in body, mind, and spirit. When combined, the benefits have even deeper, more expansive potential. There is no value more precious than having an inner wealth of resources to face into life's experiences with, and conscious movement can easily provide that type of invaluable abundance.

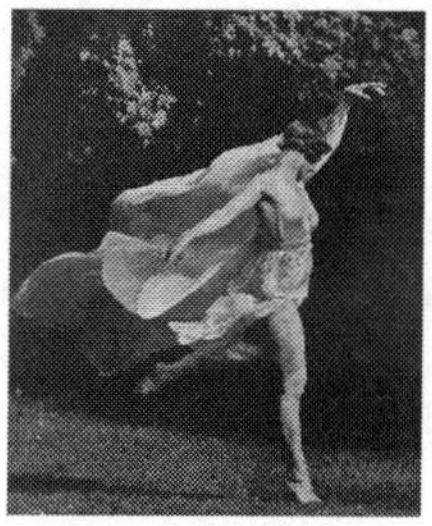
Isadora Duncan 1903

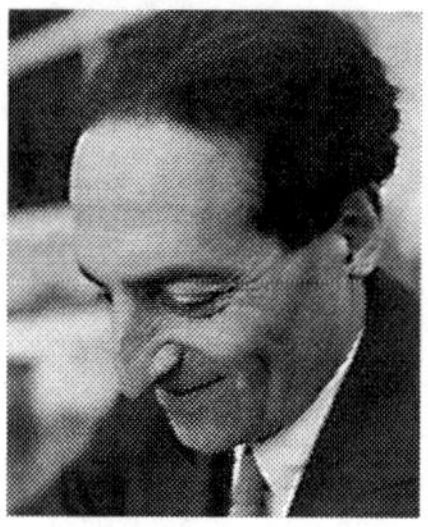
Heinrich Jacoby

Consider taking care of your cardiovascular system as it has been found to be the first system to show signs of deterioration. Consider taking care of your kidneys because they help take care of your bones, glucose metabolism, and energy (jing). Take care of your skin - your protector and gate keeper - that is connected to many types of inner skin, including the lungs, cell membrane, fascia, connective tissue, and thereby signaling processes that regulate homeostasis. Bones have a similar signaling and regulatory role and act as the main structural support and protection for vital organs and core processing coming through the spinal cord.

Appreciate that there is an uncountable amount of data being processed at the nano-molecular level every millisecond, and that your body is listening to your thoughts and feelings as part of how it will be processed and whether it will be stored. . A recent Harvard study revealed that people who meditated for just 8 weeks, 15 minutes a day, changed the genetic expression of over 172 genes. They

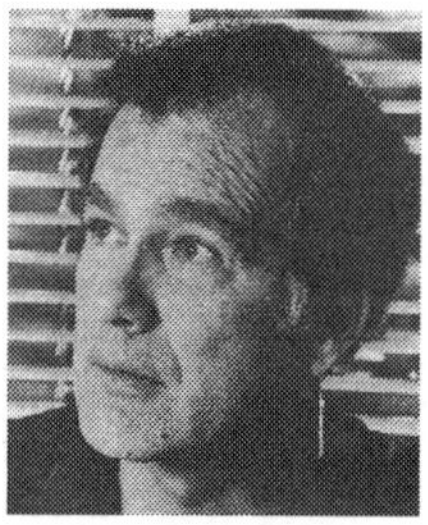
Thomas Hanna

were able to lower blood pressure, reduce inflammation and improve glucose metabolism. (Richard Knox, 2018) There are also studies that find people who are depressed or prone to negative thinking have suppressed immune responses and increased inflammation. Some researchers go as far as to say that our "genetic activity is largely determined by our thoughts, feelings, and perceptions," and effect whether normal or mutated cells are reproduced. (Trang, 2021; Dr. Mukherji, 2020; Miller, 2018)

As phenomenal as many of the man-made structures have been over time, none can parallel the intelligent, regulatory, self-correcting, multi-dimensional capabilities of the form we've been given to inhabit. It's perhaps easier to see how critical it is in a building for all of the components to be able to equalize the forces that act upon it from its own structure as well as from outer influences. It would be very helpful to view our structures and their ability to function well over time in the same way.

A key element in all living forms, as well as the key to sustaining well-being, was discovered by many of the somatic pioneers by visiting and studying more spiritual and mystical approaches from the Middle East and Africa where life is already seen to be interconnected, interdependent, and multi-dimensional. Western views of the body - as are reflected in medical practices are often, ironically and unfortunately, unhealthy. Cutting ourselves off from deeper wisdom about all of who we are and how we function as human beings has had tremendous consequences.

These simple ways of getting back in touch with life at its root are available to everyone. Both conscious movement and manual therapy practices can provide deepening awareness that awaken and enliven the body, which continues to grow in attunement. Consider becoming your own manual therapist and learning from the practitioner you've chosen to work with. Manual medicine helps to mobilize and balance tissue, fluids, and joints, which supports any form of conscious movement. The inner, awakened intelligence is either being enhanced or blocked by our choices. Your body potentially has an infinite amount of wisdom to share, as it is a gateway to the source of life - that which created the fetus and its inherent motion towards integration and health. We only need to accept the invitation to be a conscious part of the process.

Konstantin Ukhthomsky, Public Domain, via Wikimedia Commons

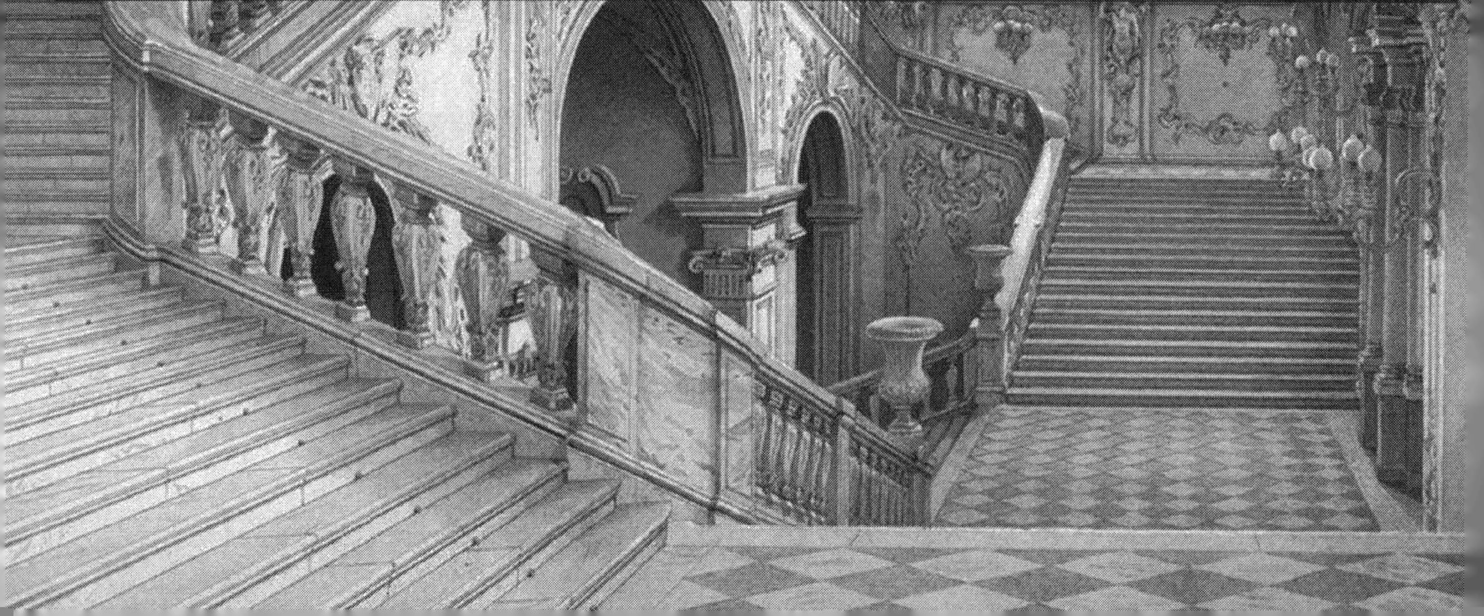

References

1. Chun-Hao Tsa, et al, *"Fracture as an Independent Risk Factor for Dementia,"* Medicine Baltimore, 2014 Nov; 93(26) e 188
2. Per M Roos, *"Osteoporosis in neurodegeneration,"* J Trace Elem Med Biol. 2014 Oct, 28: (4) 418-21)
3. Laura Gerosa and Giovanni Lombardi, *"Bone-to-Brain: A Round Trip in the Adaptation to Mechanical Stimuli,"* Frontiers of Physiology, 2021 Apr 28; 12-623893
4. Dr. Willis Haycock, Osteopathy Principles & Practices, Volume 2, 2000
5. Julie Onofrio, "The Timeline History of Massage (300BC to 100BC)," February 20, 2021
6. Ken W. S. Ashwell, *"Development of the Spinal Cord,"* The Spinal Cord, 2009
7. Yiangou, Grandy, et al, *"Cell Cycle Regulators control mesoderm specification in human pluripotent stem cells,"* JBC Article, Sept 2019
8. Bruno Bordoni and Marta Simonelli, *"The Awareness of the Fascial System,"* Cureus, 2018, Oct. 10(10)
9. (L. Wolpert, *"Positional information and the spatial pattern of cellular differen-tiation,"* Journal of Theoretical Biology, Vol. 36, Issue 1, October 1969; 1-47
10. Shoichiro Tani, et al., *"Understanding paraxial mesoderm development and sclerotome specification for skeletal repair,"* Experimental and Molecular Medicine, 2020
11. Professor James Glazier, Indiana University Department College of Arts and Sciences' Department of Physics, *"Biocomplexity researchers announce multi-scale model of early embryonic development in vertebrates,"* October 2011
12. Haibin Xi et al., *"In vivo Human Somitogenesis Guides Somite Development from hPSC's,"* Cell Report 2017 Feb. 7, 18(6) 1573-1585
13. Thomas Brade et al., *"Embryonic Heart Progenitors and Cardiogenesis,"* Perspectives in Medicine, 2013, Oct 3(10)
14. J-Marc Schleich, *"Development of the Human Heart,"* Heart Journal; 2002 May; 87 (5) 387
15. Scott F. Gilbert, Developmental Biology, 6th Edition, 2000
16. Andrew Lilly et al., *"SOXF transcription factors in cardiovascular development,"* Seminars in Cell & Developmental Biology, Vol. 63, March 2017 pgs. 50-57
17. Radha O. Joshi et al., *"Exploring the Role of Maternal Nutritional Epigenetics in Congenital Heart Disease,"* Current Developments in Nutrition, 2020 Nov. 4(11)
18. Abdalla Ahmed, et al, *"Maternal obesity persistently alters cardiac progenitor gene expression and programs adult-onset heart disease susceptibility,"* Molecular Metabolism, vol. 43, January 2021

19. Samuel T. Keating, Assam El-Osta, *"Epigenetics and Metabolism,"* Circulation Research, 2015; 116: 715-736

20. Ankur Banerjee, "Dad's smoking linked with fetal heart problems," Reuters Health, April 30, 2019

21. Rakesh K. Pai, MD, et al., *"Electrical System of the Heart,"* MyHealthAlberta, April 29, 2021

22. Corinne DeRuiter, *"Somites: Formation and Role in Developing the Body Plan,"* The Embryo Project Encyclopedia, October, 2010

23. D Šošić et al, *"Regulation of paraxis expression and somite formation by ectoderm and neural tube-derived signals,"* Developmental Biology, 1997

24. Bruder, Fink, and Kaplan, *"Mesenchymal stem cells in bone development, bone repair, and skeletal regeneration therapy,"* J Cell Biochem Nov 1994)

25. Breeland, et al., *"Embryology, Bone Ossification,"* Stat Pearls, May 8, 2021

26. Kevin Kaplan MD, et al, *"Embryology of the spine and associated congenital abnormalities,"* The Spine Journal, 5 2005; 564-576

27. Aikiko Mammoto, Tadanori Mammoto, Donald E. Ingber, "Mechanosensitive mechanisms in transcriptional regulation," J Cell Science, 2012 Jul 1; 125 (Pt 13): 3061-73

28. Yūcel Ağirdil, *"The growth plate: a physiologic review,"* EFORT Open Rev 2020 Aug; 5(8): 498-507

29. Jennifer L. Moss, Kathleen Mullan Harris, *"Impact of maternal and paternal preconception health on birth outcomes using prospective couples' data in Add Health,"* Arch Gynecology & Obstetrics, 2015 Feb: 291(2) 287-298

30. Betty R. Vohr, Elysia Poggi Davis, Christine A. Wanke and Nancy F. Krebs, "Neurodevelopment: The Impact of Nutrition and Inflammation during Preconception and Pregnancy in Low-Resource Settings", Pediatrics, April 2017, 139: 528-549

31. Zohra S. Lassi, et al., *"Preconception care: caffeine, **smoking**, alcohol, drugs and other environmental chemical/radiation exposure,"* Reproductive Health 11, Article no. S6 2014

32. Thalia R. Segal and Linda C. Guidice, *"Before the beginning: environmental exposures and reproductive and obstetrical outcomes,"* Fertil. Steril. 2019 Oct: 112(4):613-621

33. Hill & Kleinberg, *"Effects of Drugs and Chemicals on the Fetus and Newborn,"* Mayo Clinic Proceedings, October 1984; Vol. 59, Issue 10

34. Li et all, *"Prenatal epigenetics diets play protective roles against environmental pollution,"* Clinical Epigenetics, #82, 2019

35. Amal Rammah et al, *"Particle air pollution and gestational diabetes mellitus in Houston, Texas,"* Environmental Research, 2020 Nov; 190, reprinted by PubMed.gov

36. *Andrea Baccarelli and Valentina Bollati, "Epigenetics and environmental chemicals,"* Current Opinion Pediatrics, 2008 Apr: 21(2) 243-251

37. A.J. Phelan, et al., Maternal Child Health Journal, "Psychological Stress during First Pregnancy Predicts Infant Health Outcomes in the First Postnatal Year," 2015, Dec: 19(12)

38. David P. LaPlante et al, *"The effects of maternal stress and illness during pregnancy on infant temperament: Project Ice Storm,"* Pediatric Research, 2016; 79, 107-113

39. Kate Walsh et al., *"Maternal prenatal stress phenotypes associate with fetal neurodevelopment and birth outcomes,"* PNAS, November 2019; 116 (48) 23996-24005

40. Sophie Scott, *"Babies' infection risk higher if pregnant mums take antibiotics, according to new research,"* Health Magazine, Feb. 2018

41. Sayal et al., *"Prenatal Alcohol Exposure and Gender Differences in Childhood Mental Health Problems: A Longitudinal Population-Based Study,"* Pediatrics, Feb. 2007, 119 (2) 426-434

42. Richard C. Chang, et al., *"Preconception paternal alcohol exposure exerts sex-specific effects on offspring growth and long-term metabolic programming,"* Epigenetics & Chromatin, 22 January 2019, Article #9

43. Maia Szalavick, *"Unlearning Addiction,"* Volteface, 2022

44. (Adda Bjarnadóttir, MS, RDN, *"11 Foods and Beverages to Avoid During Pregnancy,"* Nutrition, August 13, 2020

45. De-Kun Li, et al, *"Exposure to Magnetic Field Non-Ionizing Radiation and the Risk of Miscarriage: A Prospective Cohort Study,"* Scientific Reports, Article number 17541, December, 2017

46. Nida Ahmed, *"Exposure to Non-ionizing Radiation during Pregnancy Increases Risk of ADHD in Offspring,"* Health Units; March 26, 2020

47. Martin L. Pall, *"Wi-Fi is an important threat to human health,"* Environmental Research, Vol. 164, July 2018

48. Sanchari Dutta, PhD, *"Does Wi-Fi Affect the Brain?"* Medical Life Sciences, April 30, 2020

49. Lap Han Tse and Yung Hou Wong, *"GPCR's in Autocrine and Paracrine Regulations,"* Frontiers in Endocrinology, 12 July 2019

50. Gilbert and Sunderland, *"Juxtacrine Signaling,"* Developmental Biology, 6th edition, 2000

51. Faber and Pereda, *"Two Forms of Electrical Transmission Between Neurons,"* Frontiers in Molecular Neuroscience, 21 November 2018

52. Saad Nagi, et al., *"Pain signaling in humans more rapid than previously known,"* Science News, July 4, 2019

53. E. Lederman, *"Facilitated Segments: a cricial review,"* CPDO, British Osteopathic Journal, 2000, 22:7-10

54. S. Finger, *"History of Neuroscience,: Charles Scott Sherrington,"* Neuro-scientifically Challeneged, 2022

55. Joseph T. Neary and Herbert Zimmerman, *"Trophic functions of nucleotides in the central nervous system,"* Trends in Neuroscience, March 11, 2009

56. Rosa M. Bruno, et al., *"Sympathetic regulaltion of vascular function in health and disease,"* Frontiers in Physiology, 24 July 2012

57. Ross Hauser, MD, *"Can cervical spine instability cause cardiovascular-like attacks, palpitations, and blood pressure problems?"* Caring Medical, June 10, 2021

58. Stephanie Hehlgans, Michael Haase, Nils Cordes, *"Signalling via integrins: implications for cell survival and anticancer strategies,"* Biochem Biophys Acta. 2007 Jan; 1775(1): 163-80

59. Olachi J. Mezu-Ndubuisi and Akhil Maheshwari, *"The role of integrins in inflammation and angiogenesis,"* Pediatric Research, 2021 89:1619-1626

60. Khalilgharibi N., Mao Y. 2021, *"To form and function: on the role of basement membrane mechanics in tissue development, homeostasis and disease,"* Open Biol. 11:200360

61. Rei Sekiguchi and Kenneth M.Yamada, *"Basement membranes in development and disease,"* Current Topics in Developmental Biol. 2018; 130:143-191

62. I.H. Chaurdy and K.I. Bland, *"Cellular mechanisms of injury after major trauma,"* British Journal of Surgery, 2009 Oct:96(10) 1097-1098

63. Thobekile S. Leyane, Sandy W. Jere, and Nicolette N. Houreld, *"Cellular Signalling and Photobiomodulation in Chronic Wound Repair,"* International Journal of Molecular Sciences, 2021, 22(20)

64. Mohammed M. Sayeed, PhD, *"Signaling Mechanisms of Altered Cellular Responses om Trauma, Burn, and Sepsis,"* Arch Surg. December 2000; 135(12) 1432-1442

65. Rafie Hamidpour et al., *"Frankincense (Boswellia Species): The Novel Physiotherapy for Drug Targeting in Cancer,"* Archives in Cancer Research, 2016, 4:1

66. Xuesheng Han, Damian Rodreguez, and Tony Parker, *"Biological activities of frankincense essential oil on human fibroblasts,"* Biochimi Open, 2017, June; 4:31-35

67. Nadja Zubecevic et al., *"Effects of Plant Lectins on Human Erythrocyte Agglutination,"* Serbian Journal of Experimental and Clinical Research, 17(3), January, 2016

68. Toshinori Suzuki, *"DNA Damage and Mutation Caused by Vital Biomolecules, Water, Nitric Oxide, and Hypochlorus Acid, Genes and Environment,"* vol. 28, No. 2 pp. 48-55, 2006

69. Muthusamy Ramesh and Arunachalam Muthuraman, *"Flavoring and Coloring Agents: Health Risks and Potential Problems,"* Natural and Artificial Flavoring Agents and food Dyes, 2018

70. Silvia Isabel Franke et al., *"Influence of orange juice over the genotoxicity induced by alkalizing agents: an in vivo analysis,"* Mutagenesis, vol. 20, Issue 4 July 2005

71. Suzanne Clancy, PhD, *"DNA Damage & Repair" Mechanisms for Maintaining DNA Integrity,"* Nature Education, 1(1):103,2008

72. Oxford University Press, *"New study shows sitting, watching TV linked to colorectal cancer risk before age 50,"* February 6, 2019

73. Shang-Ru Tsa, PhD and Michael R. Hamblin, PhD, "Biological effects and medical applications of infrared radiation," J Photochem Photobiol B., 2017 May; 170: 197-207

74. Ira Flatow, *"A Workout Can Change Your DNA,"* Talk of the Nation: Health, March 9, 2012

75. Aditi Nerurkar, *"What a Happy Cell Looks Like,"* Atlantic Magazine, February 10, 2015

76. Mark Stibich, PhD, *"Top 10 Reasons to Smile Every Day,"* VeryWell mind, April, 2021

77. J Yang, et al., "*Synchronized age-related gene expression changes across multiple tissues in humans and the link to complex diseases*," Scientific Reports 5, Article no. 15145, 2015

78. Glass, et al., "*Gene expression changes with age in skin, adipose tissue, blood and brain*," Genome Biology, 14, 2013

79. Frank & Houseley, "*Gene expression hallmarks of cellular aging*," Biogeron-tology, 19, 547-566, 2018

80. Dr. Edward Group, "*PQQ Benefits: 9 reasons It's a Key Nutrient for Healthy Aging & Energy*," Nutrition, April 3, 2019

81. National Institute on Aging (NIH) – "*Does cellular senescence hold secrets for healthier aging*?" July 13, 2021

82. Martina Rossi and Myriam Gorospe. "*Non-coding RNAs Controlling Telomere Homeostasis in Senescence and Aging*," Trends in Molecular Medicine 2020 Apr; 26(4):422-433

83. John S. Mattick and Igor V. Makunin, "*Non-coding RNA*," Human Molecular Genetics, 2006, Apr 15; 15 Spec No 1-R17-29

84. Honor Whitman, "*Scientists find way to increase length of human telomeres*," Medical News Today, January 26, 2015

85. Fyhrquist & Nilsson, "*Telomere Biology and Vascular Aging*," Early Vascular Aging, 2015

86. Zoe Corbyn, "*Elizabeth Blackburn on the telomere effect: 'It's about keeping healthier for longer'*," The Observer, January 29, 2017

87. Renee Morad, "*How Diet Can Change Your DNA*," Scientific American, June 7, 2017

88. Kristina Campbell, "*Doubts about dietary RNA*," Nature, 18 June 2020, Vol 582

89. Liz Shang, et al., "*Exogenous plant MIR168a specifically targets mammalian LDLRAP1: evidence of cross-kingdom regulation by microRNA*," Cell Research 22 107-126 (2012)

90. Baily Kirkpatrick, "*Epigenetics, Nutrition, and Our Health: How What We Eat Could Affect Tags on Our DNA*," Diet, Diseases & Disorders, Environment, News & Reviews, May 15, 2018

91. Dr. David Jockers, "*Understanding the Role of Methylation in Human Health*," DrJockers.com, January, 2022

92. Lisa Moore, Thuc Le, & Guoping Fan, "*DNA Methylation and Its Basic Function*," Neuropsychopharmacology: 38, 23-38; 2013

93. Toby Amidor, "*Are You Getting Enough Copper in Your Diet*?," US News, January 6, 2020

94. Alex Swanson, MS, "*All Health Starts in the Cell Membrane and Mitochondria*, Nutrition Genome, Dec 1, 2015

95. Dr. Aaron Ernst, "*How to Rebuild and Repair Your Cell Membranes*," May 28, 2019

96. Ornsbee, "*Food for the Cell Factory: How Fat Maintains Cellular Health*," March 20, 2020

97. Alisa Zapp Machalek, "*How Cells Eat In*," NIH, August 21, 2013)

98. Marc E. Surette, PhD, "*The science behind dietary omega-3 fatty acids*," CMAJ, 2008

99. Dr. Guy Crosby, *"As the Expert: Concerns about canola oil,"* The Nutrition Source, 2015

100. Jillian Kubala, MS, RD, *"Is Canola Oil Healthy?"* All You Need to Know," Healthline, February 7, 2019

101. Regina Bailey, "*The Purpose and Composition of Adipose Tissue*," Science, August 19, 2019

102. Bailey Kirkpatrick, *"Epigenetics, Nutrition, and Our Health: How What We Eat Could Affect Tags on Our DNA,"* What is Epigenetics, May 15, 2018

103. Nishat Fatima et al., "*Role of Flavonoids as Epigenetic Modulators in Cancer Prevention and Therapy,*" Frontiers in Genetics, 09 November 2021

104. Brian Bender, PhD, "*63 Kaempferol Rich Foods (Ranked),*" Intake Health, October 1, 2018

105. Faiz-ul Hassan et al., "*Curcumin as an Alternative Epigenetic Modulator: Mechanisms of Action and Potential Effects*," Frontiers in Genetics, June 2019

106. Angeles Carlos-Reyes et al., "*Dietary Compounds as Epigenetic Modulating Agents in Cancer*," Frontier in Genetics, March 2019

107. Noa Rivlin, et al., *"Mutations in the p53 Tumor Suppressor Gene,"* Genes Cancer, April 2011

108. Panagiota Markaki, "*Occurrence of Aflatoxin B1 in the Greek Virgin Olive Oil,*" Olives and Olive Oil in Health and Disease Prevention, pp. 406-414, Dec 2010

109. Sally Robertson, B.Sc., "*Role of Transcription Factors*," New Medical Life Sciences, Feb. 2019

110. Thanasis Mitsis, et al., *"Transcription factors and evolution: an integral part of gene expression (Review)"* World Academy of Sciences Journal, January, 2020

111. Andrew Lumsden and Anthony Graham, "*Neural Patterning: A forward role for Hedgehog*," Current Biology, Vol. 5, Issue 12, December 1995; pgs. 1347-1350

112. Cheryll Tickle and Matthew Towers, "*Sonic Hedgehog Signaling in Limb Development*," Frontiers in Cell Dev Biol., 28 Feb 2017

113. Gabriella Basile Carballo, et al., "*A highlight on Sonic hedgehog pathway,*" Cell Communication and Signaling, Article #11 (2018)

114. Yu-Chen Huang, et al., "*Targeting Sonic Hedgehog Signaling by Compounds and Derivatives from Natural Sources*," Evidence-Based Complementary Alternative Medicine, May 2013

115. Grimm, et al., "*The role of SOX family members in solid tumors and metastasis*," Seminars in Cancer Biology, Vol. 67, Part 1, December 2020, pages 122-153

116. Milena Stevanovic et al., "*SOX Transcription Factors as Important Regulators of Neuronal and Glial Differentiation during Nervous System Development and Adult Neurogenesis*," Frontier in Medical Neuroscience, 13 March 2021

117. Charles E. Murray and Gordon Keller, *"Differentiation of Embryonic Stem Cells to Clinically Relevant Populations: Lessons from Embryonic Development*," Cell, Vol. 132, Issue 4, Feb. 22, 2008; 661-680

118. Chen, Ke, Huang, Ying-Hui, and Chen, Ji-Long, "*Understanding and targeting cancer stem cells: therapeutic implications and challenges*," Acta Pharmacol Sinica 34: 2013, pgs. 732-40

119. Arpan De, et al. *"Anticancer Properties of Curcumin and Interactions with the Circadian Timing System,"* Integrative Cancer Therapies, December 8, 2019

120. Yubing Sun, et al., *"Forcing Stem Cells to Behave: A Biophysical Perspective of the Cellular Microenvironment,"* Annu Rev Biophys. 2012; 41: 519-542

121. Mariona Nadal-Ribelles, et al., *"Shaping the Transcriptional Landscape through MAPK Signaling,* Open Access, November 5, 2018

122. Duk-Hee Lee, et al., *"Neurotoxic chemicals in adipose tissue; a role in puzzling findings on obesity and dementia,"* Neurology, 2018 Jan 23; 90(4) 176-182

123. Karl Kostev, Payman Hadji, and Louis Jacob, *"Impact of Osteoporosis on the Risk of Dementia in Almost 60,000 Patients Followed in General Practices in Germany,"* J Alzheimer's Dis. 2018;65(2)401-407

124. James, et al., *"A review of the Clinical Side Effects of Bone Morphogenetic Protein-2,"* Tissue Engineering Part B, 2016 April 13

125. S. Carelli et al., *"EPO-releasing neural precursor cells promote axonal regeneration and recovery of function in spinal cord traumatic injury,"* Restorative Neurology and Neuroscience, 35 (2017) 583-599

126. Nadi Al-Sammarraie and Swapan K. Ray, *"Bone morphogenetic protein signaling in spinal cord injury,"* Neuroimmunology and Neuroinflammation, 2021; 8: 53-63

127. Samuel Stupp, Northwestern University, *"Dancing molecules successfully repair severe spinal cord injuries; After a single injection, paralyzed animals able to walk again after four weeks,"* Science News, November 21, 2021

128. Jensen, Leon-Palmer, and Townsend, *"Bone morphogenetic proteins (BMPs) in the central regulation of energy balance and adult neural plasticity,"* Metabolism, volume 123, October, 2021

129. Morrell et al., *"Targeting BMP signaling in cardiovascular disease and anemia,"* Nat. Rev. Cardiology, 2016 Feb. (13)2 106-20

130. Hua Mao, et al., *"Loss of bone morphogenetic protein-binding endothelial regulator causes insulin resistance,"* Nature Communications, 26 March 2021, Article# 1927

131. Kai Wei, Zhiwei Yin, and Yuangshen Xie, *"Roles of the kidney in the formation, remodeling, and repair of bone,"* Journal of Nephrology, 2016 March 4; 29(3) 349-357

132. Aubrey Lewis, *"The Kidneys: Root of Life,"* February, 2021

133. Xiao-Qin Wang, et al., *"From 'Kidneys Govern Bones' to Chronic Kidney Disease, Diabetes Mellitus, and Metabolic Bone Disorder: A Crosstalk Between Chinese Medicine and Modern Science,:"* Evidenced-Based Complimentary Medicine, 2016 Sept 7

134. Wang, et al., *"Sclerostin and Osteocalcin: Candidate Bone-Produced Hormones,"* Fontiers in Endocrinology, 2021 March; 12: 584147

135. Severensin and Pedersen, *"Muscle-Organ Crosstalk: The Emerging Roles of Myokines,"* Endocrine Reviews, Vol. 41, August 2020; pgs. 594-609

136. F. Patrick Ross and Angela M. Christiano, *"Nothing but skin and bone,"* Journal of Clinical Investigation, 2006 May 1

137. Houschyar et al., "*Wnt Pathway in Bone Repair and Regeneration – What We Know So Far*," Frontiers in Cell and Developmental Biology, 07 January 2019

138. Zachary Steinhart and Stephane Angers, *"Wnt signaling in development and tissue homeostasis,"* Development, 2018 June 8; 145(11)

139. Xinhong Lim and Roel Nusse, "*Wnt Signaling in Skin Development, Homeostasis, and Disease*," Cold Spring Harbor Perspectives in Biology, 2013 Feb; 5(2)

140. Jin Du et al., *"Extracellular matrix stiffness dictates Wnt expression through integrin pathway,"* Scientific Reports, Article number 20395, February, 2016

141. Heming Ge, et al., "*Extracellular Matrix Stiffness: New Areas Affecting Cell Metabolism,*" Frontiers in Oncology, 24 February 2021

142. Else M. Frohlich and Joseph L. Charest, "*Microfabricated Kidney Tissue Models*," Microfluidic Cell Culture Systems, 2013

143. Rachel Rettner, *"Meet Your Interstitium, A Newfound Organ,"* Live Science, 2018

144. Máximo-Alberto Díez-Ulloa & Ramiro Couceiro-Otero, "*Mechanical triggering of Wnt3a and beta catenin in 3D bioreactors: The role of frequency and rhythm*," Integrative Molecular Medicine, 2016

145. F. Patrick Ross and Angela M. Christiano*, "Nothing but skin and bone,"* Journal of Clinical Investigation, 2006 May 1; 116(5): 1140-1149.

146. (Sharon L. Dunn, Margaret L. Olmedo, "*Mechanotransduction: Relevance to Physical Therapist Practice – Understanding Our Ability to Affect Genetic Expression Through Mechanical Forces*," Physical Therapy, Volume 96, Issue 5; May 2016

147. Erik W. Dent & Peter W. Baas, "*Microtubules as information carriers*," Journal of Neurochemistry, April 2014

148. Jon Lieff, MD, "*Are Microtubules the Brain of the Neuron*," Cellular Intelligence, 2015

149. Pollard and Cooper, "*Actin, a Central Player in Cell Shape and Movement*," Science, 2009

150. Barbier, et al., "*Role of Tau as a Microtubule-Associated Protein: Structural and Functional Aspects*," Frontiers in Aging Neuroscience, 07 August 2019

151. Toshiya Oba et al., 2020, Kane Ando, et al., "*Cause of Alzheimer's disease traced to mutation in common enzyme*," Journal of Biological Chemistry, 24 October 2020

152. Qixiao Zhai, et al., *"Dietary Strategies for the Treatment of Cadmium and Lead Toxicity,"* Nutrients, 2015 (7) 552-571

153. Mauro W. Zappaterra and Maria K. Lehtinen, *"The cerebrospinal fluid: regulator of neurogenesis, behavior, and beyond*," Cellular and Molecular Life Sciences, March, 2012

154. John Toon, "*Mechanical forces play major role in regulating cells*," Science News; March 9, 2013

155. Bin Zheng, et al., *"Nuclear actin and actin-binding proteins in the regulation of transcription and gene expression*," FEBS Journal, 2009; 2669-2685

156. (Sham R. Iyer, et al., *"The Nucleoskeleton: Crossroad of Mechanotransduction in Skeletal Muscle",* Frontiers in Physiology, 15 October 2021

157. Meilang Xue and Christopher J. Jackson, "*Extracellular Matrix Reorganization during Wound Healing and Its Impact on Abnormal Scarring,*" Advances in Wound Care, 2015 March 1

158. Potekaev et al., "*The Role of Extracellular Matrix in Skin Wound Healing,*" Journal of Clinical Medicine, 2021

159. Fabiana Martino et al., "*Cellular Mechanotransduction: From Tension to Function,*" Frontiers in Physiology, July 5, 2018

160. Jenny Hyosun Kwon, et al., *"Exercise-Induced Myokines Can Explain the Importance of Physical Activity in the Elderly: An Overview,"* Healthcare, 1 October 2020

161. Jeffrey A. Woods, et al., *"Exercise, Inflammation and Aging,"* Aging Dis., 2012 Feb; 3(1) 130-140

162. Dilarom M. Djalilova, et al., "*Impact of Yoga on Inflammatory Biomarkers: A Systematic Review,*" Biological Research for Nursing, 2019, March 21(2): 198-209

163. Furman, et al., "*Chronic inflammation in the etiology of disease across the life span,*" Nature Medicine, December 2019

164. Stephen R. Hennigar, et al., "*Nutritional Interventions and the IL-6 response to exercise,*" The FASEB Journal, 2017

165. Pere Roca Cusachs et al., *"Cells sense their environment to explore it,"* Science News, December 13, 2017

166. Christopher Vaughan, *"Researchers find method to regrow cartilage in the joints,"* Stanford Medicine News, August 17, 2020

167. Alice J. Sophia Fox, et al., "*The Basic Science of Articular Cartilage,*" Sports Health, 2009 November

168. Kenneth Zaslav, et al., "*New Frontiers for Cartilage Repair and Protection,*" Cartilage, 3 January, 2012

169. Benjamin, et al., *"Structure-function relationship in tendons: a review,"* Journal of Anatomy, 2008

170. Xu, et al., International Journal of Molecular Sciences, 2021

Printed in Germany
by Amazon Distribution
GmbH, Leipzig

30611351R00113